Normal MRI Anatomy from Head to Toe

Guest Editor

PETER S. LIU, MD

MAGNETIC RESONANCE IMAGING CLINICS OF NORTH AMERICA

www.mri.theclinics.com

Consulting Editors
VIVIAN S. LEE, MD, PhD, MBA
LYNNE STEINBACH, MD
SURESH MUKHERJI, MD

August 2011 • Volume 19 • Number 3

SAUNDERS an imprint of ELSEVIER, Inc.

W.B. SAUNDERS COMPANY
A Division of Elsevier Inc.

1600 John F. Kennedy Boulevard • Suite 1800 • Philadelphia, Pennsylvania 19103-2899

http://www.theclinics.com

MRI CLINICS OF NORTH AMERICA Volume 19, Number 3
August 2011 ISSN 1064-9689, ISBN 13: 978-1-4557-1035-5

Editor: Barton Dudlick
Developmental Editor: Donald Mumford

Magnetic Resonance Imaging Clinics of North America (ISSN 1064-9689) is published quarterly by Elsevier Inc., 360 Park Avenue South, New York, NY 10010-1710. Months of issue are February, May, August, and November. Business and Editorial Offices: 1600 John F. Kennedy Blvd., Ste. 1800, Philadelphia, PA 19103-2899. Customer Service Office: 3251 Riverport Lane, Maryland Heights, MO 63043. Periodicals postage paid at New York, NY and additional mailing offices. Subscription prices are $309.00 per year (domestic individuals), $501.00 per year (domestic institutions), $158.00 per year (domestic students/residents), $345.00 per year (Canadian individuals), $628.00 per year (Canadian institutions), $448.00 per year (international individuals), $628.00 per year (international institutions), and $228.00 per year (international and Canadian students/residents). International air speed delivery is included in all *Clinics* subscription prices. All prices are subject to change without notice. **POSTMASTER:** Send address changes to *Magnetic Resonance Imaging Clinics*, Elsevier Health Sciences Division, Subscription Customer Service, 3251 Riverport Lane, Maryland Heights, MO 63043. Customer Service (orders, claims, online, change of address): Elsevier Health Sciences Division, Subscription Customer Service, 3251 Riverport Lane, Maryland Heights, MO 63043. Tel:1-800-654-2452 (U.S. and Canada); 314-447-8871 (outside U.S. and Canada). Fax: 314-447-8029. E-mail: journalscustomerservice-usa@elsevier.com (for print support); journalsonlinesupport-usa@elsevier.com (for online support).

Reprints. For copies of 100 or more of articles in this publication, please contact the Commercial Reprints Department, Elsevier Inc., 360 Park Avenue South, New York, NY 10010-1710. Tel.: 212-633-3812; Fax: 212-462-1935; E-mail: reprints@elsevier.com.

Magnetic Resonance Imaging Clinics of North America is covered in the *RSNA Index of Imaging Literature, MEDLINE/PubMed (Index Medicus),* and *EMBASE/Excerpta Medica.*

Printed in the United States of America.

GOAL STATEMENT

The goal of *Magnetic Resonance Imaging Clinics of North America* is to keep practicing physicians up to date with current clinical practice by providing timely articles reviewing the state of the art in patient care.

ACCREDITATION

The *Magnetic Resonance Imaging Clinics of North America* is planned and implemented in accordance with the Essential Areas and Policies of the Accreditation Council for Continuing Medical Education (ACCME) through the joint sponsorship of the University of Virginia School of Medicine and Elsevier. The University of Virginia School of Medicine is accredited by the ACCME to provide continuing medical education for physicians.

The University of Virginia School of Medicine designates this enduring material activity for a maximum of 15 *AMA PRA Category 1 Credit(s)*™ for each issue, 60 credits per year. Physicians should claim only the credit commensurate with the extent of their participation in the activity.

The American Medical Association has determined that physicians not licensed in the US who participate in this CME activity are eligible for a maximum of **15** AMA PRA Category 1 Credit(s)™ for each issue, 60 credits per year.

Credit can be earned by reading the text material, taking the CME examination online at http://www.theclinics.com/home/cme, and completing the evaluation. After taking the test, you will be required to review any and all incorrect answers. Following completion of the test and evaluation, your credit will be awarded and you may print your certificate.

FACULTY DISCLOSURE/CONFLICT OF INTEREST

The University of Virginia School of Medicine, as an ACCME accredited provider, endorses and strives to comply with the Accreditation Council for Continuing Medical Education (ACCME) Standards of Commercial Support, Commonwealth of Virginia statutes, University of Virginia policies and procedures, and associated federal and private regulations and guidelines on the need for disclosure and monitoring of proprietary and financial interests that may affect the scientific integrity and balance of content delivered in continuing medical education activities under our auspices.

The University of Virginia School of Medicine requires that all CME activities accredited through this institution be developed independently and be scientifically rigorous, balanced and objective in the presentation/discussion of its content, theories and practices.

All authors/editors participating in an accredited CME activity are expected to disclose to the readers relevant financial relationships with commercial entities occurring within the past 12 months (such as grants or research support, employee, consultant, stock holder, member of speakers bureau, etc.). The University of Virginia School of Medicine will employ appropriate mechanisms to resolve potential conflicts of interest to maintain the standards of fair and balanced education to the reader. Questions about specific strategies can be directed to the Office of Continuing Medical Education, University of Virginia School of Medicine, Charlottesville, Virginia.

The faculty and staff of the University of Virginia Office of Continuing Medical Education have no financial affiliations to disclose.

The authors/editors listed below have identified no professional or financial affiliations for themselves or their spouse/partner:

George Arnold, MD; Tessa S. Cook, MD, PhD; Eduard de Lange, MD (Test Author); Shashin Doshi, MD; Barton Dudlick, (Acquisitions Editor); Brian Ghoshhajra, MD, MBA; Waad Hanna, MD; Gaurav Jindal, MD; Usha R. Lalchandani, MBBS; Vivian S. Lee, MD, PhD, MBA (Consulting Editor); Peter S. Liu, MD (Guest Editor); David Marcantonio, MD; Michael B. Mazza, MD; Ajaykumar C. Morani, MD; Bryan Pukenas, MD; Nisha S. Ramani, MBBS; Mark Robbin, MD; Joshua A. Rubin, MD; Stephanie Simonson, MD; Joel M. Stein, MD, PhD; Vikram Venkatesh, MD; Daniel Verdini, MD; Esben S. Vogelius, MD; Saifuddin Vohra, DO; Ashish P. Wasnik, MBBS, MD; and Jeffrey R. Wesolowski, MD.

The authors/editors listed below identified the following professional or financial affiliations for themselves or their spouse/partner:

Sara C. Gavenonis, MD is an industry funded research/investigator for Hologic, Inc., ACRIN, and the Department of Defense.
Woojin Kim, MD is a stockholder for Montage Healthcare Solutions, Inc and iVirtuoso, Inc., and is a consultant for Amirsys, Inc.
Suresh K. Mukheri, MD (Consulting Editor) is a consultant for Philips.
Lynne Steinbach, MD (Consulting Editor) is a consultant for Synarc and Pfizer, Inc.

Disclosure of Discussion of non-FDA approved uses for pharmaceutical products and/or medical devices:
The University of Virginia School of Medicine, as an ACCME provider, requires that all faculty presenters identify and disclose any "off label" uses for pharmaceutical and medical device products. The University of Virginia School of Medicine recommends that each physician fully review all the available data on new products or procedures prior to instituting them with patients.

TO ENROLL

To enroll in the Magnetic Resonance Imaging Clinics of North America Continuing Medical Education program, call customer service at 1-800-654-2452 or visit us online at www.theclinics.com/home/cme. The CME program is available to subscribers for an additional fee of $196.00.

Contributors

CONSULTING EDITORS

VIVIAN S. LEE, MD, PhD, MBA
Professor of Radiology, Physiology, and
Neurosciences; Vice-Dean for Science; and
Senior Vice-President and Chief Scientific
Officer at New York University Langone
Medical Center, New York, New York

LYNNE STEINBACH, MD
Professor of Clinical Radiology and
Orthopaedic Surgery at the University of
California San Francisco, San Francisco,
California

SURESH MUKHERJI, MD
Professor and Chief of Neuroradiology and
Head and Neck Radiology; Professor of
Radiology, Otolaryngology Head Neck
Surgery, Radiation Oncology, Periodontics and
Oral Medicine, University of Michigan Health
System, Ann Arbor, Michigan

GUEST EDITOR

PETER S. LIU, MD
Clinical Assistant Professor, Departments of
Radiology and Vascular Surgery, University of
Michigan Health System, Ann Arbor, Michigan

AUTHORS

GEORGE ARNOLD, MD
Fellow, Division of Musculoskeletal Radiology,
Department of Diagnostic Radiology-Imaging
Center, William Beaumont Hospital, Royal Oak,
Michigan

TESSA S. COOK, MD, PhD
Resident, Department of Radiology, Hospital of
the University of Pennsylvania, Philadelphia,
Pennsylvania

SHASHIN DOSHI, MD
Staff Radiologist, Division of Musculoskeletal
Radiology, Department of Diagnostic
Radiology, Imaging Center, William Beaumont
Hospital, Royal Oak, Michigan

SARA C. GAVENONIS, MD
Breast Imaging, Department of Radiology,
Hospital of the University of Pennsylvania,
Philadelphia, Pennsylvania

BRIAN GHOSHHAJRA, MD, MBA
Director of Clinical Cardiac MRI, Cardiac MR
PET CT Program, Department of Radiology,
Massachusetts General Hospital, Boston,
Massachusetts

WAAD HANNA, MD
Department of Radiology, Case Western
Reserve Medical School, Cleveland, Ohio

GAURAV JINDAL, MD
Junior Faculty Member and Senior Fellow,
Division of Neuroradiology, Department of
Radiology, Hospital of the University of
Pennsylvania, Philadelphia, Pennsylvania

WOOJIN KIM, MD
Assistant Professor; Chief of Radiography,
Department of Radiology, Hospital of the
University of Pennsylvania, Philadelphia,
Pennsylvania

USHA R. LALCHANDANI, MBBS
Registrar, Department of Radiology, Grant
Medical College, Byculla, Mumbai, India

PETER S. LIU, MD
Clinical Assistant Professor, Departments
of Radiology and Vascular Surgery,
University of Michigan Health System,
Ann Arbor, Michigan

DAVID MARCANTONIO, MD
Chief, Division of Musculoskeletal Radiology;
Director, Musculoskeletal Radiology
Fellowship; Department of Diagnostic
Radiology-Imaging Center, William Beaumont
Hospital, Royal Oak, Michigan

MICHAEL B. MAZZA, MD
Clinical Lecturer II, Department of Radiology,
University of Michigan Health System,
Ann Arbor, Michigan

AJAYKUMAR C. MORANI, MD
Department of Radiology, University of
Michigan, Ann Arbor, Michigan

BRYAN PUKENAS, MD
Assistant Professor of Radiology and
Neurosurgery, Division of Neuroradiology,
Department of Radiology, Hospital of the
University of Pennsylvania, Philadelphia,
Pennsylvania

NISHA S. RAMANI, MBBS
Department of Internal Medicine, University
of Michigan, Ann Arbor, Michigan

MARK ROBBIN, MD
Program Director and Section Head of
Musculoskeletal Imaging; Assistant Professor
of Medicine, Department of Radiology,
Case Western Reserve Medical School,
Cleveland, Ohio

JOSHUA A. RUBIN, MD
Department of Radiology, University of
Michigan Medical Center, Ann Arbor, Michigan

STEPHANIE SIMONSON, MD
Assistant Professor, Department of Radiology,
Hospital of the University of Pennsylvania,
Philadelphia, Pennsylvania

JOEL M. STEIN, MD, PhD
Resident, Department of Radiology, Hospital of
the University of Pennsylvania, Philadelphia,
Pennsylvania

VIKRAM VENKATESH, MD
Cardiac MR PET CT Program, Department of
Radiology, Massachusetts General Hospital,
Boston, Massachusetts

DANIEL VERDINI, MD
Cardiac MR PET CT Program, Department of
Radiology, Massachusetts General Hospital,
Boston, Massachusetts

ESBEN S. VOGELIUS, MD
Department of Radiology, Case Western
Reserve Medical School, Cleveland, Ohio

SAIFUDDIN VOHRA, DO
Fellow, Division of Musculoskeletal Radiology,
Department of Diagnostic Radiology-Imaging
Center, William Beaumont Hospital, Royal Oak,
Michigan

ASHISH P. WASNIK, MBBS, MD
Clinical Lecturer II, Department of Radiology,
University of Michigan Health System,
Ann Arbor, Michigan

JEFFREY R. WESOLOWSKI, MD
Assistant Professor, Division of
Neuroradiology, Department of Radiology,
University of Michigan Medical Center,
Ann Arbor, Michigan

Contents

variants and their potential functional consequences. The upper extremity joints of the shoulder, elbow, and wrist are addressed separately.

New developments in musculoskeletal magnetic resonance (MR) imaging, including improved spatial resolution and MR arthrography, have led to an increasing frequency in the performance of shoulder MR imaging. As a result, radiologists' understanding of the normal and variant anatomy of the shoulder visible on MR imaging has also become more important. In this article, the authors review the normal arrangement and appearance of osseous and soft-tissue structures in the shoulder, as well as nonpathologic osseous and nonosseous variants that should be recognized.

Magnetic resonance imaging is the optimal modality for characterizing the ligaments, tendons, muscles, and neurovascular structures of the wrist and hand. Continued refinement in pulse sequence and coil design permits high-resolution examination of the many small structures and complex anatomy of this region. In this context, frequent anatomic variants and common false positives such as normal areas of high signal intensity in ligaments and tendons must be recognized to avoid misdiagnosis and improper treatment. This article discusses the osseous and soft tissue anatomy of the wrist and hand, as well as normal variants.

Magnetic resonance imaging (MRI) provides excellent delineation of the bones of the elbow and the surrounding soft tissue structures. The components of the elbow can be divided into osseous structures, the joint capsule and ligaments, muscles and tendons, and nerves. In this article, the authors review the normal anatomy and appearance of these structures on MRI as well as the anatomic variants that should be recognized and distinguished from pathologic entities.

Magnetic resonance (MR) imaging is the modality of choice for evaluating the soft tissues of the thigh and leg because of its superior soft tissue contrast resolution, multiplanar imaging capability, and lack of ionizing radiation. The superb image quality facilitates learning normal imaging anatomy, which ultimately forms the foundation of diagnostic interpretation. The purpose of this article is twofold: (1) depict normal MR anatomy throughout the thigh and leg using representative MR images, emphasizing a compartmental approach; and (2) describe and explain the rationale of standard imaging protocols.

Magnetic resonance (MR) imaging is the preferred imaging modality for evaluating internal derangement of the knee, due to its superior soft tissue contrast resolution, multiplanar imaging capability, and lack of ionizing radiation. The superb image quality facilitates learning of normal imaging anatomy and conceptualizing spatial relationships of anatomic structures, leading to improved understanding of pathologic processes, mechanisms of injury, and injury patterns, and ultimately increased diagnostic accuracy. This article depicts normal MR imaging anatomy and commonly encountered anatomic variants using representative MR images of the knee, and describes and explains the rationale of routine knee MR imaging protocol.

This article discusses anatomic relationships, anatomic variants, and MRI protocols that pertain to the foot and ankle. MR images with detailed anatomic description form the cornerstone of this article. The superb image quality will facilitate learning normal imaging anatomy, as well as conceptualizing spatial relationships of anatomic structures.

Erratum

In the article "MR Imaging of Articular Cartilage Physiology" by Choi and Gold in the May 2011 issue, credit lines for two figures were published incorrectly. The correct credit lines appear below.

Figure 11. From Xiaojuan Li, Jesus Lozano, C. Benjamin Ma, et al. Assessment of Bone Marrow Edema and the Overlying Cartilage in OA and ACL Injuries Using MR Imaging and Spectroscopic Imaging at 3T. In: Proceedings of the 14th Annual ISMRM 2006. p. 60; with permission.

Figure 30. From Stikov NA, Keenan KE, Pauly JM, et al. Bound pool fractions correlate with proteoglycan and collagen content in articular cartilage [abstract 827]. Presented at ISMRM 2010; with permission.

Magnetic Resonance Imaging Clinics of North America

FORTHCOMING ISSUES

MRI of the Newborn I
Claudia Hillenbrand, PhD, and
Thierry Huisman, MD,
Guest Editors

MRI of the Newborn II
Claudia Hillenbrand, PhD, and
Thierry Huisman, MD,
Guest Editors

RECENT ISSUES

May 2011

MRI of Cartilage
Richard Kijowski, MD, *Guest Editor*

February 2011

Diffusion Imaging: From Head to Toe
L. Celso Hygino Cruz Jr, MD,
Guest Editor

November 2010

**Normal Variants and Pitfalls in
Musculoskeletal MRI**
William B. Morrison, MD, and
Adam C. Zoga, MD,
Guest Editors

RELATED INTEREST

Endocrine Imaging
Mitchell Tublin, MD, *Guest Editor*
Radiologic Clinics of North America, May 2011

THE CLINICS ARE NOW AVAILABLE ONLINE!

Access your subscription at:
www.theclinics.com

Preface
Normal MRI Anatomy from Head to Toe

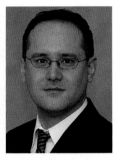

Peter S. Liu, MD
Guest Editor

Much like the central role of mathematics in science and engineering, anatomy forms a basic building block and universal language for the field of medicine. Magnetic resonance imaging (MRI) provides exquisite anatomic detail through its superior tissue contrast, flexible imaging planes, and tissue-characterization capabilities. While these imaging benefits were initially realized in the central nervous system, technological improvements have facilitated the use of MRI throughout the body, including for musculoskeletal, cardiovascular, breast, and abdominal-pelvic applications. Given the increasing scope and utilization of imaging in daily practice, the nonionizing aspect of MRI is particularly notable and may be an important incentive for its progressive integration into more clinical algorithms. Therefore, a fundamental understanding of normal anatomy as depicted on MRI is important for most radiologists.

When initially conceptualized, this issue was tasked with providing a practical guide to the normal MRI anatomy "from head to toe." Describing the innumerable anatomic features of a given body part could fill an entire journal, if not a full textbook; this is a task that would be impractical in this setting. Conversely, distilling normal anatomy down to a more clinically important subset is also a daunting task and requires careful consideration—what to include, what to exclude, when to direct the reader to an additional source. Fortunately, clinical MRI is largely driven by protocols.

Since protocols directly control what images are obtained and why the images have certain characteristics, they are central to any discussion on the MRI appearance of normal anatomy. Therefore, the body can be segmented into smaller pieces based on anatomic regions that have unique or similar imaging protocols, providing a basis for the various articles that follow. These articles are deliberately more numerous and slightly shorter in length than a typical issue. Traditional systems-based radiology subspecialties have been subdivided into several parts, including four separate areas of the central nervous system (brain, skull base, neck, and spine) and seven separate areas of the musculoskeletal system, with different articles addressing joint-specific considerations and longitudinal anatomy of the extremities as a whole. Although computed tomography (CT) is a mainstay for imaging the chest, abdomen, and pelvis, advances in MRI have led to increasing utilization in each of these body sections, particularly with novel organ-specific imaging protocols. Continued interest and adoption in these areas are likely due to increasing concerns about cumulative radiation doses from multiple CT exams. Breast MRI has also emerged as a powerful clinical tool with unique technical facets and anatomy.

Each article in this issue features a discussion of relevant protocol considerations, along with sample technical specifications from the author's institution. The normal anatomy is reviewed, highlighted by annotated figures and detailed figure legends. Important variants and clinical pitfalls are also discussed and illustrated. The goal of each article is to provide a framework for both

Magn Reson Imaging Clin N Am 19 (2011) xiii–xiv
doi:10.1016/j.mric.2011.05.016

mri.theclinics.com

anatomic knowledge and technical understanding. If further detail is required, appropriate references have been cited to allow for additional reading.

I would like to thank the contributing authors for their dedication and hard work. Each has done an outstanding job of creating a contribution that blends text and figures to reveal specific anatomy using their own individual style. Although the task of delineating normal anatomy can seem overwhelming at first, all of the contributing authors have tackled this challenge with remarkable skill and thought. Ideally, the reader will find pragmatic gains from each of the articles, whether from technical refinement, anatomic detail, or both. I hope that the knowledge gained from each article will provide a foundation for the classic radiology teaching paradigm of "you see what you know"— without understanding why the image was acquired and what normal anatomic features are present, correct identification of pathology would be impossible.

Peter S. Liu, MD
Department of Radiology
University of Michigan Health System
1500 East Medical Center Drive
Ann Arbor, MI 48109-0030, USA

E-mail address:
peterliu@umich.edu

Normal Brain Anatomy on Magnetic Resonance Imaging

Bryan Pukenas, MD

KEYWORDS

• Brain anatomy • Magnetic resonance imaging • Sagittal
• Axial

Brain magnetic resonance (MR) imaging studies provide multiple different imaging sequences in at least 2, and often 3, imaging planes. The different tissue signal characteristics and anatomic viewpoints are often complementary, and interpreting an MR imaging study of the brain can be a daunting task. The variety of pulse sequences and imaging planes makes understanding normal anatomy a necessity. Admittedly, many different approaches can be taken when interpreting images, but in this article just one approach to understanding normal anatomy is described. The normal anatomy of the brain has filled many textbooks, and a sincere effort has been made to provide a pertinent and concise reference suitable for review. Textbooks cited within the article serve as excellent references for those who wish to further their knowledge of brain anatomy.

PROTOCOL

The overwhelming advantage of MR imaging is its ability to provide images with increased signal to noise ratios. Tissue characteristics with respect to different imaging sequences provide valuable clues when interpreting an MR image of the brain. Therefore, it is important to understand the accentuated tissue features on each scan. T1-weighted images provide good tissue discrimination and, in conjunction with the postcontrast scans, allow assessment for tissue enhancement. Precontrast and postcontrast scans must be obtained with identical imaging parameters to truly assess contrast enhancement (**Table 1**). T1-weighted and T2-weighted images are complementary to each other because the

T2-weighted images are sensitive to increased water content within tissues and to differences in susceptibility between tissues. Gradient echo images are susceptible to inhomogeneities in the magnetic field, accentuating blood products, iron, calcium, and manganese within tissues. This sequence is routinely performed during evaluation for stroke and trauma because hemorrhage is well seen. Fluid-attenuated inversion recovery (FLAIR) sequence can be used to obtain T2-weighted contrast while voiding the signal from cerebrospinal fluid, allowing a pathologic process to be identified with more confidence. Diffusion-weighted (DW) imaging assesses for the ability of water to diffuse in the local cell environment, which is particularly important in stroke and tumor imaging because areas of restricted diffusion demonstrate increased signal intensity. It is paramount to compare the DW images with the source apparent diffusion coefficient (ADC) images. Areas of restricted diffusion appear dark on the ADC maps, whereas areas of facilitated diffusion appear bright.[1] Susceptibility-weighted images highlight differences in inherent tissue magnetic susceptibility and can be used for evaluation of deoxyhemoglobin in veins, hemorrhage, iron-containing tissues, and calcium deposition.[2]

IDENTIFYING THE LOBES OF THE BRAIN

The frontal lobes are located anteriorly and extend posteriorly to the central (rolandic) sulcus, which partitions the frontal and parietal lobes. Several techniques can be used to identify the central sulcus, a universal point of reference. On the axial

The author has nothing to disclose.
Division of Neuroradiology, Department of Radiology, Hospital of the University of Pennsylvania, 3400 Spruce Street, Philadelphia, PA 19104, USA
E-mail address: Bryan.Pukenas@uphs.upenn.edu

Magn Reson Imaging Clin N Am 19 (2011) 429–437
doi:10.1016/j.mric.2011.05.015

Table 1
Hospital of the University of Pennsylvania imaging parameters

Scan	Repetition Time (ms)	Echo Time (ms)	Inversion Time (ms)	Flip Angle (degrees)
1.5-T Brain MR Imaging				
Sagittal T1 spin echo	450	10	NA	90
Axial T2 turbo spin echo	5490	73	NA	150
Axial gradient echo	800	26	NA	20
Axial FLAIR	8900	141	2500	180
Axial diffusion echo planar spin echo	4000	83	NA	NA
Axial T1 precontrast spin echo	500	17	NA	90
Axial T1 postcontrast spin echo	500	17	NA	90
Coronal T1 postcontrast spin echo	500	17	NA	90
3.0-T Brain MR Imaging				
Sagittal T1 FLAIR	2100	9	896.2	150
Axial FLAIR	9000	119	2500	150
Axial T1 precontrast spin echo	700	12	NA	90
Axial T2 gradient echo	700	19.9	NA	20
Axial T2 susceptibility weighted	27	20	NA	15
Axial T2 turbo spin echo	5440	96	NA	150
Axial diffusion echo planar spin echo	6400	109	NA	NA
Axial T1 postcontrast spin echo	700	12	NA	90
Coronal T1 postcontrast spin echo	700	8.9	NA	90

Abbreviations: FLAIR, fluid-attenuated inversion recovery; NA, not available; TE, echo time; TI, inversion time; TR, repetition time.

T2-weighted images near the vertex, the central sulci can be seen as a pair of mirror image transverse grooves (**Fig. 1**), with the motor cortex always located anterior to this sulcus.[3] The superior frontal sulcus is a horizontally oriented sulcus that terminates in the obliquely oriented precentral sulcus,[4] and one can find the central sulcus as the sulcus posterior to the precentral sulcus. The precentral knob, the cortical location for hand function, is identified sitting just anterior to the central sulcus (**Fig. 2**).[5] The inferior central sulcus does not intersect the sylvian (lateral) fissure, rather it is contained by the junction of the precentral and postcentral gyri.[6] On midline sagittal MR images, the central sulcus is somewhat more difficult to identify, but it is located anterior to the marginal ramus of the cingulate sulcus (**Fig. 3**).[7]

Inferiorly, the frontal lobe is separated from the temporal lobe by the sylvian fissure, which is easily seen on both axial and sagittal images (**Fig. 4**). The middle cerebral arteries are located within the sylvian fissure and are seen as flow voids on T2-weighted images (**Fig. 5**). The parietal lobes are bound anteriorly by the central sulcus. Superficially, there is no anatomic landmark separating the parietal and occipital lobes. However, toward the midline, the parietooccipital sulcus is well seen (**Fig. 6**), demarcating their boundary.[8]

Superficial Surface Anatomy

Although there are variations of normal anatomy, the superficial surface of the brain follows a general pattern, identified best on sagittal images. Naidaich and colleagues[6] provide a thorough description of the superficial frontal and temporal lobes. The frontal lobe contains 3 horizontal gyri and the obliquely oriented precentral gyrus. The superior frontal gyrus runs horizontally, parallel to the falx and interhemispheric fissure. The middle frontal gyrus is the largest of the horizontal gyri, running parallel to the superior frontal gyrus and undulating posteriorly, where it fuses with the precentral gyrus. The superior frontal sulcus divides the superior frontal gyrus and middle frontal gyrus, and the inferior frontal sulcus divides the middle frontal gyrus and inferior frontal gyrus. The inferior frontal gyrus is triangular and is separated from the frontal pole by the frontomarginal sulcus. The superior border of the inferior frontal gyrus is

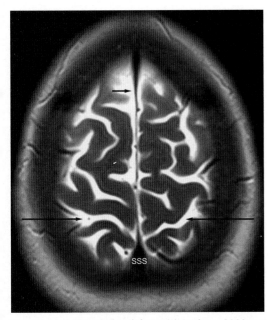

Fig. 1. Axial T2-weighted (repetition time, 3000 ms; echo time, 100 ms) image near the vertex demonstrates 2 mirror image horizontal sulci (*long black arrows*) demarcating the central sulcus. The precentral sulcus is thicker than the postcentral sulcus, a normal finding. Note the falx (*short black arrow*) and flow void within the superior sagittal sinus (SSS).

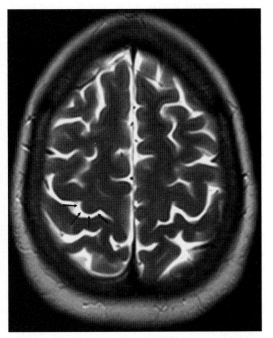

Fig. 2. Axial T2-weighted (repetition time, 3000 ms; echo time, 100 ms) image more inferior to **Fig. 1**, demonstrating the omega-shaped precentral knob (*arrows*).

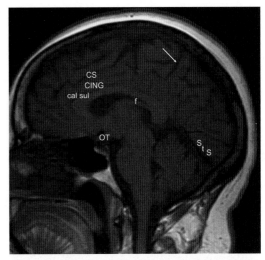

Fig. 3. Sagittal T1-weighted (repetition time, 442 ms; echo time, 9.3 ms) image in a paramidline location demonstrating the marginal sulcus (*white arrow*), cingulate sulcus (CS), callosal sulcus (cal sul), and cingulate gyrus (CING). The straight sinus flow void is also present (StS). Note also the tentorium cerebelli (*black arrow*), fornix (f), and optic tract (OT).

horizontal, whereas the inferior surface is triangular and divided into 3 parts: the pars orbitalis, pars triangularis, and pars opercularis.

The superficial temporal lobe contains 3 superficial gyri: the superior temporal gyrus, middle temporal gyrus, and inferior temporal gyrus. The

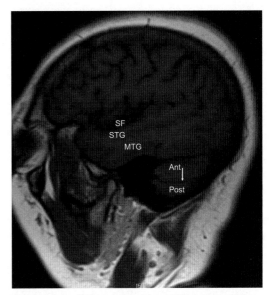

Fig. 4. Sagittal T1-weighted (repetition time, 442 ms; echo time, 9.3 ms) far-lateral image demonstrating the sylvian fissure (SF) as well as the superior temporal (STG) and middle temporal gyri (MTG). The anterior (Ant) and posterior (Post) lobes of the cerebellum are separated by the primary fissure (*white arrow*).

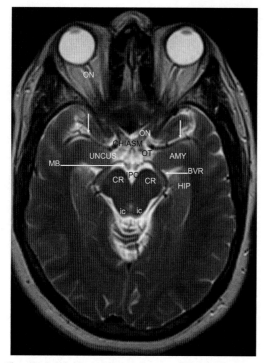

Fig. 5. Axial T2-weighted image (repetition time, 3000 ms; echo time, 100 ms) at the level of the midbrain demonstrates flow voids of the middle cerebral arteries (*vertical white arrows*) within the sylvian fissures. The optic nerve (ON), optic chiasm (CHIASM), and optic tract (OT) are well seen at this level. The interpeduncular cistern (IPC) is bounded by the crus cerebri (CR). The basal veins of Rosenthal (*white arrow*, BVR) travel around the brain stem in the ambient cistern. Note also the hippocampus (HIP), mammillary bodies (*white arrow*, MB), uncus (UNCUS), and amygdala (AMY). More posteriorly, the cerebral aqueduct (*black circle*) and inferior colliculi (ic) can be seen.

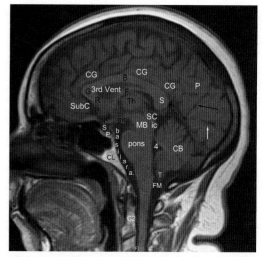

Fig. 6. Sagittal T1-weighted (repetition time, 442 ms; echo time, 9.3 ms) midline image. The rostrum (R), genu (G), body (B), and splenium (S) of the corpus callosum are well seen with the third ventricle (3rd Vent) inferior to the body. The fornix (F) is seen arching posteriorly toward the splenium. Inferior to the fornix, the thalamus (Th) is seen just lateral to the third ventricle. The fornix originates in the subiculum and terminates in the mammillary bodies (mb). The pituitary gland (P) is located in the sella (s). Superior to the sella is the optic chiasm (c). The superior colliculus (sc), along with the inferior colliculus (ic), form the quadrigeminal plate in the tectum of the midbrain (MB), posterior to the cerebral aqueduct. A flow void within the basilar artery (basilar a.) is present anterior to the belly of the pons (pons). The triangular fourth ventricle (4) is seen anterior to the cerebellum (CB). The cerebellar tonsils (T) are present in the foramen magnum (FM). The subcallosal area (subC) of the cingulate gyrus (CG) continues around the corpus callosum where it becomes the isthmus of the corpus callosum inferior to the splenium and continues as the parahippocampal gyrus (not shown). Demarcating the parietal and occipital lobes, the parietooccipital sulcus (*black arrow*) sits posterior to the precuneus (P). The calcarine sulcus (*white arrow*) divides the medial occipital lobe into the cuneus and lingual gyrus. Notice the bright signal within the clivus (CL) and C2, indicating fatty marrow.

superior temporal sulcus separates the superior and middle temporal gyri and courses parallel with the superior fontal gyrus until posteriorly, where it angles superiorly and is called the angular sulcus. The inferior temporal sulcus separates the middle temporal and inferior temporal gyri.[6]

The postcentral gyrus demarcates the anterior border of the parietal lobe and is parallel to the precentral sulcus. The intraparietal sulcus divides the parietal lobe into superior and inferior lobes. The inferior lobe is divided into the supramarginal gyrus and the appropriately named angular gyrus, which envelopes the angular sulcus and represents the posterior aspect of the inferior parietal lobe. The inferior parietal lobe can show marked left to right asymmetry.[6]

The occipital pole can be seen along the posterior superficial surface, but most occipital lobe structures are better seen on the midline sagittal views, discussed next.

Midline Structures

The easiest structure to identify on the midline sagittal image is the corpus callosum, consisting of the rostrum, genu, body, and splenium (see **Fig. 6**). The cingulate gyrus parallels the corpus callosum anteriorly until its marginal branch courses to the superior brain surface. The sulcus anterior to the marginal sulcus is named the central sulcus.

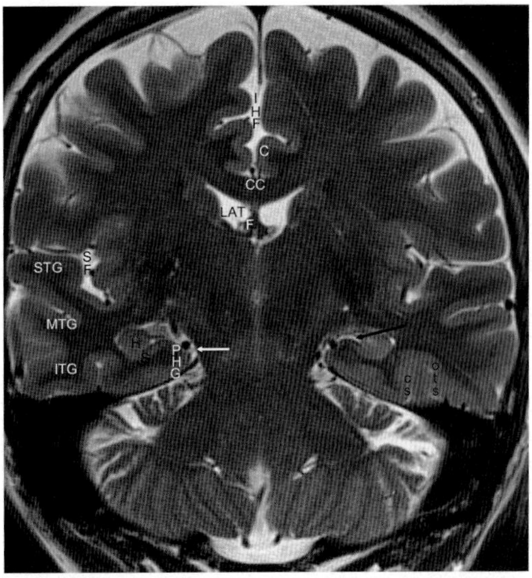

Posteriorly, the isthmus of the cingulate gyrus is located between the splenium of the corpus callosum and the anterior calcarine sulcus[9] and continues laterally as the parahippocampal gyrus where its superior border is demarcated by the hippocampal fissure. The hippocampal fissure continues above the body of the corpus callosum as the callosal sulcus (see **Fig. 3**).[10] Anteriorly, the cingulate gyrus dives under the rostrum of the corpus callosum and becomes the subcallosal area.[10] The posterior medial parietal lobe, or precuneus, is seen anterior to the parietooccipital sulcus. The calcarine sulcus divides the medial occipital lobe into the cuneus and lingual gyrus (see **Fig. 6**).

The lamina terminalis demarcates the anterior wall of the third ventricle and plays a role in cardiovascular and body fluid homeostasis.[11]

The hippocampal formation, found in the medial temporal lobe, is composed of the subiculum, the dentate gyrus, the hippocampus, and their continuations around the corpus callosum[10] and is best seen on coronal images. The parahippocampal gyrus forms the inferomedial border of the temporal lobe (**Fig. 7**). The subiculum forms the medial and superior curvature of the parahippocampal gyrus and arcs into the hippocampal fissure.[10] The hippocampal fissure is bordered superiorly by the dentate gyrus and inferiorly by the subiculum.[10] The hippocampus forms a cap on the hippocampal fissure and bulges into the medial wall and floor of the temporal horn.[10]

The fornix, a white matter tract that connects the subiculum and the mammillary bodies, originates in the subiculum where its axons travel laterally to form a thin layer of white matter along the inferomedial temporal horn.[10] The fornix continues posterior to the undersurface of the splenium, and most fibers arch upward, anterior, and inferior to the splenium to form the crura of the fornices,[10] ending in the mammillary bodies (see **Fig. 2**).

The amygdala is a gray matter structure located just lateral to the uncus and anterior to the temporal horn and remains attached to the putamen superiorly.[10] The tail of the caudate nucleus terminates in the amygdala. The anterior commissure is a white matter tract located in the anterior wall of the third ventricle at the junction of the lamina terminalis and the rostrum of the corpus callosum that connects the 2 temporal lobes and is easily seen on MR images.[12]

Deep Structures

The deep central cerebral structures located between the insula and the sagittal midline are referred to as the central core (**Fig. 8**).[13] This core

Fig. 7. Coronal T2-weighted image (repetition time, 6360 ms; echo time, 89 ms) demonstrating the inferior and medial border of the temporal lobe, the parahippocampal gyrus (PHG). The subiculum (S) and body of the hippocampus (H) are also demarcated. The hippocampal sulcus is seen on the left (*black arrow*), as are the collateral sulcus (cs) and the occipitotemporal sulcus (ots). Note the flow voids in the ambient cistern (*white arrow*) and sylvian fissure (SF). The superior, middle, and inferior temporal gyri (STG, MTG, ITG, respectively) are also seen. At this level, the bodies of the fornices (F) are present inferior to the corpus callosum (CC) and within the lateral ventricles (LAT). The cingulate gyrus (C) and interhemispheric fissure (IHF) are present in the midline.

contains, among others structures, the extreme, external, and internal capsules, the claustrum, the putamen, the globus pallidus, the caudate nucleus, the amygdala, the diencephalon, and thalamic structures. It is related to motor and sensory functions, emotion, endocrine integration, and cognition.[14] All the information passing between the brainstem and cortex passes through fibers in the central core.[15] Anteriorly, the central core gray matter consists of the caudate nucleus and, to a lesser extent, the lentiform nucleus (putamen and globus pallidus), whereas the white matter consists primarily of the anterior limb of the internal capsule.[15] More posteriorly, at the level of the foramen of Monro, the internal capsule contributes most of the white matter, whereas the lentiform nucleus contributes most of the gray matter, with a lesser contribution from the caudate nucleus.[15] At the posterior insular level, most of the gray matter contribution arises from the thalamus and the white matter from the posterior limb of the internal capsule.[15]

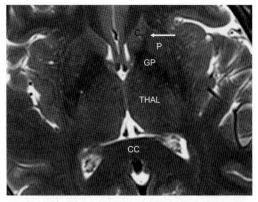

Fig. 8. Axial T2-weighted image (repetition time, 6900 ms; echo time, 96 ms) through the basal ganglia demonstrating the head of the caudate (C), anterior limb of the internal capsule (*white arrow*), putamen (P), globus pallidus (GP), thalamus (THAL), and corpus callosum (CC).

Cerebellum

The cerebellum can be divided into 4 lobes: the anterior and posterior lobes, separated by the primary fissure (see **Fig. 3**), the vermis, and the flocculonodular lobe. The inferior vermis and flocculonodular lobes help regulate balance and eye movements via interactions with the vestibular system. It is generally assumed that these regions, along with other parts of the vermis, are involved in control of the proximal trunk muscles, whereas the more lateral regions help control the distal appendicular muscles. The most lateral cerebellar hemispheres are involved in motor planning.[16] The cerebellar tonsils are located inferolaterally and herniate through the foramen magnum in patients with Chiari malformations.[17] The dentate nucleus may be seen on T1-weighted images and is located lateral to the white matter of the cerebellum.[18] There are 3 main white matter tracts connecting the cerebellum to the brainstem: the superior cerebellar peduncle (cerebellum to midbrain), middle cerebellar peduncle (pons to cerebellum), and inferior cerebellar peduncle (medulla to cerebellum).[19]

Brainstem

The brainstem, consisting of the diencephalon, mesencephalon, pons, and medulla oblongata, serves as the connection between the cerebral hemispheres, the cerebellum, and the medulla, and is responsible for the basic life functions such as breathing, heartbeat, blood pressure, consciousness, and sleep.[20] There are 3 main longitudinal divisions of the brainstem: the basis, the tectum, and the tegmentum. The motor pathway runs in the most anterior segment, the basis; the cranial nerve nuclei and somatosensory tracts are present in the tegmentum, located anterior to the fourth ventricle; and the quadrigeminal plate and superior (pons) and inferior (medulla oblongata) medullary velum form the tectum.[20,21] The pineal gland can be seen inferior to the corpus callosum on sagittal midline images.

The diencephalon contains the third ventricle and its bounding structures and is divided into 4 parts: the epithalamus, hypothalamus, subthalamus, and thalamus.[20] The epithalamus contains the trigonum habenulae, the pineal gland, and the posterior commissure.[20] The hypothalamus consists of the mammillary bodies, the tuber cinereum, the infundibulum, the hypophysis, and the optic chiasm (see **Fig. 6**).[20] The thalamus is the largest part of the diencephalon and is situated on both sides of the third ventricle (see **Figs. 6, 8** and **9**).[20] The anterior end of the thalamus forms the posterior boundary of the interventricular foramen, whereas the posterior aspect expands and overlaps the superior colliculus.[20] Medially, the posterior portion of the thalamus, the pulvinar, blends into the lateral geniculate body, which is involved in the visual pathway.[20] Beneath the pulvinar is the medial geniculate body, forming part of the auditory pathway.[20]

The midbrain connects the diencephalon to the pons and has a characteristic midline cleft, the interpeduncular cistern, which is bounded on each

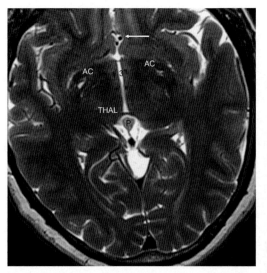

Fig. 9. Axial T2-weighted image (repetition time, 6900 ms; echo time, 96 ms) through the basal ganglia demonstrating the anterior commissure (AC), pineal gland (P), thalamus (THAL), and flow voids within the anterior cerebral arteries located in the interhemispheric fissure (*white arrow*).

side by the crus cerebri (see **Fig. 5**).[20] The tectum contains the quadrigeminal plate and lies posterior to the cerebral aqueduct. The superior colliculi contain centers for visual reflexes and connect to the superior brachium via the lateral geniculate body and the optic tract.[20] The inferior colliculi contain auditory centers and connect to the medial geniculate via the inferior brachium.[20] The fourth cranial nerves arise in the midline, below the inferior colliculi. The red nucleus is seen as areas of decreased signal intensity on T2-weighted images as a result of their high iron content (**Fig. 10**).[20] The third cranial nerve also arises from the midbrain.

The pons, named for its appearance as a bridge between the cerebellar hemispheres, has a large convex anterior surface (see **Fig. 6**) containing transverse fibers that converge to form the middle cerebellar peduncles.[20] The sixth, seventh, and eighth cranial nerves emerge from a groove at the pontomedullary junction; the trigeminal nerve also emerges from the pons.[20] The posterior pons forms the roof of the fourth ventricle and is covered by the cerebellum.[20]

The medulla oblongata connects the spinal cord and pons (**Fig. 11**). Running along both sides of the median fissure, the pyramids are composed of axons from the precentral gyrus that innervate the spinal cord gray matter (corticospinal or pyramidal tracts).[20] Lateral and posterior to the pyramids, separated by the preolivary groove, are elongated elevations formed by the olivary nuclei, the medullary olives. The ninth, tenth, eleventh, and twelfth cranial nerves are located in the

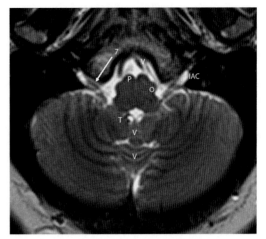

Fig. 11. Axial T2-weighted image (repetition time, 6900 ms; echo time, 96 ms) through the medulla demonstrating the medullary pyramid (P), olive (O), cerebellar tonsil (T), and cerebellar vermis (V). The seventh nerve (*arrow*, 7) is seen coursing toward the internal auditory canal (IAC).

medulla, and the rootlets of the hypoglossal nerve arise from the preolivary groove.[20]

The pituitary stalk projects inferiorly from the infundibular recess of the third ventricle, leading into the bilobed pituitary gland. The anterior lobe appears isointense to the brain on T1-weighted and T2-weighted images, although hyperintensity on T1-weighted images has been reported in pregnancy. For as yet unknown reasons, the posterior pituitary gland is hyperintense on T1-wieghted images and shows lower intensity on T2-weighted images. Injection of gadolinium results in prompt enhancement of the anterior pituitary gland and infundibulum. The normal pituitary gland has a maximal height of 8 mm in men and 9 mm in women. Immediately posterior to the pituitary, the cortical bone of the dorsum sella can be seen as a rim of hypointense signal. Posterior to this hypointensity, the fatty marrow of the clivus appears hyperintense on T1-weighted images.[1]

IMAGING NOOKS AND CRANNIES

This section provides a few anatomic insights about overlooked areas on specific sequences, namely, sagittal T1-weighted and axial T2-weighted images.

Sagittal T1

Although several anatomic features of the brain are well delineated on standard sagittal T1 images, these images also allow evaluation of the orbits and cranial marrow signal. T1-weighted images

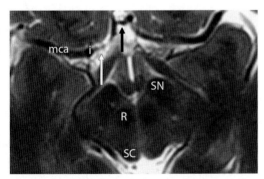

Fig. 10. Axial T2-weighted image (repetition time, 6900 ms; echo time, 96 ms) through the inferior midbrain demonstrating areas of decreased T2 signal (indicating iron deposition) within the red nucleus (R) and substantia nigra (SN). The superior colliculus is also seen at this level. Flow voids within the internal carotid artery terminus (i), middle cerebral artery (mca), anterior cerebral artery (*white arrow*), and anterior communicating artery (*black arrow*) are noted.

provide some insight into cerebrovascular structures, and normal flow voids can be visualized in the deep venous structures and dural venous sinuses.

The orbit is bounded medially by the thin-walled lamina papyracea, separating the orbit from the ethmoid air cells. The inferior boundary of the orbit, the orbital floor, also serves as the roof of the maxillary sinus,[22] whereas the orbital roof is formed by the frontal bone. The extraocular muscles, seen well on axial and sagittal T1-weighted images, show slight increase in signal intensity relative to the temporalis muscle on T1-weighted images and greater enhancement relative to the temporalis muscle after gadolinium adminstration.[23] Thus, the extraocular muscles should be evaluated on more than 1 imaging sequence when evaluating for pathologic abnormalities. The normal orbital fat demonstrates increased signal intensity on T1-weighted images and decreased signal intensity on T1-weighted fat-saturated images. When evaluating the orbital fat with frequency-selective fat suppression techniques, field inhomogeneity can contribute to incomplete fat suppression in the orbital fat. Inversion recovery techniques can be particularly useful because these sequences yield more uniform fat suppression.[24]

Conversion of red (active) marrow to yellow (inactive) marrow is a normal process usually completed by 25 years of age. Red marrow usually demonstrates a relative isointense signal compared with skeletal muscle, and yellow marrow appears hyperintense to muscle and relatively isointense to subcutaneous fat. Loevner and colleagues[25] described alterations of the normal marrow signal intensity on T1-weighted images, which may be the first indicator of a systemic disorder.

Enclosed in dural leaves, the dural venous sinuses are the major drainage pathways of the cerebral veins, and their flow voids are often seen on the sagittal T1-weighted images. However, evaluation of the dural sinuses must be performed using multiple pulse sequences. T1-weighted images are not diagnostic for sinus thrombosis because 24% to 31% of normal patients may have hypoplasia of a sinus.[26,27]

Axial T2

Although T2-weighted images provide substantial anatomic detail about the brain, these sequences also provide important detail about the intracranial vascular structures. Flow voids appear as areas of signal dropout on T2-weighted images and are normally expected for intracranial arteries. Loss of an expected flow void should key the interpreting physician to the possibility of vascular occlusion. In addition to vessel patency, flow voids on T2-weighted images may also suggest abnormalities in vascular caliber. It is not uncommon to detect middle cerebral artery aneurysms in the sylvian fissure or internal carotid artery aneurysms near the clinoids. One pitfall may occur in the case of a pneumatized clinoid process that can mimic an internal carotid artery aneurysm.

DW Imaging

As discussed earlier, DW images are exquisitely sensitive to the detection of acute infarction. In addition, these images are fat-saturated, so evaluation of calvarial lesions is aided by this sequence, particularly if there is concern for a scalp or calvarial lipoma.

SUMMARY

The exquisite detail provided by brain MR imaging scans can make interpretation simultaneously straightforward and complicated, particularly to the novice. For this reason, it is essential to become familiar with normal structures before describing the pathologic condition. This article serves as a practical reference point to further enhance knowledge of the intracranial anatomy.

REFERENCES

1. Grossman RI, Yousem DM. Neuroradiology: the requisites. 2nd edition. Philadelphia: Elsevier; 2003.
2. Atlas SW. Magnetic resonance imaging of the brain and spine, vol. 1. 4th edition. Philadelphia: Lippincott Williams & Wilkins; 2009.
3. Berger MS, Cohen WA, Ojemann GA. Correlation of motor cortex brain mapping data with magnetic resonance imaging. J Neurosurg 1990;72(3):383–7.
4. Kido DK, LeMay M, Levinson AW, et al. Computed tomographic localization of the precentral gyrus. Radiology 1980;135(2):373–7.
5. Park MC, Goldman MA, Park MJ, et al. Neuroanatomical localization of the 'precentral knob' with computed tomography imaging. Stereotact Funct Neurosurg 2007;85(4):158–61.
6. Naidich TP, Valavanis AG, Kubik S. Anatomic relationships along the low-middle convexity: part I–normal specimens and magnetic resonance imaging. Neurosurgery 1995;36(3):517–32.
7. Erbil M, Onderoglu S, Yener N, et al. Localization of the central sulcus and adjacent sulci in human: a study by MRI. Okajimas Folia Anat Jpn 1998; 75(2–3):155–62.
8. Ribas GC, Yasuda A, Ribas EC, et al. Surgical anatomy of microneurosurgical sulcal key points. Neurosurgery 2006;59(4 Suppl 2):ONS177–210 [discussion: ONS210–1].

9. Naidich TP, Daniels DL, Haughton VM, et al. Hippo-campal formation and related structures of the limbic lobe: anatomic-MR correlation. Part II. Sagittal sections. Radiology 1987;162(3):755–61.

10. Naidich TP, Daniels DL, Haughton VM, et al. Hippo-campal formation and related structures of the limbic lobe: anatomic-MR correlation. Part I. Surface features and coronal sections. Radiology 1987;162(3):747–54.

11. Johnson AK, Cunningham JT, Thunhorst RL. Integra-tive role of the lamina terminalis in the regulation of cardiovascular and body fluid homeostasis. Clin Exp Pharmacol Physiol 1996;23(2):183–91.

12. Naidich TP, Daniels DL, Pech P, et al. Anterior commissure: anatomic-MR correlation and use as a landmark in three orthogonal planes. Radiology 1986;158(2):421–9.

13. Rhoton AL Jr. The cerebrum. Anatomy. Neurosur-gery 2007;61(1 Suppl):37–118 [discussion: 118–9].

14. Choi CY, Han SR, Yee GT, et al. Central core of the cerebrum. J Neurosurg 2011;114(2):463–9.

15. Rhoton AL Jr. The cerebrum. Neurosurgery 2002; 51(4 Suppl):S1–51.

16. Blumenfeld H. Neuroanatomy through clinical cases. Sunderland (MA): Sinauer Associates; 2002.

17. Sathi S, Stieg PE. "Acquired" Chiari I malformation after multiple lumbar punctures: case report. Neuro-surgery 1993;32(2):306–9 [discussion: 309].

18. Maschke M, Weber J, Dimitrova A, et al. Age-related changes of the dentate nuclei in normal adults as re-vealed by 3D fast low angle shot (FLASH) echo sequence magnetic resonance imaging. J Neurol 2004;251(6):740–6.

19. Uchino A, Takase Y, Nomiyama K, et al. Brainstem and cerebellar changes after cerebrovascular acci-dents: magnetic resonance imaging. Eur Radiol 2006;16(3):592–7.

20. Angeles Fernandez-Gil M, Palacios-Bote R, Leo-Barahona M, et al. Anatomy of the brainstem: a gaze into the stem of life. Semin Ultrasound CT MR 2010; 31(3):196–219.

21. Smith LH, DeMyer WE. Anatomy of the brainstem. Semin Pediatr Neurol 2003;10(4):235–40.

22. Wichmann W, Muller-Forell W. Anatomy of the visual system. Eur J Radiol 2004;49(1):8–30.

23. Karakas HM, Tasali N, Cakir B. Normal magnetic resonance contrast enhancement of extraocular muscles: a quantitative analysis. Ophthalmologica 2002;216(2):85–9.

24. Brown BA, Swallow CE, Eiseman AS. MRI artifact masquerading as orbital disease. Int Ophthalmol 2001;24(6):343–7.

25. Loevner LA, Tobey JD, Yousem DM, et al. MR imaging characteristics of cranial bone marrow in adult patients with underlying systemic disorders compared with healthy control subjects. AJNR Am J Neuroradiol 2002;23(2):248–54.

26. Alper F, Kantarci M, Dane S, et al. Importance of anatomical asymmetries of transverse sinuses: an MR venographic study. Cerebrovasc Dis 2004; 18(3):236–9.

27. Ayanzen RH, Bird CR, Keller PJ, et al. Cerebral MR venography: normal anatomy and potential diag-nostic pitfalls. AJNR Am J Neuroradiol 2000;21(1): 74–8.

Skull Base, Orbits, Temporal Bone, and Cranial Nerves: Anatomy on MR Imaging

Ajaykumar C. Morani, MD[a],*, Nisha S. Ramani, MBBS[b],
Jeffrey R. Wesolowski, MD[c]

KEYWORDS

- Skull base • Orbits • Temporal bone • Cranial nerve
- MR imaging • Anatomy

Accurate delineation, diagnosis, and treatment planning of skull base lesions require knowledge of the complex anatomy of the skull base. Because the skull base is not directly accessible for clinical evaluation, imaging is critical for the diagnosis and management of skull base diseases.[1–3] Although CT is excellent for outlining the bony detail, MR imaging provides better soft tissue detail[1,4,5] and is helpful for evaluating the adjacent meninges, brain parenchyma, and bone marrow of the skull base. Thus, CT and MR imaging complement each other and are often used together for complete evaluation of skull base lesions.[1,3] This article focuses on the radiologic anatomy of the skull base pertinent to MR imaging evaluation.

PROTOCOL

At the authors' institution, conventional or fast spin-echo (FSE) T1-weighted (T1W) images in the axial and coronal planes, axial or coronal T2-weighted (T2W) images, and post–contrast-enhanced images (with and without fat suppression) are obtained in all patients with suspected skull base lesions (**Tables 1–3**). The images are obtained with higher resolution, using a smaller field of view with a slice thickness of 3 mm. Intravenous gadolinium is important to clearly delineate the extent of pathology and to detect intracranial extension, particularly meningeal involvement.[3,6,7] Fat-suppressed T1W images can be obtained if the lesion is in the vicinity of fat-containing areas, such as the orbits. However, the skull base region is extremely susceptible to artifacts from tissue inhomogeneity because of air in the adjacent paranasal sinuses. Therefore, fat-suppression technique is not always successful, particularly if the patient also has dental or craniofacial reconstruction hardware causing susceptibility artifacts and distortion.[8] To reduce the acquisition time of these high-resolution images, parallel imaging techniques (if available) can be helpful.[3] A short inversion-time inversion-recovery (STIR) sequence may be used as an alternative to fat-saturated T2W images in patients with extensive maxillofacial facial hardware. STIR provides better fat suppression but takes longer to acquire and is susceptible to pulsatile flow in adjacent vessels.[8]

For MR imaging of the cavernous sinuses, the imaging field should extend from the orbital apex

The authors have nothing to disclose.

[a] Department of Radiology, University of Michigan, 1500 East Medical Center Drive, Ann Arbor, MI 48109, USA
[b] Department of Internal Medicine, University of Michigan, 1500 East Medical Center Drive, Ann Arbor, MI 48109, USA
[c] Division of Neuroradiology, Department of Radiology, University of Michigan Medical Center, 1500 East Medical Center Drive, Room B2A205, Ann Arbor, MI 48109, USA
* Corresponding author.
E-mail address: amorani@med.umich.edu

Magn Reson Imaging Clin N Am 19 (2011) 439–456
doi:10.1016/j.mric.2011.05.006

Table 1
MR imaging of cranial nerve II (orbit)

Slice Orientation	SAG T1W HEAD	DWI HEAD	AX FLAIR HEAD	COR T2 FS	AX T1 FS W/WO	COR T1 FS W/WO	COR T1	AX T1 HEAD
Field of view (mm)	240	230	230	180	190	180	180	240
Matrix	256/512	128/256	320/512	256/512	256/512	256/512	256/512	256/512
No. of slices/location	23	24	20	40	28	40	40	24
Slice thickness/gap	4/0.5 mm	4/1 mm	6/1 mm	2/default	2/default	2/default	2/default	6/1 mm
Contrast	Pre-	Pre-	Pre-	Pre-	Pre-/Post-	Pre-/Post-	Post-	Post-
TE	10	59	125	90	10	10.6	10.6	10
TR	Shortest	Shortest	11,000	Shortest	Shortest	Shortest	Shortest	Shortest
Flip angle	—	90	—	90	90	90	90	—
Number of Excitations	1	1	1	3	2	2	2	1

Coronal coverage is from anterior globe through the optic chiasma. Axial coverage is centered over orbits. Dose of contrast media is determined according to patient weight.

Abbreviations: AX, axial; COR, coronal; DWI, diffusion weighted imaging; FLAIR, fluid attenuation inversion recovery; FS, fat saturated; SAG, sagittal; TE, echo time; TR, repetition time; W/WO, with and without.

Table 2
MR imaging of cranial nerves V and IX through XII (skull base)

Slice Orientation	SAG T1 HEAD	DWI HEAD	AX FLAIR HEAD	AX T2	AX T1	POST AX T1	AX T1 F/S	COR T1	AX T1 HEAD
Field of view (mm)	240	230	230	160	160	160	160	160	240
Matrix	304/512	128/256	320/512	336/400	224/288	224/288	224/288	224/288	256/512
No. of slices/location	21	28	25	34	34	34	34	38	25
Slice thickness/gap	5/1 mm	4/1 mm	5/1 mm	4/1 mm	4/1 mm	4/1 mm	4/1 mm	3/default	5/1 mm
Contrast	Pre-	Pre-	Pre-	Pre-	Pre-	Post-	Post-	Post-	Post-
TE	10	59	125	90	9.1	8	8	10.5	10
TR	Shortest	Shortest	11,000	Shortest	500	590	545	500	500
Flip angle	—	90	—	90	75	90	90	90	—
Number of excitations	1	1	1	1	1	3	2	4	1

Axial thin coverage is from the top of the frontal sinus to mid-C3, and from the mandible to the spinous process. Coronal coverage is from the frontal sinus to the posterior pons. Dose of contrast media is determined according to patient weight.

Table 3
MR imaging of cranial nerves VII and VIII

Slice Orientation	SAG T1 HEAD	DWI HEAD	AX FLAIR HEAD	VISTA	AX T2	AX T1 W/WO	COR T1	AX T1 HEAD
Field of view	240	230	230	180	190	190	200	240
Matrix	256/512	128/256	320/512	360/1024	256/512	256/512	256/512	256/512
No. of slices/location	19	28	20	74	18	18	18	25
Slice thickness/gap	6/1 mm	4/1 mm	6/1 mm	0.3 mm	2/default	2/default	2/default	5/1 mm
Contrast	Pre-	Pre-	Pre-	Pre-	Pre-	Pre-/Post-	Post-	Post-
TE	10	51	125	187	90	10	10.5	10
TR	Shortest	Shortest	11,000	1500	3000	500	500	500
Flip angle	—	90	—	90	90	90	90	—
Number of excitations	1	1	1	1	3	2	2	1

Coverage for thin axial and coronal slices includes internal auditory canals. VISTA images should be reformatted in both sagittal and coronal planes. Imaging of each side is performed separately.

Dose of contrast media is determined according to patient weight.

Abbreviation: VISTA, volumetric isotropic T2w aquisition.

to the prepontine cistern. Comprehensive imaging should also include routine T2W/fluid attenuated inversion recovery (FLAIR), and precontrast and postcontrast T1W sequences though the entire brain. Specific sequences through the cavernous sinuses should include 3-mm-thick postcontrast T1W slices in coronal and axial planes, with the fat-saturation technique used in at least one of these planes (see **Table 2**). Individual cranial nerves in the sinuses and adjacent cisterns may be visualized using thin-slice three-dimensional heavily T2W images (such as fast imaging using steady-state acquisition [FIESTA] or, alternatively, constructive interference in steady state [CISS]).[9]

For orbital imaging, phased-array surface coils can be used for detailed imaging of the anterior optic pathway, but these coils do not have enough penetration to image the posterior optic pathway, including the brainstem (which generally requires a standard head coil). Thus a dual-coil approach is often used for orbital MR imaging. Improvements in multichannel head coils and the increasing use of 3T scanners, however, often provide detailed imaging of both the anterior optic pathway and the posterior fossa structures, allowing for the use of a single coil.[8] Most routine orbital imaging protocols include mainly T1W and T2W spin-echo or FSE sequences, all acquired with slice thickness of 3 mm and slice gap of 1 mm. Axial or coronal T2W FSE with fat saturation and axial T1W images are acquired, followed by postcontrast axial and coronal T1W with fat saturation (see **Table 1**). To evaluate the lacrimal system, MR dacryocystography can be obtained through filling the lacrimal sac and nasolacrimal duct with a dilute mixture of gadolinium-containing contrast agent administered typically via cannulation of the lacrimal canaliculi.[8]

MR imaging of the temporal bone always covers imaging of the internal auditory canal, cerebellopontine angle, and the labyrinth (see **Table 3**). Three-millimeter-thick conventional spin-echo or attenuation recovery T1W images provide good imaging of the labyrinth. However, currently 2-mm spin-echo or 1-mm gradient-echo T1W images are used to show different turns of the cochlea, vestibule, semicircular canals, and, in several cases, the endolymphatic sac. Neurovascular structures in the internal auditory canal (IAC) and cerebellopontine angle are well seen on these images. Fat-suppressed coronal T1W spin-echo images can also be used while imaging the temporal bone to eliminate the high T1 signal intensity of the fatty bone marrow in the walls of the internal auditory canal.

For detailed evaluation of the labyrinth, 0.5- to 0.7-mm heavily T2W gradient echo or FSE three-dimensional images are very useful and provide high contrast between the cerebrospinal fluid, intralabyrinthine fluid, nerves, and the bone. These sequences are very useful to evaluate the facial nerve and the three branches of the vestibulocochlear nerves in the internal auditory canal. Submillimeter images can also distinguish between the scala tympani and scala vestibuli/scala media. High-resolution images of both inner ears can be acquired with a good signal-to-noise ratio using a small field of view (95 mm) and a matrix of 192 × 256. Multiplanar three-dimensional reconstructions and virtual images of the fluid-containing membranous labyrinth can be obtained using these small field of view images. Contiguous three-dimensional intraluminal view can be displayed with virtual otoscopy.

Vascular time-of-flight MR angiography images should also be used, particularly in patients with pulsatile tinnitus. On these images, arteries are hyperintense in appearance, whereas the nerves and veins remain hypointense. These images can also be used to show neurovascular conflicts, vascular tumors, or vascular malformations in relation to the temporal bone.[10]

Axial T2/FLAIR images of the brain are also used to complete the study of temporal bone MR imaging, mainly to exclude intra-axial lesions. If a central lesion is suspected as the cause of vertigo or sensorineural hearing loss, 4-mm-thick heavily T2W spin-echo images through the brainstem are also acquired. The myelinated structures can be easily seen on these heavily T2W images, from which the location of the nuclei and the vestibulocochlear pathways can be presumed.[10] The location of the nuclei of other cranial nerves can also be presumed using the same principle.

ANATOMY

The anterior, middle, and posterior cranial fossae are the three naturally contoured regions forming the skull base when seen from above. However, no defined boundaries correspond to these fossae when seen from below. The anterior skull base is formed by the frontal bone and sinus, along with the roof of the ethmoid sinuses, nasal cavity, and orbits. The central skull base is formed predominantly by the sphenoid bone, and the posterior skull base is formed by temporal and occipital bones.[1]

Bones forming the skull base contain normal fatty marrow, which appears hyperintense on T1W images without fat suppression, and loses signal on fat-saturated images. The marrow also normally appears dark on fat-saturated T2W images, which increases the conspicuity of the skull base bony lesions.[1] The cortical bones contain nonmobile protons similar to the air in the adjacent paranasal sinuses, hence these appear as signal voids on all of the MR pulse sequences.[8] Although cortical erosion is more confidently diagnosed on CT, infiltration of the marrow spaces is better delineated on MR imaging. CT often underestimates the frequency and extent of skull base involvement.[1] However, the skull base bones may not have a medullary cavity and therefore marrow fat. For example, the orbital roof and ethmoid sinuses do not have marrow cavities, whereas the clivus has a marrow cavity normally containing abundant fat.[11] However, in the pediatric age group, the marrow may still be hematopoietic and not replaced by fat, appearing relatively hypointense on T1W imaging.[3,11]

ANTERIOR SKULL BASE

The anterior skull base forms the floor of the anterior skull and includes the roof of the ethmoid sinuses, the nasal cavity, and the orbits (**Figs. 1** and **2**). Anteriorly, it is bounded by the posterior wall of the frontal sinus and its posterior margin is formed by the lesser wing of the sphenoid bone.[1,3] Medially along the anterior skull base, the thin cribriform plate of the ethmoid bone and lateral fovea ethmoidalis constitute the roof of the nasal cavity and ethmoid sinuses. The cribriform plate possesses multiple small perforations transmitting olfactory nerves from the nasal mucosa to the olfactory bulb (see **Fig. 1**). The middle nasal turbinate is delicately attached to inferior surface of the cribriform plate. The anterior ethmoid artery enters the anterior cranial fossa from the ethmoid sinus through the lateral lamella of the cribriform plate before reentering the nose. Laterally, the anterior skull base is bounded by the orbital plates of the frontal bone, which form the orbital roof and roof of the ethmoid sinuses. The orbital plate of the frontal bone is actually the largest area of the anterior skull base. Although the cribriform plate forms the weak part of anterior skull base and the site of common bony injuries, erosions, and cerebrospinal fluid (CSF) leaks, the orbital roof is thick and sturdy with relative resistance to these changes.[1,3]

CENTRAL SKULL BASE

The sphenoid bone forms most of the central skull base and floor of the middle cranial fossa. Its anterior border is formed by the greater wings of the sphenoid bone, and the posterior border is formed by the anterior surface of the petrous temporal bone. The medial part of the central skull base is formed by the body of the sphenoid bone, with the cavernous sinuses on either side; the lateral

aspect of the central skull base is constituted by the squamous temporal bone. The central large depression in the sphenoid body is called the *sella turcica*.[1,12] The roof of the sella turcica is formed by a fold of dura called *diaphragma sella*, which is perforated to allow passage of the pituitary stalk or infundibulum (see **Fig. 1**).

The pituitary gland is composed of two lobes that are distinct anatomically, embryologically, and physiologically. The anterior lobe is the larger part, constituting 75% of the pituitary volume, and is also called the *adenohypophysis*. It appears homogenous and isointense to gray matter on T1W and T2W images. The posterior lobe of the pituitary occupies the posterior third of the sella turcica and is also called the *neurohypophysis*. The so-called posterior pituitary bright spot is the hyperintense signal of the neurohypophysis on T1W images because of the proteinaceous antidiuretic hormone complex.[12,13] The posterior pituitary enhances before the anterior pituitary during dynamic imaging, because it has a direct blood supply via the meningohypophyseal artery.[13] The sphenoid sinus is located inferior to the sella turcica and its degree of pneumatization is variable. The internal carotid artery and cranial nerve V2 (maxillary division) frequently groove the lateral wall of sphenoid sinus during their course through the cavernous sinus.[1] The posterior sloping portion of the sphenoid bone is called the *clivus*, which forms the roof of the nasopharynx along its inferior surface.[1,12]

The cavernous sinuses are located on either side of the sphenoid bone. They form the lateral walls of the pituitary fossa or sella.[1,9,12] Each cavernous sinus contains the internal carotid arteries as the most medial structure called the carotid trigone, and cranial nerves III, IV, and VI and the first (ophthalmic-V1) and second (maxillary-V2) divisions of cranial nerve V. Cranial nerve VI runs in the center of the cavernous sinus adjacent to the internal carotid artery, whereas the other nerves run in the lateral wall of the cavernous sinus (oculomotor trigone). The cavernous sinus is actually a multiseptate space, which shows intense contrast enhancement of the slower-flowing venous blood. The internal carotid artery appears as a signal void structure on the standard MR imaging sequences and appears hyperintense on time-of-flight and other bright blood MR sequences.[8] Because of intense background enhancement, detection of intracavernous lesions is challenging. T2W images without fat saturation often provide better contrast resolution between the cavernous sinus and intracavernous lesions, and hence should be included to evaluate the cavernous sinus pathologies.[8] Sometimes the

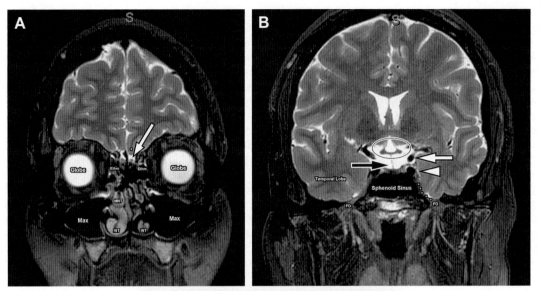

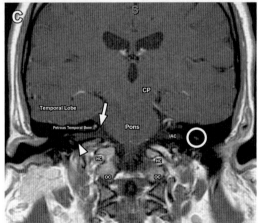

Fig. 1. Coronal fat-suppressed T2W images of the anterior (*A*) and central (*B*) skull base, and coronal T1W post-contrast image of the posterior skull base (*C*). (*A*) At the level of the maxillary sinuses (Max) and optic globes (Globe), the cranial nerves I are well seen (*arrow*) just inferior to the gyrus rectus (*asterisk*). The ethmoid sinuses (Ethm) are located slightly inferiorly and laterally, whereas the middle and inferior nasal turbinates (MNT, INT) are located more inferiorly. (*B*) At the level of the sella turcica, the optic chiasm is noted (*ellipse*), with the pituitary infundibulum (*black arrow*) present just inferior. The internal carotid artery flow voids are denoted by the white arrowhead (cavernous segment) and arrow (paraclinoid segment). The third division of the trigeminal nerve is noted to course inferior and lateral to the cavernous sinus (*asterisks*) as it heads toward the foramen ovale (FO). (*C*) At the level of the posterior skull base, the internal auditory canal (IAC) is seen with the lateral fundus (*arrowhead*) and medial porus acusticus (*arrow*) noted. More inferiorly, the hypoglossal canals (HC) and occipital condyles (OC) are seen. The posterior skull base is intimately associated with the pons and the cerebral peduncle (CP). Note the enhancing tympanic segment of the left cranial nerve VII (*circled*), which is a normal finding.

sinuses may contain fatty deposits, which are normal and may be more prominent in obese patients, those with Cushing syndrome, or patients receiving steroids.[9] Individual cranial nerves in the sinuses may be visualized using thin-slice three-dimensional heavily T2W images (such CISS or FIESTA).[9]

The optic canal, superior orbital fissure, foramen rotundum, foramen ovale, foramen spinosum, and vidian canal are found within the sphenoid bone

and form part of the central skull base.[1,14] The optic canal is the only canal that passes through the lesser wing of sphenoid. It transmits cranial nerve II and the ophthalmic artery. The lesser wing is attached to the sphenoid body with two roots, which form the roof, lateral wall, and floor of the optic canal. The sphenoid body forms the medial wall of the optic canal. The inferior root of lesser wing or the optic strut separates the optic canal from the superior orbital fissure. The superior

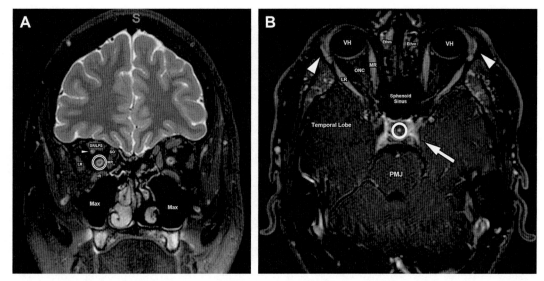

Fig. 2. Orbital coronal T2W imaging with fat saturation (*A*) and axial T1 postcontrast fat-saturated image (*B*). (*A*) The conal muscles are well seen, namely the inferior, medial, and lateral recti (IR, MR, LR), as are the superior oblique (SO) and the superior rectus/levator palpebrae superioris complex (SR/LPS). Intraconally, the optic nerve complex is noted, with the T2 hypointense (white matter tract) cranial nerve II surrounded by T2 bright cerebrospinal fluid (*circled*). The superior ophthalmic vein is noted just inferior to the superior rectus (*arrowhead*). (*B*) On postcontrast fat-suppressed imaging, the vitreous humor of the optic globe remains hypointense (VH), whereas the recti muscles (MR, LR) enhance avidly. The optic nerve complex (ONC) remains hypointense. However, the lacrimal glands enhance avidly (*arrowheads*). More posteriorly, the pituitary stalk (*circle*) and the densely enhancing cavernous sinus (*arrow*) just anterior to the pontomedullary junction (PMJ) can be seen.

orbital fissure is formed by the lesser wing of the sphenoid bone superiorly, the greater wing inferiorly, and the sphenoid body medially. This fissure transmits cranial nerves III, IV, VI, and V1. The optic canal and the superior orbital fissure together form the orbital apex, one of the important transition zones between intracranial and extracranial contents.[1]

The foramen rotundum is seen inferior to the superior orbital fissure and it transmits cranial nerve V2. This foramen connects the cavernous sinus in the middle cranial fossa to the pterygopalatine fossa.[1,15] The vidians canal is located at the junction of the pterygoid process and the sphenoid body. It connects the pterygopalatine fossa anteriorly and the foramen lacerum posteriorly. The vidian canal transmits the vidian artery, which is a branch of the maxillary artery, and also transmits the vidian nerve, which is formed by the greater superficial petrosal nerve and the deep petrosal nerve.[1] The fibrocartilage that plugs the foramen lacerum is one of the most resistant tissues to tumor infiltration.[1]

Fat is helpful in the evaluation of bones and the foramina of the central skull base, which are easily seen on T1W images without fat saturation, particularly in the coronal plane. The earliest sign of involvement of these foramina or bones by any malignant, infiltrative, or infective process is the obliteration of the normal fat content or normal fat planes, especially when compared from opposite side.[1,16,17] Obliteration of the high fat signal intensity on T1W MR images is actually the key sign of impending perineural spread by the malignancies at the skull base.[18]

The foramen ovale transmits cranial nerve V3 and is located in the posterolateral aspect of the greater wing in the central skull base (see **Fig. 1**). It connects the middle cranial fossa and the masticator space. The foraminal size can be variable on either side and also in different patients, but usually it should not differ by more than 4 mm on the two sides in an individual. Foramen spinosum is another foramen of the central skull base, located posterolateral to the foramen ovale and usually less than 2 mm in diameter. It transmits the middle meningeal artery. If the diameter of foramen spinosum exceeds 5 mm, a middle meningeal artery abnormality must be ruled out.[19] Conversely, if absent, a persistent stapedial artery must be suspected.

POSTERIOR SKULL BASE

The posterior surface of the clivus forms the anterior portion of the posterior skull base and posterior cranial fossa. The clivus is formed from fusion of the basisphenoid and basiocciput. It extends from the foramen magnum inferodorsally to the dorsum sellae superoventrally. The lateral portion of posterior skull base is formed by the posterior surface of the petrous temporal bone superiorly and the condylar part of the occipital bone inferiorly. The posterior portion of the posterior cranial fossa and posterior skull base is constituted by the mastoid temporal bone and the squamous occipital bone. The foramen magnum is entirely formed within the occipital bone.[1] The junction between the petrous temporal bone anterolaterally and the occipital bone posteromedially is called the *petro-occipital suture*.

The jugular foramen is seen at the posterior end of petro-occipital suture.[1,20] Its appearance varies depending on the level of the imaging sections, because it courses anteriorly, then laterally, and finally inferiorly through the skull base[1] into the carotid space. The right jugular foramen is larger than the left in 75% of the population.[21] Anteriorly, the caroticojugular spine, a bony ridge, separates the jugular foramen from the inferior carotid opening. Medially, an osseous bar called the *jugular tubercle* is an important landmark separating the jugular foramen from the hypoglossal canal.[1,21] Pars nervosa forms the anteromedial compartment, and the pars vascularis forms the posterolateral compartment of the jugular foramen. These compartments are separated by a dividing fibrous or bony septum. Pars nervosa is smaller and more consistent in size, and transmits cranial nerve IX (glossopharyngeal nerve) with its tympanic branch (Jacobson nerve) and the inferior petrosal sinus. The inferior petrosal sinus forms a multichannel confluence with the sigmoid sinus in the pars nervosa and empties into the jugular bulb.[21] The pars vascularis is larger and more variable in size, transmitting the internal jugular vein, cranial nerve X (vagus nerve) with its auricular branch (Arnold nerve), cranial nerve XI (accessory nerve), and the posterior meningeal artery,[1,21–23] a branch of ascending pharyngeal artery supplying the posterior fossa meninges.[21]

The appearance of the jugular foramen is anatomically variable, and sometimes both cranial nerves IX and X traverse through the pars nervosa.[21] Cranial nerves in the jugular foramen cannot be seen on conventional MR imaging sequences, but may be well seen on the contrast-enhanced three-dimensional fast imaging using steady-state acquisition, which provides high contrast and spatial resolution.[21] The most common pseudolesion of the jugular foramen on MR imaging results from the complex flow pattern within a normal jugular bulb, which may be misinterpreted as intraluminal thrombus or a glomus tumor. This pseudolesion can produce intermediate signal or high signal on postcontrast T1W images. T2W images in these cases should show lack of flow artifact. If still unclear, MR venography can help resolve the issue. Another potential pitfall is a large or high jugular fossa caused by normal variation in size and symmetry, which may be mistaken as a sign of a space-occupying lesion. When the roof of the jugular bulb is seen above the level of inferior margin of the cochlear basal turn, it is called a *high-riding jugular bulb*, which is more common on the right side. It compromises the exposure during translabyrinthine surgery and during surgery for cerebellopontine angle lesions.[21]

ORBITS

Contents of the orbit are located within a bony pyramid. Its roof is formed by the orbital plate of the frontal bone. The lacrimal gland lies in the lacrimal fossa, a recess of the frontal bone anterolaterally in the orbit. The lateral orbital wall is formed by the orbital surface of zygomatic bone and the greater wing of sphenoid bone. From anterior to posterior, the medial orbital wall is formed by the maxillary bone, lacrimal bone, lamina papyracea of the ethmoid bone, and lesser wing of the sphenoid. The lacrimal sac lies in the fossa along the anteromedial orbital wall.

The orbital floor is formed by the zygomatic, maxilla, and the palatine bones. The infraorbital groove containing the infraorbital nerve traverses the orbital floor, ending in the infraorbital canal and foramen. If the distal portion of the infraorbital canal is not formed, the infraorbital nerve may traverse through the underlying maxillary sinus. In these cases, it is vulnerable to any sinus surgery or sinus pathology.[24] The zygomatic branch of cranial nerve V2 also traverses within the orbital floor and divides into the zygomaticofacial and zygomaticotemporal nerve, which emerge through the respective foramina in the face. These foramina are sometimes seen on high-resolution T1W MR imaging. Similarly, the anterior and posterior ethmoidal foramina transmitting the corresponding ethmoidal vessel and nerve may be seen medially between the frontal bone and the lamina papyracea or within the frontal bone.[24] The optic canal transmits cranial nerve II and the ophthalmic artery. The inferior root of lesser wing or the optic strut separates the optic canal from the superior orbital fissure. The superior orbital fissure is formed by the lesser wing of the sphenoid bone superiorly, the greater wing inferiorly, and the sphenoid body medially. This fissure transmits the cranial nerves III, IV, VI, and V1.[1,24]

High-signal marrow of the optic strut may be seen separating the optic nerve within the optic canal from cranial nerve III and other cranial nerves in the superior orbital fissure on high-resolution T1W MR imaging.[24] The inferior orbital fissure lies between the orbital floor and the greater wing of sphenoid, and communicates with the pterygopalatine fossa and masticator space.[24] The optic canal and the superior orbital fissure together form the orbital apex, one of the important transition zones between intracranial and extracranial contents.[1]

Fat-saturated pulse sequences allow better assessment of the lacrimal glands, optic nerves, and fatty reticulum of the orbit. However, this technique may be suboptimal if the patient has hardware as previously described. STIR images, if used as an alternative to fat-saturated T2W images because of dental or craniofacial hardware, may show better fat suppression, but will be susceptible to eye movements as they take a longer time to acquire.[8] The lacrimal glands appear hypointense compared with the surrounding orbital fat on T1W images, whereas they are slightly hyperintense to muscle on T2W images and show homogenous contrast enhancement (see **Fig. 2**). MR imaging itself is not always sufficient for reliable assessment of the lacrimal canaliculi, lacrimal sac, and nasolacrimal duct, for which MR dacryocystography may be useful.[8] The ophthalmic artery accompanies cranial nerve II in the optic canal. Its retinal artery branch traverses within cranial nerve II, and other branches accompany the corresponding nerves in the orbit. Intraorbital arteries are generally beyond the resolution of conventional MR imaging, although larger vascular lesions may show flow voids and partly may be seen on time-of-flight MR angiography images.[8] The superior ophthalmic vein is larger and more consistently visualized on both coronal and axial imaging. It lies lateral to the superior oblique muscle anteriorly, and passes posteriorly beneath the superior muscle complex where it can be seen on coronal imaging. It is supplied by the facial vein and drains via the superior orbital fissures into the cavernous sinus, providing an important route for the spread of thrombosis from the face in cases of orbital cellulitis or facial infection.[24]

The extraocular muscles consist of four rectus muscles, two oblique muscles, and one levator palpebrae superioris, in each orbit. These muscles are particularly well seen on coronal MR imaging (see **Fig. 2**), and appear hypointense to orbital fat on T1W and T2W images.[8] These muscles enhance intensely after contrast because of the absence of a blood–tissue barrier.[24] The medial, lateral, superior, and inferior rectus muscles and superior oblique muscle originate at the annulus of Zinn at the optic foramen. Rectus muscles insert directly on the globe behind the limbus, whereas the superior oblique passes through the tendinous sling (trochlea) posterior to superior orbital margin before it inserts into the sclera in the middle of the globe. The inferior oblique muscle arises from the orbital floor posterior to the lacrimal sac and then traverses beneath the inferior rectus, medial to the lateral rectus, and inserts into the sclera adjacent to superior oblique. Because the superior rectus and levator palpebrae are not seen discretely from one another, these are often referred to together as the superior muscle complex on imaging.[24]

Divisions of cranial nerve III (oculomotor nerve) supply the superior, medial, and inferior rectus muscles and the inferior oblique along with a motor root to ciliary ganglion. The abducens nerve, cranial nerve VI, supplies the lateral rectus and the trochlear nerve supplies the superior oblique. Cranial nerve V1 (ophthalmic nerve) divides into three branches in the distal cavernous sinus before entry into the orbit. These branches are the frontal, lacrimal, and nasociliary nerves. Supraorbital and supratrochlear (medial) branches of the frontal nerve traverse just above the superior muscle complex with the accompanying artery. The lacrimal nerves lie in the lateral portion of the orbit, superior to the lateral rectus muscle. The nasociliary nerve crosses from lateral to medial side above the optic nerve to reach the superior surface of medial rectus, where it may be seen on high-resolution T1W images.[24]

The aqueous and vitreous humor in the ocular globe appear isointense to CSF on all the pulse sequences. In the globe, T2W images are used to evaluate lesions in the vitreous and aqueous chambers, whereas precontrast and postcontrast T1W images are used to evaluate the uveoretinal structures. The optic nerve-sheath complex, as the name suggests, includes the central cranial nerve II and surrounding sheath (dura and arachnoid), which contains CSF communicating with the subarachnoid space. MR imaging distinguishes the nerve, the dura, and the subarachnoid space on T2W and contrast-enhanced T1W MR imaging (see **Fig. 2**).[24]

Cranial nerve II is generally isointense to cerebral white matter and the surrounding extraocular muscles on T1W and T2W images.[8] MR imaging is not the preferred modality for assessing orbital fractures, calcifications, and wooden foreign bodies, for which CT is very useful. Finally, imaging of orbits is incomplete without evaluation of the cranial nerves III through VI and the cavernous sinus through which they traverse.

be excluded. Brainstem and cisternal segments are evaluated using 4-mm slices. Contrast-enhanced 0.625-mm T1W fast-field echo slices are obtained when evaluating through the cerebellopontine angle, internal auditory canal, and the jugular foramina.

Cranial Nerve I

Olfactory epithelium is present in the upper one-fifth of the nasal cavity and covers the septal and lateral surface of this cavity. Dendrites of the bipolar olfactory neurons reach the epithelial surface, and its unmyelinated axons, which are grouped in bundles called *filia*, pass through the openings in the cribriform plate to reach the olfactory bulb. Some of these filia, which together constitute cranial nerve I (olfactory), are sometimes seen on high-resolution T2W images. The olfactory bulb and tract are located in the olfactory sulcus between the gyrus rectus and medial orbital gyrus and are seen on coronal T2W or T1W images (see **Fig. 1**). These are actually the extensions of the brain and not truly cranial nerves. The olfactory tract divides posteriorly into the lateral, intermediate, and medial stria in front of the anterior perforated substance on high-resolution T2W images. The lateral stria terminates in the piriform lobe and connects to the orbital frontal cortex (highest center for olfactory discrimination) via the thalamus. The intermediate stria reach the intermediate cortical olfactory area, which is a small focus of gray matter at the level of the anterior perforated substance. Some axons in the medial stria reach the septal area via the diagonal band, whereas others reach the contralateral olfactory tract via the anterior commissure across the midline.

Cranial Nerve II

Cranial nerve II (optic nerve) is also an extension of the brain and not a true cranial nerve. It can be divided into several segments: intraocular, intraorbital, intracanalicular, and intracranial. The optic pathway then continues in the optic chiasm and optic tracts, which further extend to the optic radiation and visual cortex, which are discussed elsewhere in this issue. The axons of the retinal ganglion cells form the intraocular optic nerve, which is difficult to visualize. The intraorbital segment runs from the ocular globe to the orbital apex in the intraconal orbit. The subarachnoid CSF space surrounding the intraorbital nerve is contiguous with the suprasellar cistern. The nerve and surrounding CSF are best visualized on heavily T2W or STIR images (see **Fig. 2**). The central retinal artery, with its accompanying vein, runs within the distal 1 cm of the intraorbital segment just behind the globe. The intracanalicular segment, as the name suggests, is located in the optic canal along with the ophthalmic artery (inferior to the nerve) and is best seen on MR images. The intracranial segment (covered by only pia matter) is approximately 1 cm long and extends from the optic canal to the optic chiasm. The optic chiasm is X-shaped and located anterior to the pituitary stalk, and is best seen on reformatted three-dimensional T1W images, such as three-dimensional fast-field echo, magnetization prepared rapid gradient echo (MPRAGE), or T2W images like DRIVE and balanced fast-field echo. In the chiasm, fibers from the temporal hemiretina continue uncrossed into the ipsilateral optic tract, whereas fibers from the nasal hemiretina continue into the contralateral optic tract after crossing the midline. Each optic tract divides into a smaller medial root carrying only 10% of its fibers and a larger root carrying 90% of fibers. The medial root terminates in the medial geniculate body, and the lateral root terminates in the lateral geniculate body. The optic tracts are better seen on high-resolution T2W or FLAIR images.

Cranial Nerve III

The cranial nerve III (oculomotor nuclear) complex is located in the periaqueductal gray matter. The fascicular segment of the nerve courses through the midbrain anterolaterally to emerge medial to the cerebral peduncle (**Fig. 4**). The cisternal segment starts in the interpeduncular cistern and then courses below the posterior cerebral and above the superior cerebellar artery. Further anteriorly, it continues below the posterior communicating artery to pierce the dural roof of the cavernous sinus. This segment is best seen on high-resolution heavily T2W images and is also large enough to be seen on T1W images. The cavernous segment of the nerve runs in the lateral wall of the cavernous sinus and is highest in position superolateral to the cavernous internal carotid artery. It lies medial to cranial nerve IV in the anterior-most portion of the cavernous sinus but becomes inferomedial to it in the superior orbital fissure. Cranial nerve III courses through the cavernous sinus and is best seen on coronal contrast-enhanced high-resolution T1W imaging, and reportedly also on contrast-enhanced heavily T2W imaging. The nerve divides into the superior and inferior divisions within the superior orbital fissure. The superior division innervates the superior rectus and levator palpebrae. The inferior division supplies the inferior rectus, medial rectus, and inferior oblique muscles. These branches can

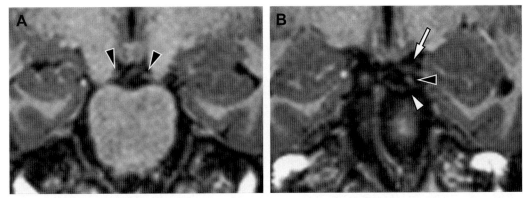

Fig. 4. T1W thin-section coronal images along the interpeduncular cistern (*A, B*). (*A*) At the level of the peduncles, cranial nerves III can be seen exiting the midbrain (*black arrowheads*). (*B*) More anteriorly, the left nerve is noted to travel between the posterior cerebral artery (*white arrow*) and the superior cerebellar artery (*white arrowhead*).

again be well seen on high-resolution coronal T1W images. Parasympathetic fibers in the nerve continue via the branch to the inferior oblique muscle to reach the ciliary ganglion, which gives rise to postganglionic parasympathetic fibers in the short ciliary nerves.

Cranial Nerve IV

Cranial nerve IV (trochlear) nucleus is situated inferior to the cranial nerve III complex at the level of the inferior colliculus, ventral to the aqueduct and posterior to the medial longitudinal fasciculus. Its fascicular segments cross the midline at the level of superior medullary velum before exiting the midbrain along the dorsal surface just caudal to the inferior colliculus. After exiting the brainstem, its cisternal segment runs in a nearly horizontal mediolateral direction to reach the free edge of the tentorium and then courses anteriorly around the brainstem. It passes through the gap between the superior cerebral artery and superior cerebellar artery, lateral to the cranial nerve III. Its course proximal to the cavernous sinus is usually only seen on high-field-strength (3T) FIESTA- or CISS-style imaging.[26] The cavernous segment of the nerve is also seen in lateral wall of the cavernous sinus adjacent to cranial nerve III, as described previously. It enters the orbit through the superior orbital fissure and supplies the superior oblique muscle.

Cranial Nerve V

The nuclei of cranial nerve V (trigeminal) are numerous and a full discussion of them is beyond the extent of this article. The cisternal or preganglionic segment of the nerve leaves from the midpons, also called the root entry zone. It is composed of sensory and motor roots. It courses anterosuperiorly through the prepontine cistern,

over the tip of the petrous apex, and then enters the CSF-filled Meckel cave. It is best seen on heavily T2W images but can also be seen on high-resolution T1W images (**Fig. 5**). The preganglionic segment of the nerve ends in the gasserian ganglion in Meckel cave; the postganglionic fibers exit through the three divisions of trigeminal nerve. The motor root passes under the gasserian ganglion and exits through the foramen ovale.

Ophthalmic: first division (V1)

V1 is seen in the lateral wall of the cavernous sinus, inferior to the fourth nerve and lateral to the sixth nerve. It is larger than these cranial nerves and is better seen on coronal contrast-enhanced high-resolution T1W images through the cavernous sinus. It then enters the superior orbital fissure, where it divides into frontal, lacrimal, and nasociliary nerves with sensory nerve supply from the globe, nose, forehead, and scalp.

Maxillary: second division (V2)

V2 courses in the wall of the floor of the cavernous sinus and exits the skull through the foramen rotundum, and is best seen on coronal images. The nerve continues through the upper part of the pterygopalatine fossa and then reaches the orbit through the inferior orbital fissure to terminate in the infraorbital nerve. In the pterygopalatine fossa, it gives off several side branches: the posterior superior alveolar nerve, the zygomatic nerve, and two nerves to the pterygopalatine ganglion. The infraorbital nerve exits the infraorbital foramen after giving off the anterior superior alveolar nerve, which runs in the lateral nasal wall.

Mandibular: third division (V3)

V3 immediately exits the skull inferiorly through the foramen ovale without coursing through the

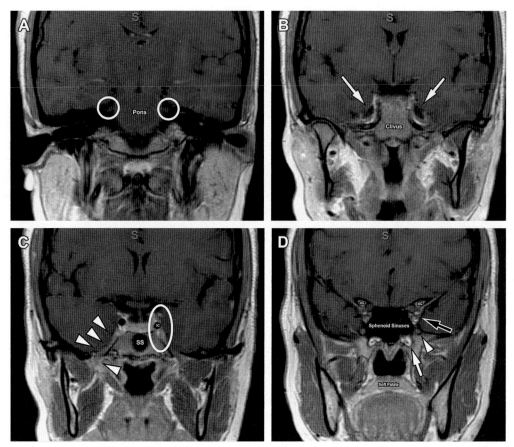

Fig. 5. Coronal T1W postcontrast images of cranial nerve V from posterior to anterior. (*A*) At the level of the pons, the exiting cranial nerve V roots are well seen (*circled*). (*B*) More anteriorly, the trigeminal nerves/ganglia are noted within the Meckel caves (*arrows*). (*C*) The cavernous sinuses are now visualized (*circled*). Note the internal carotid flow void (IC) and the descending and exiting mandibular division (V3) of the trigeminal nerve (*arrowheads*). SS, sphenoid sinus. (*D*) At the orbital apex, the contents of the superior orbital fissure can be seen (*black arrow*). The foramen rotundum and vidians canal are denoted by the white arrowhead and arrow, respectively. AC, anterior clinoid process.

cavernous sinus. The motor root joins it in the foramen and then both continue to the masticator space. Its further detailed course below the skull base is beyond the scope of this article. It has a few salient features. The enhancing venous plexus around the nerve just under the skull base allows the area of the buccal and anterior deep temporal nerve, major mandibular branch, and the posterior extension of the nerve corresponding to the area of the otic ganglion, auriculotemporal nerve origin, and meningeal branch to be distinguished. On sagittal postcontrast high-resolution T1W images, V3 can be seen in the oval foramen dividing into the lingual and inferior alveolar branches at the level of the internal maxillary artery. The middle meningeal artery, which passes through an opening in the auriculotemporal nerve just below the skull base, is seen as a contrast-enhanced structure surrounded by a nerve with a low signal intensity. The inferior alveolar nerve can be seen in its canal within the mandible, and the lingual nerve can always be seen in the pterygomandibular fat pad, located just behind and medial to the posterior free edge of the mylohyoid muscle on T1W images.[27]

Cranial Nerve VI

Cranial nerve VI (abducens) is a pure motor nerve and innervates only the lateral rectus muscle, which abducts the eye. Its nucleus is located in the middle of the pons. The fascicular segment of the nerve travels through the pontine tegmentum to leave anteriorly at the lower border of the pons. Its cisternal segment crosses the prepontine cistern and follows an anterolateral superior course to reach posterior aspect of the clivus

(Fig. 6). This segment is best seen in the axial plane on heavily T2W images, and also on coronal STIR and T1W images. The nerve then pierces the dura to enter the Dorello canal, a channel between two dural layers through the basilar venous plexus. Contrast-enhanced time-of-flight MR angiography images or three-dimensional fast-field echo images are useful for seeing the signal void of the nerve within the enhancing venous plexus at the level of the Dorello canal. The nerve then runs over the petrous apex and enters the cavernous sinus just above the Meckel cave. It continues within the cavernous sinus itself, in contrast to other cranial nerves that run in the cavernous sinus walls. It then enters the orbit through the superior orbital fissure to supply the lateral rectus. The cavernous and extracranial segments are best seen on gadolinium-enhanced high-resolution T1W images.[27]

Cranial Nerve VII

The cranial nerve VII loops around the nucleus of cranial nerve VI in the pons, creating the facial colliculus in the floor of the fourth ventricle. It then continues anterolaterally and exits the brainstem together with the intermediate nerve at the lower border of the pons. The cisternal segment of both nerves traverse through the cerebellopontine angle. These nerves are better seen on heavily T2W images. The sensory and parasympathetic fibers are carried in the nervus intermedius, which is located just posterior to the nerve proper (carrying motor fibers). The intracanalicular portion of cranial nerve VII is seen in the anterosuperior part of the IAC. Cisternal and the intracanalicular portions of the nerve and nervus intermedius can be distinguished on high-resolution T2W images, especially at 3T. The intratemporal segment of the nerve begins at the fundus of the IAC, where it enters the labyrinthine part of the facial nerve canal. It runs anterior to reach geniculate ganglion, which gives off the greater superficial petrosal nerve carrying the parasympathetic fibers anteromedially for lacrimation.

From the geniculate ganglion, the nerve continues posteriorly in the tympanic segment canal under the lateral semicircular canal to reach the posterior genu, where it turns inferiorly as the mastoid segment (see Fig. 3). It supplies the stapedius muscle and also carries taste fibers from the anterior tongue received from the lingual nerve through the chorda tympani nerve. These branches of the nerve are not seen on MR imaging. The extracranial segment of cranial nerve VII begins after it leaves the stylomastoid foramen and enters the posterior parotid. It may be seen along the proximal-most extracranial segment on high-resolution T1W images, but is no longer visible beyond this in the parotid. Its position may be assumed, because it normally courses just lateral to the retromandibular vein. If needed, microscopic coils and strong gradients may be used to visualize the intraparotid course of nerve. Finally, the nerve divides into motor end branches supplying the muscles of facial expression; the platysma, buccinator, stylohyoid, and occipitalis muscles; and the posterior belly of the digastric muscle.[27] The temporal bone portion of the facial nerve and the greater superficial petrosal nerve can show normal but mild enhancement throughout, except in the cisternal and canalicular segments.[28]

Cranial Nerve VIII

Cranial nerve VIII is composed of a cochlear and a vestibular nerve. Both are sensory nerves and are formed by the bipolar neurons. The bipolar neurons of the cochlear nerve are located in the spiral ganglion within the modiolus of the cochlea. Peripheral fibers of these neurons are connected to the organ of Corti in the scala media of the cochlea, and the central fibers join to form the cochlear nerve proper. The cochlear nerve enters the IAC through an opening in the anteroinferior part of the fundus of the IAC and remains in the anteroinferior quadrant of the IAC. It is joined by the superior and inferior vestibular nerves near the porus acusticus to form the vestibulocochlear nerve or cranial nerve VIII, which crosses the cerebellopontine angle posterior to cranial nerve VII to reach the lateral pontomedullary junction ending in cochlear nuclei.

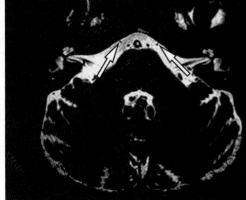

Fig. 6. Axial CISS image shows cranial nerve VI ascending within the prepontine cistern (arrows), B, basilar artery.

Bipolar neurons of the vestibular nerve are located in the Scarpa ganglion. Its peripheral fibers connect the maculae in the utricle and saccule, and the three cristae in the three ampullae of the semicircular canals with the four vestibular nuclei in the lower pons. Its multiple fibers pass though the foramina in the fundus of the IAC to form the superior and inferior vestibular nerves. The superior vestibular nerve courses in the posterosuperior quadrant and the inferior vestibular nerve in the posteroinferior quadrant of the IAC, respectively. These join to form a single vestibular nerve in porus acusticus and, further medially, join with the cochlear division to form the eighth cranial nerve. Generally, within the cerebellopontine angle, cranial nerve VII is approximately half the size of VIII (see **Fig. 3**). A subtle thickening can often be seen on the vestibular nerves in the IAC where the common vestibular branch splits into a superior and inferior branch. This thickening corresponds with the Scarpa ganglion. Sometimes connecting fibers are seen between cranial nerve VII and the vestibular nerves on high-resolution T2W images.

Cranial Nerve IX

The nuclei for cranial nerve IX (glossopharyngeal nerve) are located in the upper and middle medulla. The nerve leaves the brainstem in the postolivary sulcus and courses anterolaterally together with cranial nerves X and XI, which are located just caudal to cranial nerve IX (**Fig. 7**).[26] It then enters the pars nervosa of the jugular foramen, where its superior and inferior ganglia are also located. Cranial nerve IX can be seen and distinguished from remaining structures in the foramen on high-resolution gadolinium-enhanced fast-field echo or time-of-flight images. The nerve then enters the carotid space and courses lateral to the carotid artery, stylopharyngeus, and the palatine tonsil to reach the posterior part of sublingual space as the lingual nerve.

Cranial Nerve X

Cranial nerve X (vagus) is a parasympathetic nerve supplying the head, neck, thoracic region, and abdominal viscera, and has motor function to the soft palate, pharyngeal constrictor muscle, larynx, and palatoglossus muscles. It also carries sensory information from the viscera, external ear, and tympanic membrane, and taste from the epiglottis. The nerve exits the brainstem just below cranial nerve IX and courses with this nerve to reach the pars vasculosa of the jugular foramen (see **Fig. 7**).[26] The superior vagal ganglion is located in the jugular foramen, and the inferior vagal ganglion is located just below the skull base. The Arnold nerve branches off from the superior cervical ganglion and carries sensory information from the external ear. The other branches of cranial nerve X include the pharyngeal branches, the superior laryngeal nerve, and the recurrent laryngeal nerve, which ascends in the tracheoesophageal groove after looping around the subclavian artery on the right, or passes through the aortopulmonary window on the left side. The cisternal segment is well seen on high-resolution heavily T2W images. The foraminal and extracranial segments can be well seen on high-resolution T1W fast-field echo or time-of-flight images. Cranial nerve X appears relatively thicker than cranial nerves IX and XI.

Cranial Nerve XI

Cranial nerve XI is a pure motor nerve, innervating the sternocleidomastoid and trapezius muscles. It is formed from the bulbar and spinal motor fibers. The spinal fibers arise from the spinal motor nucleus lateral to the anterior horns of the cervical spinal cord from the C1 to C5 vertebral levels. The spinal fibers exit the cord from its lateral surface between the anterior and posterior nerve roots. These fibers form an ascending nerve, which

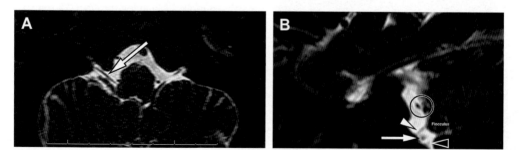

Fig. 7. Axial and coronal reformatted CISS images at the skull base (*A, B*). (*A*) Note the course of cranial nerve X as it heads from the medulla to the jugular foramen (*arrow*). (*B*) This is well demonstrated on the sagittal reformats, where the nerve (*arrow*) travels between the cranial nerve IX superiorly (*white arrowhead*) and cranial nerve XI inferiorly (*black arrowhead*). The cranial nerve VII/VIII complex is circled.

reaches the jugular foramen after passing through the foramen magnum. The bulbar cisternal segment is located just below cranial nerve X (see **Fig. 7**).[26] The bulbar and spinal fibers join in the lateral part of basal cistern. The nerve then passes through the pars vasculosa of the jugular foramen and then enters the carotid space below the skull base.

Cranial Nerve XII

Cranial nerve XII is a motor nerve, innervating the intrinsic and extrinsic tongue musculature. Its nucleus is located in the lower medulla, producing a slight bulge into the fourth ventricle called the *hypoglossal eminence*. Its fascicular segment traverses anterolaterally and exits from the brainstem from the preolivary sulcus. It emerges as a series of rootlets, which converge to form one or two root nerves. This (cisternal) segment is well seen on thin high-resolution T2W images. It then enters the skull base at the hypoglossal canal (see **Fig. 1**). On contrast-enhanced T1W three-dimensional fast-field echo images through the hypoglossal canal, this nerve can be seen as a gray arch from its entrance in the hypoglossal canal down to the upper carotid space, in the background of surrounding hyperintensity from the enhancing veins. The nerve leaves the carotid space at the inferior margin of the posterior belly of the digastric muscle, coursing lateral to the carotid bifurcation and the hypoglossus muscle to reach the tongue.[27]

SUMMARY

The skull base is a complex region with multiple compartments and components, susceptible to a multitude of disease processes. Cross-sectional imaging, particularly MR imaging, is vital in interrogating these spaces, because they are not easily evaluated clinically. Therefore, knowledge of the normal appearance of this area on MR imaging is a prerequisite for evaluating pathologic processes within it.

REFERENCES

1. Chong VF, Khoo JB, Fan YF. Imaging of the nasopharynx and skull base. Neuroimaging Clin N Am 2004;14(4):695–719.
2. Ginsberg LE, Pruett SW, Chen MY, et al. Skull-base foramina of the middle cranial fossa: reassessment of normal variation with high-resolution CT. AJNR Am J Neuroradiol 1994;15(2):283–91.
3. Parmar H, Gujar S, Shah G, et al. Imaging of the anterior skull base. Neuroimaging Clin N Am 2009; 19(3):427–39.
4. Ginsberg LE. Neoplastic diseases affecting the central skull base: CT and MR imaging. AJR Am J Roentgenol 1992;159(3):581–9.
5. Eisen MD, Yousem DM, Montone KT, et al. Use of preoperative MR to predict dural, perineural, and venous sinus invasion of skull base tumors. AJNR Am J Neuroradiol 1996;17(10):1937–45.
6. Borges A. Skull base tumours part I: imaging technique, anatomy and anterior skull base tumours. Eur J Radiol 2008;66(3):338–47.
7. Glenn LW. Innovations in neuroimaging of skull base pathology. Otolaryngol Clin North Am 2005;38(4): 613–29.
8. Conneely MF, Hacein-Bey L, Jay WM. Magnetic resonance imaging of the orbit. Semin Ophthalmol 2008;23(3):179–89.
9. Razek AA, Castillo M. Imaging lesions of the cavernous sinus. AJNR Am J Neuroradiol 2009; 30(3):444–52.
10. Mark AS, Casselman JW. Magnetic resonance imaging of the brain and spine. Philadelphia: Lippincott Williams & Wilkins; 2002.
11. Curtin HD. Magnetic resonance imaging of the brain and spine. Philadelphia: Lippincott Williams & Wilkins; 2002.
12. Johnsen DE, Woodruff WW, Allen IS, et al. MR imaging of the sellar and juxtasellar regions. Radiographics 1991;11(5):727–58.
13. Colombo N, Berry I, Kucharczyk J, et al. Posterior pituitary gland: appearance on MR images in normal and pathologic states. Radiology 1987;165(2): 481–5.
14. Chong VF, Fan YF, Tng CH. Pictorial review: radiology of the sphenoid bone. Clin Radiol 1998; 53(12):882–93.
15. Borges A, Casselman J. Imaging the trigeminal nerve. Eur J Radiol 2010;74(2):323–40.
16. Chong VF, Fan YF, Mukherji SK. Carcinoma of the nasopharynx. Semin Ultrasound CT MR 1998; 19(6):449–62.
17. Chong VF, Fan YF. Pterygopalatine fossa and maxillary nerve infiltration in nasopharyngeal carcinoma. Head Neck 1997;19(2):121–5.
18. Curtin HD. Detection of perineural spread: fat is a friend. AJNR Am J Neuroradiol 1998;19(8):1385–6.
19. Sondheimer MK. Radiology of the skull base and brain. New York: Mosby; 1971.
20. Chong VF, Fan YF. Radiology of the jugular foramen. Clin Radiol 1998;53(6):405–16.
21. Ong CK, Fook-Hin Chong V. Imaging of jugular foramen. Neuroimaging Clin N Am 2009;19(3): 469–82.
22. Rubinstein D, Burton BS, Walker AL. The anatomy of the inferior petrosal sinus, glossopharyngeal nerve, vagus nerve, and accessory nerve in the jugular foramen. AJNR Am J Neuroradiol 1995;16(1): 185–94.

23. Saleh E, Naguib M, Aristegui M, et al. Lower skull base: anatomic study with surgical implications. Ann Otol Rhinol Laryngol 1995;104(1):57–61.

24. Aviv RI, Casselman J. Orbital imaging: part 1. Normal anatomy. Clin Radiol 2005;60(3):279–87.

25. Davidson HC. Imaging evaluation of sensorineural hearing loss. Semin Ultrasound CT MR 2001;22(3):229–49.

26. Sheth S, Branstetter B, Escott E. Appearance of normal cranial nerves on steady-state free precession MR images. Radiographics 2009;29:1045–55.

27. Casselman J, Mermuys K, Delanote J, et al. MRI of the cranial nerves–more than meets the eye: technical considerations and advanced anatomy. Neuroimaging Clin N Am 2008;18(2):197–231, preceding x.

28. Gebarski SS, Telian SA, Niparko JK. Enhancement along the normal facial nerve in the facial canal: MR imaging and anatomic correlation. Radiology 1992;183(2):391–4.

Neck MR Imaging Anatomy

Joshua A. Rubin, MD[a],*, Jeffrey R. Wesolowski, MD[b]

KEYWORDS

- MR imaging • Neck anatomy • Neck MRI
- Imaging of the neck

The anatomy of the neck can be daunting for both radiologists and clinicians alike. Although small, the neck contains many vital structures. Therefore, mastery of its radiologic anatomy is essential for physicians evaluating for pathology. Magnetic resonance imaging (MR imaging) has become a vital tool to diagnose many disease processes affecting the neck region. Similar to computed tomography (CT), MR imaging has the advantage of cross-sectional imaging. Unlike CT, however, MR imaging does not require the use of intravenous contrast material to add soft tissue contrast, as the intrinsic signal characteristics of the interrogated tissues can often provide inherent differentiation.[1] Moreover, when gadolinium contrast is required for MR imaging, it is generally considered safer than iodinated contrast used for CT, with a lower incidence of anaphylaxis and renal nephrotoxicity in patients with impaired renal function.[2]

Additionally, MR imaging does not carry the burden of radiation exposure, which can become problematic for patients undergoing multiple CT scans throughout life, particularly considering the relative radiosensitivity of the thyroid gland. To spare ionizing radiation exposure, MR imaging of the neck can be performed in children, who are especially sensitive to the effects of repeated exposure. However, in very young children, general anesthesia is typically administered to prevent significant motion degradation. Therefore, the risks and benefits of MR imaging in young children must be weighed accordingly. MR imaging is advantageous in that multiplanar imaging can be easily performed without needing to reposition the patient, allowing for improved differentiation of masses, vessels, and soft tissue.[2]

The suprahyoid neck is best imaged by MR imaging, as it is less affected by dental amalgam as compared with CT. Ultrasound may be used to evaluate the carotid arteries and thyroid gland, but cannot penetrate deeply enough to evaluate the visceral structures of the neck. Since the advent of MR imaging, serial improvements in spatial resolution and protocol technique have allowed for proper evaluation of normal anatomy, as well as the full array of pathology. This article describes the protocols used at our institution and the normal neck anatomy seen with current MR imaging techniques. Correlative imaging examples are provided as well.

Many systems are used for classifying and organizing the neck structures. This article approaches the neck from a neck space perspective. The neck space concept is a commonly used method to assist radiologists in organizing the neck and establishing appropriate differential diagnoses for pathology discovered within a specific space of the neck.[3] For imaging purposes, the boundaries of the neck are considered to be the mandible and the mylohyoid muscles anterosuperiorly, the base of the skull posterosuperiorly, the scapulae posteroinferiorly, and the thoracic inlet (sternum, first ribs, first thoracic vertebra) centrally at the inferior aspect.[4]

The authors have nothing to disclose.
[a] Department of Radiology, University of Michigan Medical Center, 1500 East Medical Center Drive, Room B1D502C, Ann Arbor, MI 48019, USA
[b] Division of Neuroradiology, Department of Radiology, University of Michigan Medical Center, 1500 East Medical Center Drive, Room B2A205, Ann Arbor, MI 48109, USA
* Corresponding author.
E-mail address: josrubin@med.umich.edu

Magn Reson Imaging Clin N Am 19 (2011) 457–473
doi:10.1016/j.mric.2011.05.003
1064-9689/11/$ – see front matter

PROTOCOL

Most neck MR imaging examinations performed at our institution follow a standard "General Neck" protocol, typically performed on a 1.5-Tesla magnet, although 3.0-Telsa examinations can provided increased spatial and contrast resolution (**Table 1**). For all neck imaging, the patient is placed head first and supine into the magnet. A neurovascular array coil is placed on the patient. We use a 20-cm to 23-cm field of view (FOV), 5-mm to 6-mm slice thickness, and 1-mm to 2-mm interscan spacing. A wide range of matrices are used (see **Table 1**). First, a sagittal T1 sequence is obtained using a spin-echo pulse sequence from the clivus to the thoracic inlet, providing information about the pre-epiglottic space and the nasopharynx. Next, axial fluid-attenuated inversion recovery (FLAIR) and diffusion sequences are obtained through the entire brain. Then, an axial T2 fat-saturated fast spin-echo (FSE) sequence is performed from the clivus to the thoracic inlet, followed by an axial T1 FLAIR sequence, which is the best sequence for establishing anatomic relationships and identifying pathology within fat.[2] FSE imaging provides the added benefit of a relatively short acquisition time limiting motion degradation, reduced magnetic susceptibility artifacts, and improved patient tolerance.[5,6] Moreover, spin-echo techniques have high signal-to-noise ratios and therefore superior spatial resolution, as compared with inversion recovery sequences.[1] Next, an axial dynamic spoiled gradient sequence is obtained from the skull base to the bottom of the hyoid bone following the administration of intravenous gadolinium. Then, sequential postcontrast axial T1 FLAIR and axial T1 fat-saturated images are obtained from the clivus to the thoracic inlet. Fat saturation assists in elucidating adenopathy, as well as enhancing mass lesions, which may otherwise be obscured by bright fat.[7] Finally, an axial T1 postcontrast sequence is obtained through the brain.

Our institution also offers a "Larynx" protocol with a smaller FOV (18–20 cm) and smaller slice thickness (3–5 mm as compared with 5–6 mm for the general neck protocol). This sequence also provides smaller interscan spacing (0.5–1.5 mm). First, a sagittal T1 sequence is performed followed by axial T1 and T2 sequences. These images are obtained from the bottom of the pituitary gland to the thoracic inlet. Next, the axial T1 larynx sequence is performed from the hyoid bone to the thoracic inlet followed by postcontrast axial T1 fat-saturated images, both at 3-mm slice thickness. Finally, delayed axial T1 postcontrast standard and fat-saturated sequences are obtained

at 5-mm slice thickness. A 256 × 256 matrix is used for the infrahyoid neck to increase the signal-to-noise ratio (**Table 2**). The neck surface coil is vital to infrahyoid neck imaging, as is adequate motion suppression.

Additional "nasopharynx" T1 spin-echo precontrast and postcontrast sequences are obtained in the coronal plane using the thinner slice thickness and interscan spacing described previously (see **Table 1**).

Typically, imaging of the suprahyoid neck requires only a standard head coil, whereas the infrahyoid neck requires a dedicated neck coil. The use of surface coils may improve spatial resolution, but at the cost of anatomic coverage.[2] Water bags may be placed on either side of the patient's neck to reduce magnetic susceptibility artifact.[6]

ANATOMY

The hyoid bone is used as a landmark to divide the neck into the suprahyoid and infrahyoid neck (**Fig. 1**A). The suprahyoid neck can be further subdivided into the following spaces: parapharyngeal space, pharyngeal mucosal space, masticator space, parotid space, sublingual and submandibular spaces, and the buccal space. There are spaces that are common to both the suprahyoid and infrahyoid neck, including the carotid space, retropharyngeal/danger space, perivertebral space, and the posterior cervical space. Finally, the visceral space is located solely within the infrahyoid neck.

Deep cervical fascial planes are used to divide the neck further into deep fascial spaces. The deep cervical fascia is made up of 3 layers: a superficial layer, a middle layer, and a deep layer. The spatial resolution of MR imaging does not allow direct visualization of the fascia itself, but knowledge of the fascial layer's course provides a manner by which to divide the neck into the deep fascial spaces with cross-sectional imaging.[7,8] Of note, the superficial fascial layer is a separate layer not included within the 3 sublayers of the deep cervical fascia and consists of the subcutaneous tissues of the head and neck.[3] The platysma and muscles of facial expression are embedded within this fascial layer, along with vessels, superficial lymph nodes, and cutaneous nerves.[7]

NODAL ANATOMY

An understanding of cervical lymph node anatomy is vital to the staging of head and neck cancers. Lymph nodes can be described as being submental-submandibular (level IA and IB), located along the internal jugular chain (levels II, III, IV), spinal accessory chain (level VA-VB), or the anterior

Table 1
General neck

1.5 Tesla	T1, SE	Diffusion Brain	T2-FLAIR	T2-Fat Sat, FSE	T1-FLAIR	Dynamic SPGR	T1-FLAIR	T1-Fat Sat, SE	T1, SE Brain	T1, SE[a]	T1, SE[a]
TR, ms	600	10,000	10,000	3000–5000	1600–2500	230–305	1600–2500	500–700	500–700	500–700	450–700
TE, ms	Min.Full	Minimum	100	98	24	In Phase	24	Minimum	Min.Full	19.23	19.23
TI, ms	—	—	2200	—	—	90	—	—	—	—	—
Slice, mm	5	6	6	5–6	5–6	4–5	5–6	5–6	6	3	3
Interscan spacing, mm	1.5	0	1.5	1.5–2	1.5–2	1	1.5–2	1.5–2	1.5	0.5	0.5
Gadolinium	Pre	Pre	Pre	Pre	Pre	Post	Post	Post	Post	Pre	Post
Acquired planes	Sagittal	Axial	Axial	Axial	Axial	Axial	Axial	Axial	Axial	Coronal	Coronal
Matrix, freq.	512	128	256	512	256	256	512	256	256	256	256
Matrix, phase	256	128	192	256	192	128	256	192	192	256	256
FOV, cm	20	22	23	20	20	20	20	23	20	20	20
Signal Averages	2NEX	1NEX	1NEX	3NEX	3NEX	1NEX	3NEX	2NEX	1NEX	2NEX	2NEX

Abbreviations: FLAIR, fluid attenuation inversion recovery; FOV, field of view; FSE, fast spin echo; SE, spin echo; SPGR, spoiled gradient recalled.
[a] Part of the nasopharynx protocol, imaged from posterior globe to posterior spinal cord in anteroposterior dimension and the top of frontal sinus to C1 in craniocaudal dimension.

Table 2
Larynx

1.5 Tesla	T1, SE	T1, SE	T2, SE	T1, SE	T1-Fat Sat, SE	T1, SE	T1-Fat Sat, SE
TR, ms	625	500–700	3000–5000	400–500	600–750	625	575
TE, ms	Minimum Full	Minimum	102	Minimum Full	Minimum	Minimum Full	Minimum
TI, ms	—	—	—	—	—	—	—
Slice, mm	4	5	5	3	3	5	5
Interscan spacing, mm	1	1.5	1.5	0.5	0.5	1.5	1.5
Gadolinium	Pre	Pre	Pre	Pre	Post	Post	Post
Acquired planes	Sagittal	Axial	Axial	Axial	Axial	Axial	Axial
Matrix, freq.	512	448	448	256	512	448	512
Matrix, phase	256	256	256	256	256	256	256
FOV, cm	20	18	18	18	18	18	18
Signal averages	2NEX	2NEX	3NEX	2NEX	2NEX	2NEX	2NEX

Abbreviations: FOV, field of view; SE, spin echo.

cervical chain (level VI). Lymph nodes are also noted in the parotid group, retropharyngeal group, and facial group.[8]

Level I lymph nodes include those nodes anterior to the posterior edge of the submandibular gland, but above the hyoid bone and below the mylohyoid muscle. Level IA nodes lie between the medial margins of the anterior bellies of the digastric muscles, whereas level IB nodes lie posterior and lateral to the anterior bellies. Level II nodes lie in front of the sternocleidomastoid muscle and posterior to the submandibular gland. Level II extends from the skull base to the hyoid bone. Level III extends from the hyoid bone to the cricoid cartilage arch. Level IV extends from the cricoid cartilage arch to the level of the clavicle. These level IV nodes are in front of the sternocleidomastoid muscle. Of note, the medial aspect of the internal and common carotid artery is the landmark separating levels III and IV, respectively, from level VI nodes. Level V extends from the skull base at the posterior attachment of the sternocleidomastoid muscle to the level of the clavicles. Level V nodes are posterior to the sternocleidomastoid muscle superiorly and anterior to the trapezius muscle. The cricoid cartilage arch separates level VA superiorly from level VB inferiorly. Level VI nodes lie inferior to the hyoid bone and superior to the sternal manubrium, centrally within the neck, medial to the common and internal carotid arteries, also known as the visceral nodes. Level VII nodes are caudal to the manubrium but medial to the common carotid arteries. A lymph node should not be considered to be supraclavicular if a portion of the clavicle is not included on the same axial slice; rather, this node would be level IV or VB.[9] Normal lymph nodes typically contain a fatty hilum and are isointense to muscle to T1-weighted sequences and hyperintense to muscle on T2-weighted sequences.[10] Normal lymph nodes should be less than 10 mm in maximum diameter.[8] Despite the superior soft tissue contrast and multiplanar capabilities of MR imaging, CT is most frequently used to evaluate cervical lymph nodes. The use of dextran-coated ultrasmall superparamagnetic iron oxide can be used as a lymph node contrast agent. Normal nodes would be expected to accumulate the agent, whereas pathologic nodes would not.[2]

PARAPHARYNGEAL SPACE

The parapharyngeal space can be thought of as a landmark for evaluating neck pathology. This is because the parapharyngeal space is made up mostly of T1-hyperintense fat that is easily depicted on routine MR images of the neck. The nomenclature of the parapharyngeal space can be confusing and therefore requires a brief discussion. When referring to the parapharyngeal space in this article, we are speaking of the prestyloid parapharyngeal space. Classically, anatomists describe the parapharyngeal space as having a prestyloid and a poststyloid component. The poststyloid component is also known as the carotid space.[3,11] We refer to the poststyloid parapharyngeal space as the carotid space and discuss this space in greater detail later in this article. The parapharyngeal space extends from the skull base to the hyoid bone and is bound by the masticator and parotid spaces laterally. The space is not bound by its own fascia and communicates freely with the submandibular space inferiorly.[7,8] Fat, branches of the mandibular division of cranial nerve (CN) V, and vascular structures, including the internal maxillary artery, the ascending pharyngeal artery, and the pharyngeal venous plexus, are included in the crescent-shaped parapharyngeal space. An imaging pitfall of which to be aware is that of the normal asymmetry of the pterygoid venous plexus, which can mimic a vascular mass. This pseudomass would be found along the medial border of the lateral pterygoid muscle and enhance on T1-weighted fat-suppressed images (see **Fig. 1C; Fig. 2E**).[8]

MUCOSAL SPACE

The pharyngeal mucosal space is located on the airway side of the middle layer of the deep cervical fascia.[7,12] Essentially, this space is made up of the mucosal surface structures of the nasopharynx, oropharynx, and hypopharynx. The pharyngeal mucosal space extends from the skull base to the cricoid cartilage. The retropharyngeal space is directly posterior to the pharyngeal mucosal space, as there is no fascial layer on the airway side of pharyngeal mucosal space.[12] The parapharyngeal space is closely associated with the lateral aspect of the pharyngeal mucosal space. Structures intrinsic to the mucosal space include mucosa, Waldeyer lymphatic ring (adenoids, faucial tonsils, lingual tonsils), superior and middle constrictor muscles, pharyngobasilar fascia, minor salivary glands, salpingopharyngeus muscle, levator palatini muscle, and the torus tubarius. It should be noted that normal variations in the thickness of the mucosal surface are expected. Therefore, close attention must be paid to the preservation of adjacent fat planes to avoid a pseudotumor pitfall.[7] Close contact with the referring clinician is essential, as many superficial mucosal lesions are easily visualized on clinical examination but may not be apparent on MR imaging. The T1-weighted high signal of the parapharyngeal space is noted on either side of the pharyngeal mucosal space. The tonsils should appear symmetric and demonstrate high signal on T2-weighted sequences but similar signal to muscle on T1-weighted sequences (see **Fig. 1D**).[13]

MASTICATOR SPACE

As suggested by the name, the muscles of mastication are contained within the masticator space. The aforementioned muscles include the medial and lateral pterygoid, temporalis, and the masseter, which is the largest muscle. Also included in the masticator space is the mandibular branch of the trigeminal nerve as it passes through the foramen ovale, as well as the ramus and posterior body of the mandible.[3] The inferior alveolar vein and artery and branches of the internal maxillary artery course within the masticator space. The superficial layer of the deep cervical fascia splits along the inferior mandible, creating a sling, which encloses the masticator space.[14] The inferior extent of the masticator space is the undersurface of the posterior mandibular body, where the medial pterygoid and masseter attach. The superior extent continues quite cephalad to the parietal calvarium where the temporalis muscle attaches. Therefore, analysis of this space requires attention to the suprazygomatic aspect as well. The masticator space is bound by the buccal space anteriorly, the parapharyngeal space posteromedially, and the parotid space posteriorly (see **Fig. 1B**).

Three pseudomasses of the masticator space exist. An asymmetric accessory parotid gland is found in up to 21% of the general population and is found on the surface of the masseter, but should follow the same intensity as the adjacent parotid gland.[8] Benign masseteric hypertrophy is usually associated with teeth grinding and appears as homogeneous enlargement of one or both masseters. After injury or surgery, V_3 branch denervation atrophy occurs unilaterally, causing increased fat and mass of the muscles of mastication, creating a pitfall of a pseudomass on the unaffected side. The radiologist should remain aware of this phenomenon in all of the neck spaces containing muscle. Normal muscles appear mildly hypointense and homogeneous on T1-weighted images. The muscle tendons have very low intrinsic signal, thereby providing contrast with nearby muscles and fat (see **Figs. 1B–D and 2B, C**).[15]

BUCCAL SPACE

The buccal space is a small space anterior to the masseter muscle, medial to the parotid space, and lateral to the buccinator muscle.[2,3,16] At its anterior aspect, the buccal space is separated from the subcutaneous tissues of the face by a plane of superficial muscles of facial expression. No complete fascial covering separates the buccal space from adjacent spaces (see **Figs. 1C and 2B, C**).There is no well-defined superior or inferior boundary of the buccal space.[16] Adipose tissue, known as the buccal fat pad, comprises most of the buccal space; however, other contents include minor salivary gland tissue, the distal portion of the parotid duct, lymph nodes, facial vein, buccal artery, and branches of CNs V and VI.[3,8]

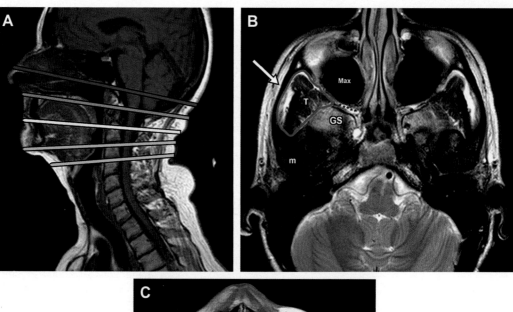

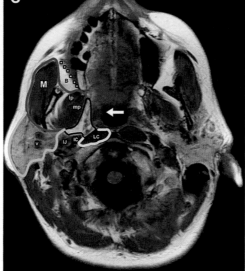

Fig. 1. Suprahyoid neck anatomy: (*A*) Sagittal T1-weighted midline image of the neck demarcating the level of the hyoid bone (*blue line*), separating the suprahyoid neck above from the infrahyoid neck below. Other colored lines demarcate the various levels listed below (*red line, B; orange line, C; yellow line, D; green line, E*). (*B*) Axial T2-weighted image at the skull base: the cephaled-most aspect of the masticator space (*red outline*) extends superior to the zygomatic arch (*arrow*). Any disease process that occurs in this space warrants evaluation superiorly to the aponeurosis of the temporalis muscle (T) along the calvarium. GS, greater wing of sphenoid; Max, maxillary sinus; m, mandible; asterisk, pterygopalatine fossa. (*C*) Axial T1-weighted image more inferiorly at the alveolar ridge: The parapharyngeal space (PPS, *black outline*) is readily apparent as a T1 hyperintense region, relating to its fat content. Anterolateral is the masticator space (*red border*) containing the masseter (M), lateral pterygoid (lp), and medial pterygoid (mp) muscles. The buccal space is located just anterior to the masticator space (B, asterisk border). Lateral to the parapharyngeal space is the parotid space (*green border*), which encompasses the isointense gland itself along with the retromandibular vein (v) within the substance of the parotid parenchyma. The carotid space encompassing the internal carotid artery (IC) and internal jugular vein (IJ) provides an additional lateral border to the PPS. Note the T1 isointense mucosal space medial to the PPS, including the torus tubaris (*arrow*). Posteriorly is the perivertebral space (*yellow border*) containing the longus colli muscle. (*D*) Axial T2-weighted image more inferiorly at the level of the oropharynx: Note the continuation of the masticator space (*red outline*) containing the mandible (m) and masseter (M). The parotid (*green border*) and parapharyngeal spaces have tapered down. The perivertebral space (*yellow outline*) is again noted, located just dorsal to the retropharyngeal space (*blue border*). Ton, palatine tonsils; IJ, internal jugular vein; IC, internal carotid artery; v, retromandibular vein; LC, longus colli. (*E*) Axial T1-weighted image at the level of the submandibular glands and hyoid bone (labeled): As the other suprahyoid neck spaces continue to taper down, the submandibular space appears (*orange outline*). This is bordered medially and superiorly by the isointense mylohyoid muscle (labeled) and contains the submandibular gland (labeled) as well as fat. The median raphe of the tongue is denoted by an arrow and the epiglottic valecula can be seen posteriorly (v).

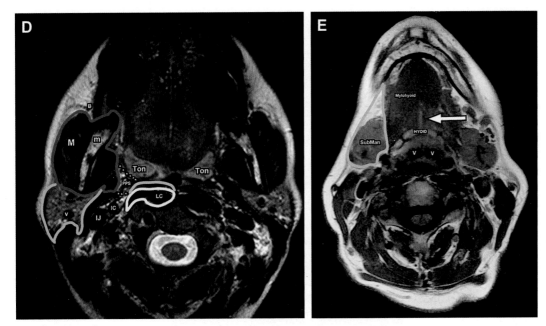

Fig. 1. (*continued*)

PAROTID SPACE

The parotid space contains the parotid gland, which is divided into superficial and deep lobes by the facial nerve. The facial nerve is just lateral to the retromandibular vein, which is commonly easier to locate on routine MR imaging.[3,7,8] The superficial layer of the deep cervical fascia surrounds the parotid space, similar to the masticator space. Within this space, the parotid gland, facial nerve, retromandibular vein, external carotid artery, lymph nodes, and parotid (Stentsen) ducts can be found. The external carotid artery is just medial to the retromandibular vein. The parotid space extends from the external auditory canal/mastoid tip superiorly to just below the angle of the mandible, known as the parotid tail.[17] The parotid tail inserts between the platysma and the sternocleidomastoid muscle. The posterior belly of the digastric muscle separates the parotid space from the carotid space posteromedially. The parapharyngeal space is directly medial to the parotid space (see **Figs. 1**C, D, and **2**E). Of note, MR imaging has limited utility when searching for parotid duct pathology, such as calculi, for which CT is more appropriate.

SUBLINGUAL SPACE

The sublingual space is a potential space between the mylohyoid muscle and the tongue musculature.[7,8,18] Otolaryngologists commonly refer to the sublingual space as the "floor of the mouth."

The mylohyoid muscle separates the sublingual space inferolaterally from the submandibular space.[19] The genioglossus/geniohyoid complex forms the medial border of the sublingual space. Anteriorly, the space is bordered by the mandible. There is direct communication with the submandibular space and the parapharyngeal space at the posterior aspect of the sublingual space (see **Fig. 2**A, D). No fascial layer encapsulates the sublingual space. The sublingual space contents include the anterior extension of the hyoglossus muscle; CNs IX and XII; the lingual nerve, artery, and vein; and the sublingual gland and ducts, as well as the deep portion of the submandibular gland and ducts.[3,8]

SUBMANDIBULAR SPACE

The submandibular space is located below the mandible, inferior to the mylohyoid muscle, in contrast with the sublingual space, which is superior to the mylohyoid muscle. As stated previously, it is important to note that the posterior submandibular space is in direct communication with the posterior sublingual space and the parapharyngeal space. The hyoid bone marks the inferior aspect of the submandibular space, making the submandibular space the most caudal space within the suprahyoid neck (see **Fig. 1**E). The anterior belly of the digastric muscle; the superficial submandibular gland; the submandibular and submental lymph nodes; the facial artery, vein, and

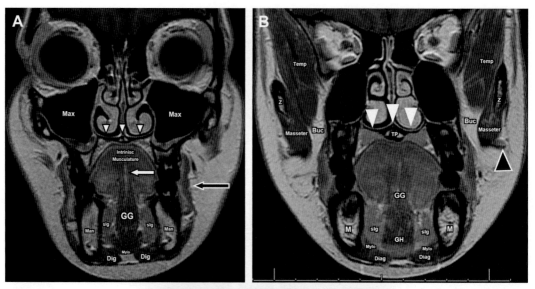

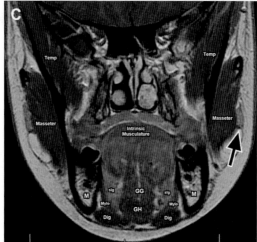

Fig. 2. Coronal T1-weighted imaging of the suprahyoid neck at several levels. (*A*) Just dorsal to the mandibular mentum, the sublingual glands (slg) are present between the mylohyoid (mylo) and genioglossus (GG) muscles. They are of increased signal intensity in comparison with muscle. Inferior to the mylohyoid muscle is the anterior belly of the digastric (Dig). The fatty T1-hyperintense median raphe of the tongue is present superiorly between the genioglossus muscles (*white arrow*). Just inferior to the hard palate (*white arrowheads*), which is hyperintense because of marrow fat, is the apposed tongue surface with intrinsic musculature (labeled) noted. The buccal mucosa and buccinator musculature are noted along the lateral border of the oral cavity (*black arrow*). Max, maxillary sinus. (*B, C*) More posteriorly, the masticator space is noted with the masseter (Masseter) and temporalis (Temp) muscles now identified (labeled) along with the T1 hyperintense zygomatic arch (Z). The buccal fat/space is well demonstrated (Buc) and the geniohyoid muscle (GH) is noted along the floor of the mouth. Stensen duct is present lateral to the buccal mucosa (*black arrowhead*) and the parotid gland comes into view (*black arrow*). (*D*) At the level of the nasal choana, the oral cavity structures are again well seen, including the mylohyoid muscle, which divides the submandibular space inferiorly from the sublingual space superiorly. The hyoglossus muscle is noted along the lateral margin of the tongue, providing the medial margin of the sublingual space. Within the masticator space, the medial and lateral pterygoids are identifiable (mp, lp). The soft palate (labeled) is also now noted. (*E*) At the level of the mandibular rami, the submandibular glands (SMG) are visualized inferiorly as are the parotid glands (PG) superiorly. Posterior and medial to the masticator space is the fat-filled, T1-hyperintense parapharyngeal space (PPS). The longus colli (LC) muscles of the prevertebral space are well seen, as are the lingual (labeled) and palatine tonsils (PT).

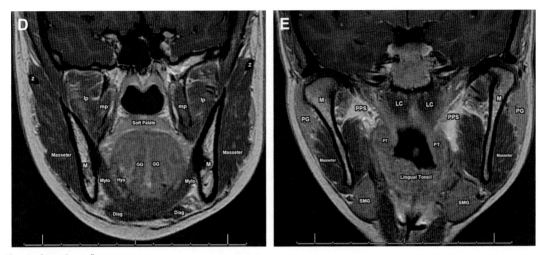

Fig. 2. (*continued*)

nerve; as well as the inferior loop of CN XII are located within the submandibular space.[3,8] The submandibular space is enclosed by the superficial layer of the deep cervical fascia. All of the aforementioned salivary glands are typically intermediate in intensity (brighter than muscle but darker than fat) on T1-weighted images in the young and increase in fat content with age; however, only the parotid gland increases in signal intensity on MR imaging.[20] The glands remain bright relative to muscle on T2-weighted sequences, may be either heterogeneous or homogeneous, and avidly enhance.[4,8,20,21] Studies have shown that salivary gland size decreases with age as well.[20] MR imaging is especially advantageous over CT in evaluating the sublingual and submandibular spaces, as there is no streak artifact from the dental amalgam. Infrequently, dental amalgam with high ferrous content can distort signal.

RETROPHARYNX AND PERIVERTEBRAL SPACE

The retropharyngeal space is just posterior to the pharynx, bordered by the visceral/buccopharyngeal fascia (middle layer of the deep cervical fascia) anteriorly and the prevertebral fascia (deep layer of the deep cervical fascia) posteriorly. The retropharyngeal space is medial to the carotid space and extends from the skull base to the level of approximately T3. The pharyngeal mucosal space is anterior to the retropharyngeal space, whereas the perivertebral space lies posteriorly (see **Fig. 1**D). To complicate this space further, the alar fascia, which is a very thin anterior component of the prevertebral fascia, actually divides the retropharyngeal space into anterior and posterior compartments as well as provides a lateral border

for the retropharyngeal space. The posterior compartment is commonly referred to as the "danger space" because it extends from the skull base to the diaphragm, thereby providing a pathway for spread of head and neck infections into the posterior mediastinum.[3,7,8] However, because of the thin nature of the alar fascia, many anatomists consider the retropharyngeal space to be singular. The retropharyngeal space proper empties into the danger space inferiorly.[22] The danger space and the retropharyngeal space cannot be distinguished with imaging. Fat and lymph nodes are contained within the retropharyngeal space in the suprahyoid neck and only fat is noted below the level of the hyoid bone.[7,23] In the suprahyoid neck, the lymph nodes are separated into lateral and medial groups. Normal lateral lymph nodes, also known as the nodes of Rouvier, are frequently visualized on MR imaging as being of homogeneous signal intensity smaller than 10 mm in size.[23] The retropharyngeal space should appear as a thin line of fat on cross-sectional imaging.[8] A tortuous carotid artery projects medially into the lateral retropharyngeal space and can cause a pseudomass.

The perivertebral space is bounded by the prevertebral fascia, also known as the deep layer of the deep cervical fascia. It can be thought of as having 2 components: the prevertebral portion of the space (anterior to the vertebral transverse process) and the paraspinal portion of the space (posterior to the vertebral transverse process). The perivertebral space extends from the skull base to the level of T4 in the posterior mediastinum.[24] Some anatomists feel that this space actually extends to the coccyx.[7] The prevertebral portion is directly posterior to the

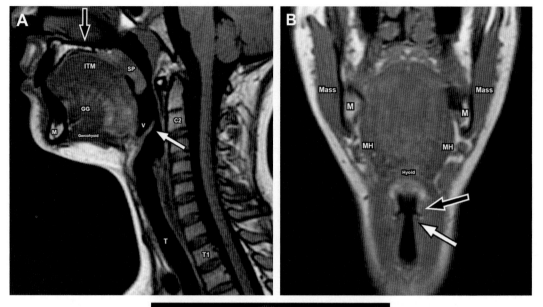

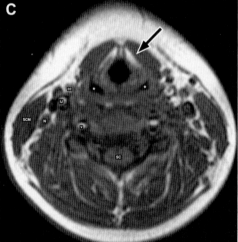

Fig. 3. Imaging of the infrahyoid neck. (*A*) Sagittal T1-weighted image demonstrates the geniohyoid (labeled) and genioglossus (GG) muscles along the floor of the mouth, attaching to the T1-hyperintense mandible (M). The intrinsic tongue muscles (ITM) lie essentially apposed to the hard (*black arrow*) and soft (SP) palates. The epiglottis (*white arrow*) lies posterior to the vallecula (v). The air-filled T1-hypointense trachea (T) is noted inferiorly. Posteriorly, the vertebrae are noted (C2 and T1 labeled). (*B*) Coronal T1-weighted image highlights the false (*black arrow*) and true (*white arrow*) vocal cords, with a small amount of T1-hyperintense fat noted along the false cord. The hyoid bone is visualized (labeled) and the mylohyoid (MH), mandible (M), and masseter (Mass) muscle are seen. (*C, D*) Axial T1-weighted image through the larynx. Superior image (*C*) demonstrates the false vocal cords (*black arrow*) with the paired, air-filled T1 hypointense pyriform sinuses noted posteriorly (*asterisk*). Subjacent to the sternocleidomastoid muscle are the common carotid artery (cc), internal jugular vein (IJ), and jugular chain lymph nodes (N). The vertebral artery (v) is noted traversing the foramen transversarium, whereas the spinal cord (SC) is noted posteriorly. Inferiorly, (*D*) the true cords (v) are noted with a portion of the cricoid cartilage seen posteriorly (C). (*E*) Axial T2-weighted fat-suppressed image at the same level. Most of the neck tissues lose signal. A few small nodes are again present (*circled*) and a venous plexus is noted along the spinal column (*arrowhead*). The T2-hyperintense cerebrospinal fluid surrounds the spinal cord. (*F*) Axial T1-weighted image at the level of the thyroid gland (Thy). The thyroid borders the trachea and the esophagus (E). The brachial plexus (*asterisk*) is noted traveling between the anterior (AS) and middle (MS) scalene muscles.

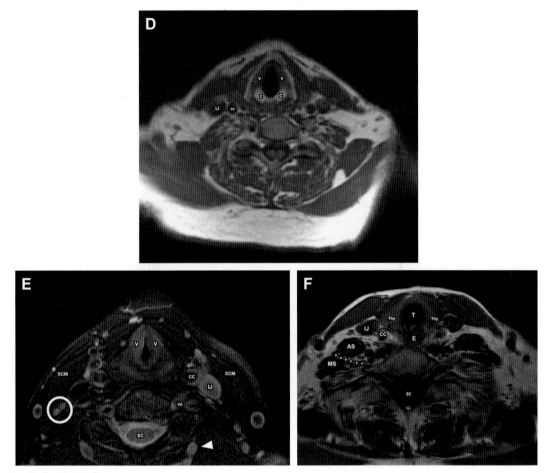

Fig. 3. (*continued*)

retropharyngeal space and/or danger space. The carotid space is just anterolateral, whereas the posterior cervical space is just lateral to the prevertebral portion of the perivertebral space (see **Figs. 1**C, D and **2**E).Contents of the prevertebral portion include the vertebral body, vertebral artery and vein, the phrenic nerve, brachial plexus roots, scalene muscles, and prevertebral muscles. The paraspinal portion contains the paraspinal muscles and the posterior elements of the vertebral body.[8]

CAROTID AND VISCERAL SPACES

The carotid space is enclosed by the carotid sheath, which is formed by all 3 layers of the deep cervical fascia. Of note, the carotid sheath is also known as the poststyloid parapharyngeal space, as previously discussed. The carotid space extends from the aortic arch to the skull base and contains the carotid artery, the internal jugular vein, CNs IX to XII in the suprahyoid region (with only CN X continuing in the infrahyoid neck), lymph nodes, and portions of the sympathetic plexus.[7] Near the skull base, the vagus nerve (CN X) lies medial to both the internal carotid artery and internal jugular vein, but as it travels caudally, it shifts posteriorly to lie between the common carotid artery and the internal jugular vein. The carotid bifurcation is at approximately the level of the hyoid bone. The internal jugular vein typically courses posterolaterally to the carotid artery. The carotid space is bounded by the parotid space laterally, the retropharyngeal and perivertebral space medially, the parapharyngeal space anteriorly, and the posterior cervical space posterolaterally (see **Fig. 1**C, D).[7] The alar fascia separates the carotid space from the retropharyngeal space.

POSTERIOR CERVICAL SPACE

The posterior cervical space lies within the posterolateral neck and is formed by complex fascial boundaries. This space begins as a small component superiorly at the level of the mastoid tip and then becomes more pronounced as it descends to the level of the clavicle. The space is just deep and posterior to the sternocleidomastoid muscle.[8,25] Fat, CN XI, level V lymph nodes, brachial plexus, and the dorsal scapular nerve are contained within the posterior cervical space. The carotid space is just anteromedial to the posterior cervical space. The lateral aspect of the prevertebral portion of the perivertebral space is deep to the anterior portion of the posterior cervical space. The posterior portion of the posterior cervical space has the paraspinal portion of the perivertebral space just deep to it. The posterior cervical space is best visualized at its infrahyoid component because of the large amount of T1 hyperintense fat.[7]

INFRAHYOID NECK

The infrahyoid neck extends from the hyoid bone to the thoracic inlet. The middle layer of the deep cervical fascia encircles the neck viscera and is referred to as the visceral fascia in the infrahyoid neck as opposed to the buccopharyngeal fascia in the suprahyoid neck. The deep layer of the deep cervical fascia encapsulates the prevertebral, paraspinal, and scalene muscles along with the vertebrae, brachial plexus, vertebral arteries and veins, and phrenic nerve. As previously described, the carotid, retropharyngeal/danger, perivertebral, and posterior cervical space involve both the suprahyoid and infrahyoid neck. Only the visceral space, with its many components, lies solely within the infrahyoid neck.[8,10] Cross-sectional imaging should always be extended to the level of the carina when assessing for visceral space pathology. It is not uncommon for MR imaging evaluation of the infrahyoid neck to be limited by motion artifact secondary to patient motion from breathing, coughing, or swallowing.[8]

Enclosed by the middle layer of the deep cervical fascia, the visceral space extends from the hyoid bone to the superior mediastinum, with the carotid space and retropharyngeal space lateral and posterior to it, respectively. The visceral space contains the thyroid gland, the parathyroid glands, the cervical trachea, the cervical esophagus, the recurrent laryngeal nerves, and the paratracheal lymph nodes. The hypopharynx and larynx are also included.[8,26] The normal thyroid gland appears slightly hyperintense to muscle on T1-weighted images, hyperintense to muscle on T2-weighted images, and should be homogeneous (**Fig. 3**F). Normal thyroid homogeneously enhances following the administration of gadolinium.[27] The variable pyramidal process extending superiorly from the isthmus should not be

mistaken for a mass. Cross-sectional imaging is performed secondary to scintigraphy or ultrasound in the setting of clinical hyperparathyroidism to evaluate the parathyroid glands, which, if normal, are difficult to see on MR imaging, but follow characteristics similar to the thyroid gland; however, their most common locations are important to note.[4] Most frequently, there are 4 parathyroid glands, 2 of which are closely approximated to the posterior middle third of the thyroid gland, representing the less variable superior glands. The inferior glands, which are more variable and can be seen as far as the pericardium, most commonly are located lateral to the lower pole of the thyroid gland.

The caudal continuation of the pharyngeal mucosal space is known as the hypopharynx, between the oropharynx and the esophagus, extending from the hyoid bone to the cricopharyngeus muscle. The hypopharynx consists of 3 regions, the pyriform sinus, the posterior wall, and the postcricoid region.[28] The postcricoid region forms the anterior wall of the lower hypopharynx, representing the interface between the hypopharynx and the anteriorly located larynx.[13] Pharyngeal plexus nerves provide motor and sensory functions to the hypopharynx and are composed of branches of CN IX and CN X. Three tissues in the hypopharynx can be differentiated: fat, muscle, and lymphoid tissue. Muscle in the hypopharynx, as elsewhere, has a low/intermediate T1-weighted signal, with low T2-weighted signal intensity.[4] The T1-weighted sequence is ideal for differentiating hyperintense fat from isointense muscle; T2-weighted sequences are ideal for differentiating muscle from more hyperintense lymphoid tissue. A pitfall, however, is that most tumors and lymphoid tissue cannot be differentiated on MR imaging.[13]

LARYNX

The larynx is a very complex structure, best evaluated with coronal imaging. The larynx is the junction of the upper and lower airway, providing airway maintenance and preventing aspiration. The presence of the vocal cords provides phonation.[28] The larynx is bounded and protected by the thyroid and cricoid cartilages. The endolarynx consists of the supraglottis, glottis, and subglottis. The supraglottis extends from the tip of the epiglottis to the laryngeal ventricle and contains the false vocal cords, which represent the mucosal surfaces of the laryngeal vestibule. The valleculae are just above and anterior to the epiglottis, whereas the laryngeal vestibule is just below the epiglottis (see **Fig. 3**A). The supraglottis is separated from the pyriform sinuses of the hypopharynx by the aryepiglottic folds.[8] The glottis consists of the true vocal cords as well as the anterior and posterior commissures. The true vocal cords are thyroarytenoid muscles, and can be seen when the cricoid and arytenoid cartilage are included in the same image. In quiet respiration, the true vocal cords should be relaxed/abducted. On breath-hold images, the true vocal cords should be adducted/opposed. The space between the false and true vocal cords is the laryngeal ventricle (see **Fig. 3**B–D). The subglottis extends from the undersurface of the true vocal cords to the inferior surface of the cricoid cartilage. The cervical esophagus begins at the level of the cricoid cartilage. The paraglottic and preepiglottic spaces serve as landmarks on MR imaging because of their fat content. The paraglottic spaces are paired, just lateral to the false and true vocal cords. They merge into the pre-epiglottic space superiorly, which is a single C-shaped fatty region posterior to the hyoid bone, bound by the epiglottis posteriorly.[8] Imaging of the hypopharynx and larynx must be correlated with clinical endoscopic examination, as MR imaging can be limited for the evaluation of lesions of the mucosa, which do not invade. The epiglottis and velleculae are best seen on the sagittal sequence. The coronal sequence is ideal for evaluation of the true vocal cord, which because of its muscular nature, can be easily contrasted against the high-signal fat of the false vocal cord immediately superior on T1-weighted images.[29] The pre-epiglottic space can be seen just above the anterior commissure. Evaluation of the subglottic region can be performed on the same slices as the true vocal cord. Because cartilage can ossify with time, the appearance is variable on MR imaging. Nonossified thyroid and arytenoid cartilage is dark on both T1-weighted and T2-weighted images, whereas ossified cartilage is hyperintense on T1-weighted sequences secondary to the presence of fat in the medullary space. The simplest way to identify the vocal cord level on axial images is to recognize a region of airway narrowing with high T1-weighted signal at the false cord level and the low T1-weighted signal of muscle at the true cord level.[29]

NECK VASCULATURE

The major extracranial neck vessels are vertical in orientation, of which the common carotid artery and the internal jugular vein are the largest. The right common carotid artery originates at the bifurcation of the inominate artery near the sternoclavicular joint, ascends within the carotid sheath deep to the sternocleidomastoid muscle in the lower neck, and then becomes more superficial,

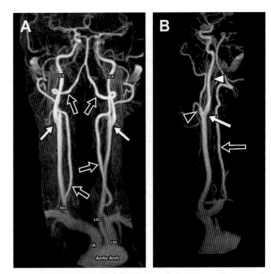

Fig. 4. Contrast-enhanced MR angiogram of the neck was obtained and presented as MIP images (*A*, anteroposterior view; *B*, oblique). The aortic arch most commonly gives rise to 3 great vessels: the inominate (or brachiocephalic) artery (IA), the left subclavian artery (LSA), and the left common carotid artery (LCC). The right common carotid artery (RCC) arises off of the inominate distally. Both common carotids travel anteriorly within the carotid space of the neck and bifurcate (*white arrows*) at approximately the level of the hyoid bone into external (*black arrowhead*) and internal carotid arteries (ICA, *white arrowhead*). The vertebral arteries (*black arrows*) are typically the first branches off of the subclavian arteries and ascend posteriorly along the transverse foramina, entering the skull base through the foramen magnum.

although still medial to the muscle in the upper neck. The left common carotid artery follows a similar course after arising directly from the aortic arch. The common carotid artery bifurcates into

Table 3 Magnetic resonance angiography carotid		
1.5 Tesla	**2D Phase Contrast**	**Contrast-Enhanced Carotid 20cc**
TR, ms	33	—
TE, ms	—	Minimum
Flip angle	20	45
Matrix, freq.	256	384
Matrix, phase	128	192
Slice, mm	30–50	1.6–2.0
Interscan spacing, mm	0	0
FOV, cm	35	24–28
Signal averages	1NEX	1NEX

Abbreviation: FOV, field of view.

the internal and external carotid artery at the level of the hyoid bone. The carotid bulb is considered to be the most proximal portion of the internal carotid artery, where it appears slightly focally dilated.[30] The internal carotid artery lies posterolateral to the external carotid artery. No branches arise from the internal carotid artery throughout its course in the neck (**Fig. 4**). The internal carotid artery courses within the carotid sheath, whereas the branching external carotid artery lies anterior to the carotid sheath.

The internal jugular vein courses within the carotid sheath and is usually larger in size as compared with the artery. Typically, the right side is larger than the left. The internal jugular vein originates in the skull base as a continuation of the sigmoid sinus. The vein begins posterolateral to the internal carotid and common carotid artery

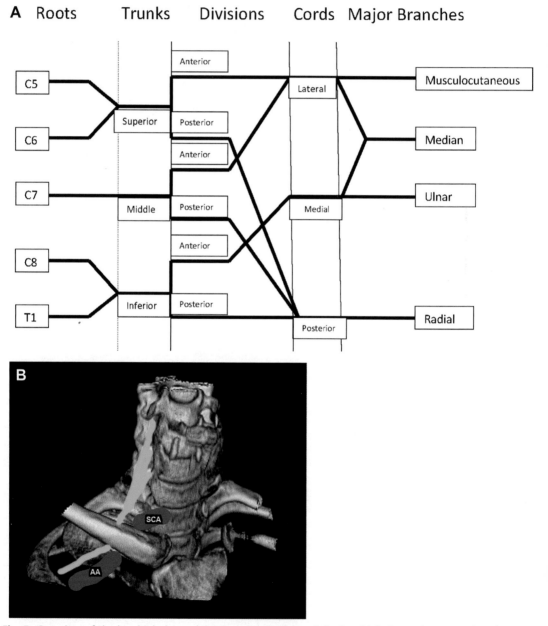

Fig. 5. Overview of the brachial plexus. (*A*) Schematic diagram of the brachial plexus demonstrating the roots, trunks, divisions, cords, and major nerve branches as well as the various divergences and convergences that occur along their courses. (*B*) Volume-rendered image of the right brachial plexus. The course of the plexus is shown in green as the individual roots descend from the neural foramina and converge. The plexus travels along the right subclavian (SCA) and axillary (AA) arteries.

superiorly and then gradually becomes anterolateral as it descends. The internal jugular vein joins the subclavian vein to form the brachiocephalic vein. The external jugular vein forms at the angle of the mandible from the retromandibular and posterior auricular vein, descends between the platysma and the sternocleidomastoid, and empties into the subclavian vein.[4,7] Many variants in venous vascular anatomy, however, exist.

The vertebral arteries originate from the subclavian arteries and ascend posterior to the scalene muscles, typically entering the foramina transversaria at approximately C6, eventually entering the skull at the foramen magnum (see **Fig. 4**). The subclavian artery itself courses between the anterior and middle scalene muscles, along with the brachial plexus, eventually reaching the axilla and becoming the axillary artery.[4,7]

The neck vessels can be differentiated from similarly shaped lymph nodes by the presence of flow voids and the continuous nature of vessels on serial axial slices on MR imaging. Gadolinium-enhanced MR angiography can produce high signal-to-noise ratio images, obtained within a single breath-hold. Time-of-flight MR angiography does not require the use of contrast and is dependent on high flow of vessels. Phase-contrast MR angiography also does not require the use of contrast, is dependent on flow, and can provide flow velocity information. When performing MR angiography of the neck arteries at our institution, we use a neurovascular array coil and obtain sagittal 2-dimensional phase-contrast imaging followed by coronal dynamic contrast-enhanced 3-dimensional (3D) imaging. For MR venography, a 3D gadolinium-enhanced sequence is obtained in the coronal plane. We also perform time-of-flight and phase-contrast MR venography (**Table 3**).

BRACHIAL PLEXUS

MR imaging is the preferred modality to evaluate the brachial plexus because of its inherent soft tissue contrast differentiation and multiplanar capabilities.[31] The ventral rami of C5-T1 form the brachial plexus. Shortly after exiting the spine,

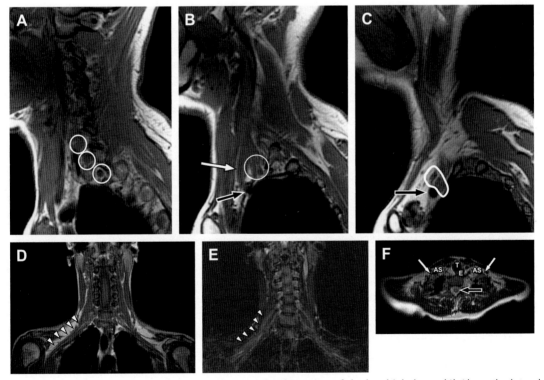

Fig. 6. Brachial plexus imaging. (*A–C*) Sagittal T1-weighted imaging of the brachial plexus. (*A*) Along the lateral aspect of the cervical spine, the originating nerve roots can be seen as they exit the neural foramina (*circles*). (*B*) As the plexus forms (*circled*), it can be seen posterior to the anterior scalene muscle (*white arrow*) and superior to the subclavian artery (*black arrow*). (*C*) Laterally, the plexus (*circled*) is best seen superior to the axillary artery (*black arrow*). (*D, E*) Coronal T1-weighted (*D*) and STIR (*E*) imaging of the plexus. Note the plexus descending through the thoracic inlet (*white arrowheads*). (*F*) Axial T2-weighted image at the thoracic inlet demonstrates bilateral plexi (*white arrows*) traveling posterior to the anterior scalene (AS). Midline trachea (T) and esophagus (E) are present and the spinal cord is noted centrally (*black arrow*).

Table 4
Brachial plexus

1.5 Tesla	STIR, FSE	T2, FRFSE	T1, SE	T1, SE	T1, SE	T1, SE	SPGR, FS
TR, ms	4000	3000–5000	500–700	500–700	500–700	500–700	165
TE, ms	34	85	Minimum	Minimum	Minimum	Minimum	In Phase
TI, ms	165	—	—	—	—	—	—
Slice, mm	4	4	4	4	4	4	4
Interscan spacing, mm	1	1	1	1	1	1	1
Gadolinium	No	No	No	No	No/Yes	Yes	Yes
Acquired planes	Coronal	Axial	Axial	Sagittal	Coronal	Axial	Coronal
Matrix, freq.	256	384	512	384	448	512	384
Matrix, phase	160	224	256	224	256	256	256
FOV, cm	34–36	32–34	32–34	24	34–36	32–34	34–36
Signal averages	2NEX	3NEX	2NEX	2NEX	2NEX	2NEX	2NEX

Abbreviations: FOV, field of view; FRFSE, fast relaxation fast spin echo; FS, fat saturated; SE, spin echo; SPGR, spoiled gradient recalled; STIR, short tau inversion recovery.

the nerves enter the scalene triangle, which is bound by the anterior scalene muscle anteriorly and the middle scalene muscle posteriorly. The 3 trunks (upper, middle, lower) of the brachial plexus are formed at the lateral border of the scalene triangle. The roots and trunks comprise the supraclavicular brachial plexus (**Fig. 5**). Just before the brachial plexus passes posterior to the clavicle, the trunks divide into an anterior and posterior division, known as the retroclavicular brachial plexus. At the infraclavicular brachial plexus, 3 cords are formed just lateral to the outer border of the first rib. Finally, just lateral to the pectoralis muscle, in the axilla, the cords divide into the 5 terminal branches: musculocutaneous nerve, ulnar nerve, radial nerve, median nerve, and axillary nerve.[31–33] In keeping with the spatial description of the neck, the brachial plexus originates in the prevertebral portion of the perivertebral space, courses between the anterior and medial scalene muscles, enters the posterior cervical space, and then continues inferolaterally into the axillary apex (**Fig. 6**). The brachial plexus courses superior and posterior to the subclavian artery and vein.[8,34] Brachial plexus nerves are isointense or slightly hypointense to muscle on T1-weighted and T2-weighted images. Normal nerves do not enhance, but mild perineural enhancement can be expected because of the presence of vasa vasorum. The normal nerves are round/ovoid in shape, which are homogeneous and interspersed with fibrofatty connective tissue. The sagittal plane allows for nerves to be seen in cross section, the axial plane permits evaluation of the exiting nerve roots, and the coronal plane demonstrates the nerves in long axis. The coronal plane can show the ventral rami, trunks, divisions, and cords all in one plane and allows for comparison with the contralateral side.[31,32] Typically, oblique sequences are acquired in an attempt to include all components. At our institution, we use coronal Short Tau Inversion Recovery (STIR), axial T2 sequence, and axial T1 sequence. Next, a sagittal T1 sequence is performed on the affected side. Then, coronal and axial T1 postcontrast images are obtained followed by a coronal spoiled gradient fat-saturated postcontrast sequence (**Table 4**).

SUMMARY

Imaging of the head and neck is extremely complex. An understanding of the fascial spaces is essential for the radiologist to distinguish normal anatomy from pathology. Knowledge of the fascial spaces allows one to formulate a differential diagnosis after localizing pathology to a specific space within the neck. Thorough review of the literature, textbooks, and images will prepare the radiologist to recognize all normal anatomy on MR imaging; this article strives to serve as a foundation.

REFERENCES

1. Stark DD, Moss AA, Gamsu G, et al. Magnetic resonance imaging of the neck. Part I: normal anatomy. Radiology 1984;150(2):447–54.
2. Wippold FJ 2nd. Head and neck imaging: the role of CT and MRI. J Magn Reson Imaging 2007;25(3): 453–65.
3. Mukherji SK, Castillo M. A simplified approach to the spaces of the suprahyoid neck. Radiol Clin North Am 1998;36(5):761–80, v.

4. Branstetter BF 4th, Weissman JL. Normal anatomy of the neck with CT and MR imaging correlation. Radiol Clin North Am 2000;38(5):925–40, ix.

5. Sharafuddin MJ, Diemer DP, Levine RS, et al. A comparison of MR sequences for lesions of the parotid gland. AJNR Am J Neuroradiol 1995;16(9):1895–902.

6. Sigal R. Infrahyoid neck. Radiol Clin North Am 1998;36(5):781–99, v.

7. Williams DW 3rd. An imager's guide to normal neck anatomy. Semin Ultrasound CT MR 1997;18(3):157–81.

8. Harnsberger HR. Handbook of head and neck imaging. St Louis (MO): Mosby; 1995.

9. Som PM, Curtin HD, Mancuso AA. Imaging-based nodal classification for evaluation of neck metastatic adenopathy. AJR Am J Roentgenol 2000;174(3):837–44.

10. Shah RR, Lewin JS. Imaging of the infrahyoid neck. Neuroimaging Clin N Am 1998;8(1):219–34.

11. Chong VF, Mukherji SK, Goh CH. The suprahyoid neck: normal and pathological anatomy. J Laryngol Otol 1999;113(6):501–8.

12. Harnsberger HR. Suprahyoid and infrahyoid neck—pharyngeal mucosal space. In: Harnsberger HR, Wiggins RH, Hudgins PA, et al, editors. Diagnostic imaging: head and neck. 1st edition. Salt Lake City (UT): Amirsys; 2004. p. III-1-1, III-1-2.

13. Mukherji SK. Pharynx. In: Som PM, Curtin HD, editors. Head and neck imaging. 4th edition. St Louis (MO): Mosby; 2003. p. 1466–76.

14. Harnsberger HR. Suprahyoid and infrahyoid neck—masticator space. In: Harnsberger HR, Wiggins RH, Hudgins PA, et al, editors. Diagnostic imaging: head and neck. 1st edition. Salt Lake City (UT): Amirsys; 2004. p. III-6-2, III-6-3.

15. Schellhas KP. MR imaging of muscles of mastication. AJR Am J Roentgenol 1989;153(4):847–55.

16. Kim HC, Han MH, Moon MH, et al. CT and MR imaging of the buccal space: normal anatomy and abnormalities. Korean J Radiol 2005;6(1):22–30.

17. Harnsberger HR. Suprahyoid and infrahyoid neck—parotid space. In: Harnsberger HR, Wiggins RH, Hudgins PA, et al, editors. Diagnostic imaging: head and neck. 1st edition. Salt Lake City (UT): Amirsys; 2004. p. III-7-2, III-7-3.

18. Macdonald AJ, Harnsberger HR. Suprahyoid and infrahyoid neck—oral cavity. In: Harnsberger HR, Wiggins RH, Hudgins PA, et al, editors. Diagnostic imaging: head and neck. 1st edition. Salt Lake City (UT): Amirsys; 2004. p. III-4-2, III-4-5.

19. Otonari-Yamamoto M, Nakajima K, Tsuji Y, et al. Imaging of the mylohyoid muscle: separation of submandibular and sublingual spaces. AJR Am J Roentgenol 2010;194(5):W431–8.

20. Sumi M, Izumi M, Yonetsu K, et al. Sublingual gland: MR features of normal and diseased states. AJR Am J Roentgenol 1999;172(3):717–22.

21. Som PM, Curtin HD. Fascia and spaces of the neck. In: Som PM, Curtin HD, editors. Head and neck imaging. 4th edition. St Louis (MO): Mosby; 2003. p. 1805–26.

22. Harnsberger HR. Suprahyoid and infrahyoid neck—retropharyngeal space. In: Harnsberger HR, Wiggins RH, Hudgins PA, et al, editors. Diagnostic imaging: head and neck. 1st edition. Salt Lake City (UT): Amirsys; 2004. p. III-9-2, III-9-3.

23. Davis WL, Harnsberger HR, Smoker WR, et al. Retropharyngeal space: evaluation of normal anatomy and diseases with CT and MR imaging. Radiology 1990;174(1):59–64.

24. Harnsberger HR. Suprahyoid and infrahyoid neck—perivertebral space. In: Harnsberger HR, Wiggins RH, Hudgins PA, et al, editors. Diagnostic imaging: head and neck. 1st edition. Salt Lake City (UT): Amirsys; 2004. p. III-10-2, III-10-3.

25. Harnsberger HR. Suprahyoid and infrahyoid neck—posterior cervical space. In: Harnsberger HR, Wiggins RH, Hudgins PA, et al, editors. Diagnostic imaging: head and neck. 1st edition. Salt Lake City (UT): Amirsys; 2004. p. III-12-2, III-12-3.

26. Harnsberger HR. Suprahyoid and infrahyoid neck—visceral space. In: Harnsberger HR, Wiggins RH, Hudgins PA, et al, editors. Diagnostic imaging: head and neck. 1st edition. Salt Lake City (UT): Amirsys; 2004. p. III-11-2, III-11-3.

27. Loevner LA. Thyroid and parathyroid glands: anatomy and pathology. In: Som PM, Curtin HD, editors. Head and neck imaging. 4th edition. St Louis (MO): Mosby; 2003. p. 2138–41.

28. Salzman KL, Harnsberger HR. Suprahyoid and infrahyoid neck—hypopharynx, larynx, and cervical trachea. In: Harnsberger HR, Wiggins RH, Hudgins PA, et al, editors. Diagnostic imaging: head and neck. 1st edition. Salt Lake City (UT): Amirsys; 2004. p. III-3-2, III-3-5.

29. Curtin HD. Larynx. In: Som PM, Curtin HD, editors. Head and neck imaging. 4th edition. St Louis (MO): Mosby; 2003. p. 1596–614.

30. Osborn AG, Jacobs JM. Normal gross and angiographic anatomy of the craniocervical vasculature. In: Osborn AG, Jacobs JM, editors. Diagnostic cerebral angiography. 2nd edition. Philadelphia: Lippincott Williams & Wilkins; 1999. p. 58–9.

31. van Es HW. MRI of the brachial plexus. Eur Radiol 2001;11(2):325–36.

32. Sureka J, Cherian RA, Alexander M, et al. MRI of brachial plexopathies. Clin Radiol 2009;64(2):208–18.

33. Reede DL, Holliday RA. Brachial plexus. In: Som PM, Curtin HD, editors. Head and neck imaging. 4th edition. St Louis (MO): Mosby; 2003. p. 2216–21.

34. Aralasmak A, Karaali K, Cevikol C, et al. MR imaging findings in brachial plexopathy with thoracic outlet syndrome. AJNR Am J Neuroradiol 2010;31(3):410–7.

Normal Spinal Anatomy on Magnetic Resonance Imaging

Gaurav Jindal, MD*, Bryan Pukenas, MD

KEYWORDS

- Normal spine MRI • Normal spinal anatomy
- Normal MRI anatomy • Spine MRI • Spinal MRI
- Spinal anatomy • MRI anatomy

Over the past few decades, spinal magnetic resonance imaging (MR imaging) has largely replaced computed tomography (CT) and CT myelography in the assessment of intraspinal pathology at institutions where MR imaging is available. Given its high contrast resolution, MR imaging allows the differentiation of the several adjacent structures comprising the spine. This article illustrates normal spinal anatomy as defined by MR imaging, describes commonly used spinal MR imaging protocols (**Tables 1–3**), and discusses associated common artifacts.

SPINAL MR IMAGING TECHNIQUES

Sagittal and axial magnetic resonance images should be acquired through the cervical, thoracic, and lumbar segments of the spine, as they are generally considered complementary, and imaging the spine in only one plane may result in misinterpretation. The addition of coronal images may also be useful, especially in patients with scoliosis. Stacked axial images and/or angled images through the discs can be obtained, often useful when the indication for imaging is pain, degenerative change, and/or radiculopathy.[1] Although imaging in the axial plane is a matter of personal preference, using only angled axial images through the discs may be inadequate, as portions of the spinal canal will not be imaged axially. Slice thickness from 3 to 4 mm is generally optimal for imaging of the spine. Axial gradient-echo images

through the cervical spine are typically 2 mm thick.[2]

To depict the fine anatomic detail in the spine, high spatial resolution is a priority because of the small size of the cervical spine relative to the human body and because of the relatively superficial position of the spine within the human body. The use of surface coils, typically phased array receiver coils, helps to maximize signal-to-noise ratio and spatial resolution. Increasing phase-encoding steps results in a larger matrix and higher spatial resolution as a result but also leads to increased imaging acquisition time, which increases the possibility of motion-related image degradation. Among the other factors affecting spinal imaging are matrix size, field of view, gradient moment nulling motion compensation, pulse triggering and gating, band width, and phase-encoding axis.[3]

The pulse sequences used are determined by the clinical indications for the examination based on the following major categories: degenerative disease including radicular symptomatology, trauma, cord compression/bony metastases, and infection.[4] Spin-echo and fast spin-echo sequences are the most common sequences used in spinal MR imaging. Short tau inversion recovery (STIR) imaging is useful to assess the bone marrow[5] and in cases of infectious,[6] inflammatory,[7] and neoplastic[8] lesions. STIR imaging is also useful in the workup of trauma, to assess for ligamentous injury[9] and changes from hemorrhage

The authors have nothing to disclose.
Division of Neuroradiology, Department of Radiology, Hospital of the University of Pennsylvania, 3400 Spruce Street, Philadelphia, PA 19103, USA
* Corresponding author.
E-mail address: drjindal@gmail.com

Magn Reson Imaging Clin N Am 19 (2011) 475–488
doi:10.1016/j.mric.2011.05.013

Table 1
Cervical spine MR imaging protocols

Sequence	Localizer	FLAIR	T2	T2	GRE	T1	T1	STIR	Enhanced T1	Enhanced T1
Plane	3 plane	Sagittal	Sagittal	Axial	Axial	Sagittal	Axial	Sagittal	Sagittal	Axial
Coil type	Neck	Neck	Neck	Neck	Neck	Neck	Neck	Neck	Neck	Neck
Thickness, mm	10	3	3	3	3	3	3	3	3	3
TR, ms	24	1700	3530	4210	32	653	649	4400	653	649
TE, ms	6	12	106	111	14	10	11	74	10	11
Flip angle	30	150	180	150	5	170	150	150	170	150
NEX	1	1	2	2	1	2	2	1	2	2
Matrix	128 × 256	250 × 384	269 × 384	240 × 320	216 × 320	269 × 384	205 × 256	192 × 256	269 × 384	205 × 256
FOV read, mm	300	260	240	200	200	240	240	240	240	240
FOV phase, mm	100	100	100	75	75	200	100	100	100	100
Comments								Trauma, Mets	If indicated	If indicated

Abbreviations: FLAIR, fluid-attenuated inversion-recovery imaging; FOV, field of view; GRE, gradient-recalled echo; Mets, metastases; NEX, number of excitations; STIR, short tau inversion recovery; TE, echo time; TR, repetition time.

Table 2
Thoracic spine MR imaging protocols

Sequence	Localizer	T1	T2	T2	STIR	Enhanced T1	Enhanced T1
Plane	3 plane	Sagittal	Sagittal	Axial	Sagittal	Sagittal	Axial
Coil type	Spine	Spine	Spine	Spine	Spine	Spine	Spine
Thickness	10	4	4		4	4	4
TR, ms	20	641	3000	7360	3220	670	579
TE, ms	6	17	100	106	74	14	13
Flip angle	30	180	150	150	180	150	130
NEX	1	1	2	1	2	2	2
Matrix	128 × 256	256 × 256	307 × 384	192 × 256	256 × 256	269 × 384	230 × 256
FOV read, mm	380	300	320	200	320	320	200
FOV phase, mm	100	100	100	100	100	100	100
Comments					Trauma, Mets	If indicated	If indicated

Abbreviations: FOV, field of view; Mets, metastases; STIR, short tau inversion recovery; TE, echo time; TR, repetition time.

and/or edema. Contrast-enhanced imaging should be used, unless contraindicated, for indications including evaluation of the postoperative spine, suspected infection, or intradural or nontraumatic cord lesions.[10] Abnormalities within the epidural space identified during unenhanced evaluation for metastases and/or cord compression can be better delineated using contrast-enhanced images.[10]

Gradient-recalled echo (GRE), or gradient-echo, sequences allow for delineation of bone and disk margins, provide excellent contrast between the spinal cord and surrounding subarachnoid space, and allow clear visualization of the neural foramina and exiting nerve roots. Gradient-echo axial images are used in the cervical and thoracic spine to detect spinal canal and foraminal stenoses[11] and serve as an important complement to long repetition time spin-echo imaging, given faster acquisition time of GRE. As a result, GRE images are less susceptible to patient motion artifact. Although signal-to-noise ratio is increased with

Table 3
Lumbar spine MR imaging protocols

Sequence	Localizer	T1 FLAIR	T2	T2	T1	STIR	Enhanced T1	Enhanced T1
Plane	3 plane	Sagittal	Sagittal	Axial	Axial	Sagittal	Sagittal	Axial
Coil type	Spine	Spine	Spine	Spine	Spine	Spine	Spine	Spine
Thickness	10	4	4	4	4	4	4	4
TR, ms	3.27	1600	3150	4250	500	4560	657	539
TE, ms	1.64	12	95	106	14	79	12	14
Flip angle	55	150	180	150	90	180	90	90
NEX	2	1	2	1	1	2	2	1
Matrix	115 × 256	256 × 256	256 × 256	218 × 256	205 × 256	192 × 256	192 × 256	192 × 256
FOV read, mm	450	280	280	200	200	280	280	200
FOV phase, mm	100	100	100	100	100	100	75	100
Comments						Trauma, Mets	If indicated	If indicated

Abbreviations: FLAIR, fluid-attenuated inversion-recovery imaging; FOV, field of view; Mets, metastases; STIR, short tau inversion recovery; TE, echo time; TR, repetition time.

GRE, fat is of low signal intensity on GRE sequences compared with T1-weighted spin-echo imaging; as a result, morphologic detail defined by fat is not as well demonstrated on GRE images as on spin-echo images.[12]

Proton density images can be obtained simultaneously (TR 2000 to 3000 milliseconds or greater, TE 20 to 90 milliseconds) when obtaining T1-weighted images and can also be derived from an earlier (first) echo while generating T2-weighted images. Proton density images of the spine are not routinely obtained but can provide valuable information concerning normal and pathologic spinal morphology.[5]

NORMAL SPINAL ANATOMY BASICS

The cervical spine comprises the first 7 superior vertebrae of the spinal column. The first and second segments of the cervical spine are unique. The other cervical vertebrae are similar in size and configuration. The first segment, C1, also known as the atlas, is ring shaped and composed of anterior and posterior arches and lateral articular masses. It lacks a central vertebral body. The second segment, C2, also known as the axis, is also ring shaped and has a superiorly oriented odontoid process, also known as the dens, which lies posterior to the anterior arch of C1. The normal distance between the dens and anterior arch of C1 is approximately 3 mm in adults and 4 mm in children.[13] There are prominent tubercles along the medial aspects of the lateral masses of C1 from which extend the transverse portion of the cruciate/cruciform ligament, ie, the transverse ligament, which confines the odontoid process of C2 posteriorly and delineates the anterior and posterior compartments. This relationship allows free rotation of C1 on C2 and provides for stability during upper cervical spinal flexion, extension, and lateral bending. The transverse ligament is covered posteriorly by the tectorial membrane. The alar ligaments are paired winglike structures connecting the lateral aspects of the odontoid process with the occipital condyles. The thin apical ligament of the odontoid process directly anchors the tip of the odontoid process to the clivus in the anterior aspect of the foramen magnum. The tip of the odontoid process is anterior to the lower medulla. A line of low T1-weighted signal intensity seen through the base of the dens represents the subdental synchondrosis, present in many healthy individuals; it may be distinguished from a fracture because the synchondrosis does not extend to the adjacent cortical bone (**Figs. 1** and **2**).

Unique to the cervical spine, the bilateral uncovertebral joints, also referred to as Luschka joints,

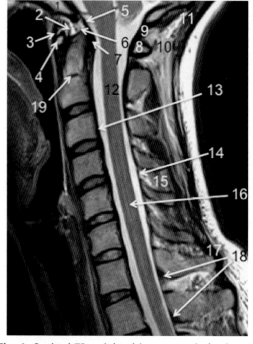

Fig. 1. Sagittal T2-weighted image, cervical spine. 1, Clivus; 2, Atlanto-occipital ligament; 3, Anterior longitudinal ligament; 4, Anterior arch C1; 5, Superior fascicle of cruciform ligament/tectorial membrane; 6, Apical ligament; 7, Transverse ligament (of cruciform ligament); 8, Posterior arch C1; 9, Posterior occipital-atlantal membrane; 10, Nuchal ligament; 11, Semispinalis capitis muscle; 12, Cervical spinal cord; 13, Posterior longitudinal ligament/anterior thecal sac dura; 14, Posterior dural sac; 15, Interspinous ligament; 16, Gray matter along central canal; 17, Supraspinous ligament; 18, Ligamentum flavum; 19, Dental synchondrosis (disc anlage).

are formed by articulation of the uncinate process of the inferior vertebral body with the uncus of the superior vertebral body (see **Fig. 2**; **Figs. 3** and **4**). The uncus is a cup-shaped groove on the posterior/inferior aspect of each cervical vertebral body (except C1), whereas the uncinate processes are located bilaterally on the posterosuperior aspects of the cervical vertebral bodies (except for C1 and C2). The cervical vertebrae also form transverse foramina bilaterally through which the vertebral arteries pass. Although the C7 vertebral body forms transverse foramina, the vertebral arteries usually enter the foramina at C6. The vertebral arteries are seen as circular low-signal structures owing to the flow-void phenomenon (see **Fig. 3B**). The spinous processes of the cervical spine are short and have bifid tips. Compared with the lumbar disks, the disks of the cervical and thoracic spine are much thinner and the outermost portion of the anulus is not as thick.

The cervical spine is depicted in images in **Figs. 1–5** and **Fig. 6**.

Given the anterolateral-directed obliquity of the cervical neural foramina, oblique sagittal views are required to view cross-sectional sagittal anatomy of the neural foramina of the cervical spine.[14,15] These images are obtained by using an axial image to first assess optimal angulation of the oblique sagittal plane through the foramina.

Throughout the spine, the intervertebral canals, or neural foramina, contain the nerve root and its sleeve, the dorsal root ganglion, fat, and blood vessels. The neural foramina are bounded anteriorly by the vertebral bodies and disc, superiorly and inferiorly by the pedicles, and posteriorly by the facet joints which are covered by the ligamentum flavum (see **Fig. 3**).[16] The segmental osseous structures of the spine include the vertebral bodies and their appendages, including the pedicles, the articular pillars, laminae, and transverse and spinous processes. The major ligaments of the spine are the anterior longitudinal ligament, posterior longitudinal ligament, and ligamentum flavum (**Fig. 7**).[16] The spinal canal contains the thecal sac enclosed by the dura mater and surrounded by the epidural space, which contains epidural fat and a large venous plexus. Within the thecal sac are the spinal cord, conus medullaris, and cauda equina, surrounding by freely flowing cerebrospinal fluid (CSF) within the subarachnoid space. The conus medullaris normally terminates near the L1 vertebral level.[16] In the supine position,

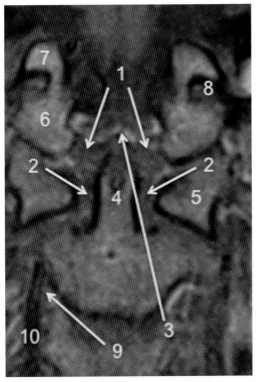

Fig. 2. Coronal T1-weighted image, craniocervical junction. 1, Alar ligament; 2, Transverse ligament (of cruciform ligament); 3, Apical ligament; 4, Dens; 5, Lateral mass C1; 6, Occipital condyle; 7, Jugular tubercle of occipital bone; 8, Hypoglossal canal; 9, Uncinate process C3; 10, Vertebral artery.

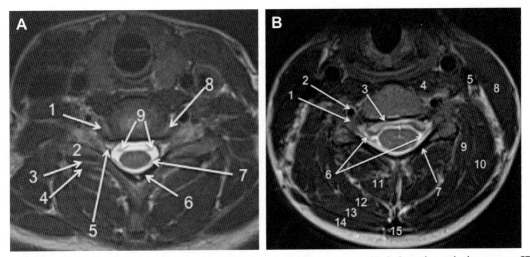

Fig. 3. (*A*) Axial T2-weighted image, lower cervical spine. 1, Uncinate process C7; 2, Superior articular process C7; 3, Apophyseal (facet) joint; 4, Inferior articular process C6; 5, Foraminal vein; 6, Ligamentum flavum/cortex of lamina; 7, Dorsal rootlet C7; 8, Uncovertebral joint; 9, Ventral rootlets C7. (*B*) Axial T2-weighted image, mid cervical spine. 1, Dorsal root ganglion; 2, Vertebral artery; 3, Posterior longitudinal ligament/anterior thecal sac dura; 4, Longus colli muscle; 5, Internal jugular vein; 6, Dorsal rootlets; 7, Lamina; 8, Sternocleidomastoid muscle; 9, Longissimus capitis muscle; 10, Levator scapulae muscle; 11, Semispinalis colli muscle; 12, Semispinalis capitis muscle; 13, Splenius capitis muscle; 14, Trapezius muscle; 15, Nuchal ligament.

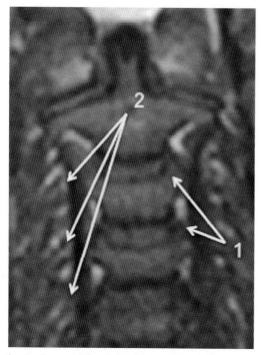

Fig. 4. Coronal T1-weighted image, cervical spine. 1, Uncinate processes; 2, Segmental spinal veins and nerve roots.

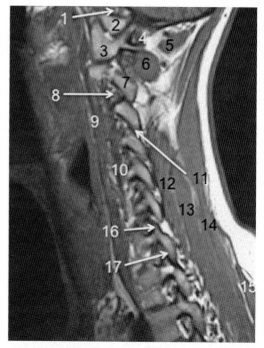

Fig. 5. Parasagittal T1-weighted image, cervical spine. 1, Hypoglossal canal; 2, Occipital condyle; 3, Lateral mass C1; 4, Vertebral artery; 5, Rectus capitis posterior major muscle; 6, Obliquus capitis inferior muscle; 7, Articular pillar C2; 8, C3 dorsal root ganglion; 9, Longus coli (cervicis) muscle; 10, Vertebral artery; 11, Apophyseal (facet) joint C3-4; 12, Multifidis muscle; 13, Semispinalis cervicis muscle; 14, Splenius capitis muscle; 15, Trapezius muscle; 16, Superior articular process; 17, Inferior articular process.

the nerve roots of the cauda equina in the lumbar spine are clustered in the dependant/posterior aspect of the spinal canal (**Figs. 8** and **9**).

The posterior border of nearly all of the vertebral bodies is flat or slightly concave when viewed in axial section and the discs do not normally extend beyond the margins of the adjacent vertebral bodies.[16] However, with exaggerated extension, 1-mm to 2-mm budging may occur in some histologically normal disks.[17–19] The posterior margins of the discs tend to be slightly concave in the upper lumbar spine, straight at the L4/5 level, and slightly convex at the lumbosacral spinal junction. This appearance should not be confused with pathologic bulging. The axial appearance of the L5 vertebral body is biconcave shaped, and iliolumbar ligaments emanate laterally from L5, characteristics that allow distinction of this vertebral segment from others when viewed in the axial plane (see **Fig. 9**). The spinal canal is round in the upper lumbar region and transitions to a triangular configuration in the lower lumbar region. Posterior epidural fat is consistently present in the posterior part of the spinal canal, whereas the anterior epidural fat is most prominent in the L5-S1 region (see **Fig. 8**).[16]

The bony canals of the neural foramina are normally well seen en face in the lumbar region using standard sagittal images (**Fig. 10**) because the orientation of the neural foramina in the lumbar spine is nearly directly lateral as opposed to the anterolateral angle of the neural foramina of the cervical spine. This is in distinction to the anterior obliquity required to optimally visualize the neural foramina of the cervical spine in the sagittal plane.

NORMAL SPINAL ANATOMY, T1-WEIGHTED MR IMAGING

T1-weighted images (TR 300 to 500 milliseconds, TE 20 to 30 milliseconds) in the sagittal plane are obtained as the preliminary survey pulse sequence for analyzing the cervical, thoracic, and lumbar spine. Sagittal and axial T1-weighed sequences provide the anatomic detail with which to begin a survey of the spine.

On T1-weighted images, high signal intensity is demonstrated in mature bone marrow and the epidural fat. Normal bone marrow signal is usually homogeneous but may be heterogeneous and

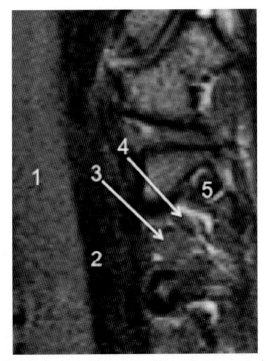

Fig. 6. Coronal oblique T1-weighted image, cervical spine. 1, Cervical spinal cord; 2, Subarachnoid space; 3, Dorsal root ganglion; 4, Superior foraminal vein; 5, Vertebral artery.

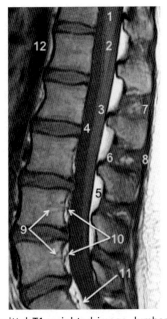

Fig. 8. Sagittal T1-weighted image, lumbar spine. 1, Spinal cord; 2, Conus medullaris; 3, Cauda equina; 4, Subarachnoid space; 5, Posterior epidural fat; 6, Ligamentum flavum; 7, Interspinous ligament; 8, Supraspinous ligament; 9, Basivertebral venous plexus; 10, Epidural venous plexus; 11, Anterior epidural fat; 12, Aorta.

normally changes with aging.[20] The basivertebral venous channel is seen on the midline sagittal images as high signal within the posterior aspect of the vertebral body owing to fat surrounding the vein (see **Fig. 8**).[10] Peripherally, bone marrow

is surrounded by low signal, proton-poor cortical bone, making it indistinguishable from the adjacent low T1-weighted signal intensity of the annulus fibrosus, spinal ligaments, and dura (**Fig. 6**).[21] The relatively poor distinction between

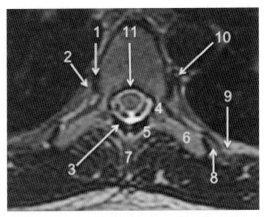

Fig. 7. Axial T2-weighted image, thoracic spine. 1, Costovertebral joint; 2, Head of rib; 3, Ligamentum flavum; 4, Pedicle; 5, Lamina; 6, Transverse process; 7, Spinous process; 8, Costotransverse joint; 9, Tubercle of rib; 10, Hemiazygous vein; 11, Posterior longitudinal ligament.

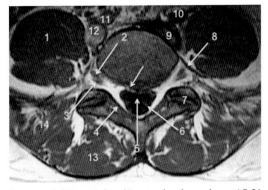

Fig. 9. Axial T1-weighted image, lumbar spine at L5-S1. 1, Psoas muscle; 2, L5 nerve root, ventral ramus; 3, L5 nerve root, dorsal ramus; 4, Ligamentum flavum; 5, Subarachnoid space; 6, Nerve roots of cauda equina; 7, Facet joint; 8, Iliolumbar ligament (signifies L5 vertebral level); 9, Left external iliac vein; 10, Left external iliac artery; 11, Right external iliac artery; 12, Right external iliac vein; 13, Transversospinalis (multifidis) muscle; 14, Erector spinae muscle group.

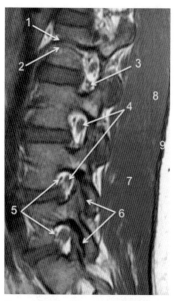

Fig. 10. Parasagittal T1-weighted image, lumbar spine. 1, Lumbar vein; 2, Lumbar artery; 3, Inferior foraminal veins; 4, Dorsal root ganglia; 5, Superior foraminal veins; 6, Facet joints; 7, Transversospinalis (multifidis) muscle; 8, Erector spinae muscle group; 9, Thoracolumbar fascia, posterior layer.

these structures on spin-echo imaging of the cervical and thoracic spine is attributable to little anterior epidural fat compared with that in the lumbar spine (see **Figs. 6** and **8**). Spin-echo imaging often also poorly differentiates cortical osteophytes from disc material. The anterior and posterior longitudinal ligaments adhere to the fibers of the annulus and will appear on midsagittal images as an uninterrupted band of very low signal intensity on all pulse sequences (see **Figs. 8** and **10**).[21]

The intervertebral discs demonstrate slightly less signal than the adjacent vertebral bodies and differentiation of the centrally located nucleus pulposis and peripheral annulus fibrosis of the discs cannot be made precisely on T1-weighted images (see **Figs. 8** and **10**).

Cerebrospinal fluid demonstrates low signal on T1-weighted images and provides contrast with the adjacent, relatively higher signal intensity spinal cord and nerve roots within the spinal canal. The periphery of the spinal canal is lined by high signal-intensity epidural fat (see **Fig. 9**). The nerve roots and dorsal ganglia occupy the upper portion of the neural foramina, also referred to as the subpedicular notch (see **Fig. 10**), and appear as rounded low-signal structures surrounded by high signal fat in the neural foramina. The nerve roots can be followed through the neural foramina on sagittal images. Epidural veins appear as signal

voids anterosuperior to the nerves. It is important to distinguish the ventral internal longitudinal vein from the adjacent nerve and ganglion (see **Figs. 6, 9** and **10**). Each intervertebral canal can be divided arbitrarily into superior and inferior portions. The superior portion of the canal contains the dorsal root ganglion, veins, and epidural fat. The inferior portion contains the nerves, which lie below the disk level close to the superior articular process of the facet joint.[2]

The facet joints appear as linear structures with intermediate signal owing to the presence intra-articular hyaline cartilage and synovial fluid (see **Fig. 9**).[22] The facet joint is formed by the concave surface of the superior articular process and the convex surface of the inferior articular process (see **Fig. 10**). The superior facet is located antero-laterally and faces posteromedially. The inferior facet is located posteromedially and faces antero-laterally. This differs in the cervical spine where the superior and inferior articular processes are fused on either or both sides to form articular pillars, columns of bone that project laterally from the junction of the pedicle and lamina. The bony processes of the spine are better delineated on CT as compared with MR imaging. The ligamentum flava, which bilaterally cover the inner surface of the lamina and the anterior aspects of the facet, joints, are intermediate in signal intensity and are distinguishable from the adjacent high-signal central epidural fat and adjacent peripheral low-signal lamina (see **Fig. 9**; **Fig. 11**).

NORMAL SPINAL ANATOMY, T2-WEIGHTED MR IMAGING

The parameters of T2-weighted imaging include a TR of 2000 to 3000 milliseconds and a TE of 60 to 120 milliseconds; the acquisition time is 2 to 3 times longer than that of T1-weighted imaging, rendering T2-weighted imaging more susceptible to motion artifact and greater noise.

In general, T2-weighted images reveal greater contrast differentiation among structures in comparison with T1-weighted images. With T2 weighting, the proton-poor cortical bone demonstrates low signal intensity and the bone marrow remains fairly high in signal intensity because of its fat content. The basivertebral veins may be of even higher signal intensity because of flow phenomena and should not be mistaken for a fracture (**Fig. 12**). The channel of the basivertebral vein is usually of intermediate signal on the T2-weighted image. The normally hydrated nucleus pulposus composed of water and proteoglycans shows high T2-weighted signal centrally with lower signal from the less-hydrated annulus fibrosis (see

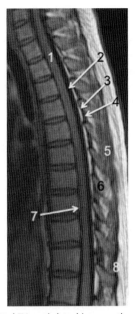

Fig. 11. Sagittal T1-weighted image, thoracic spine. 1, Thoracic spinal cord; 2, Subarachnoid space; 3, Posterior epidural fat; 4, Ligamentum flavum; 5, Transversospinalis (multifidus) muscle; 6, Spinous process; 7, Epidural vein; 8, Supraspinous ligament.

Fig. 12). The annulus fibrosis is composed of fibrocartilage centrally, whereas the outer fibers are made of concentrically oriented collagen fibers. The annulus is anchored to the adjacent vertebral bodies by Sharpey fibers, which are normally not visible by MR imaging.

CSF demonstrates high signal intensity because of its long T2-weighted relaxation time, which allows sensitive identification of surrounding intraspinal structures such as the spinal cord and nerve roots that are intermediate in signal intensity (see **Fig. 12; Figs. 13–15**). When the patient is supine, as in most cases of spinal imaging, the midthoracic spinal cord is positioned within the central/anterior aspect of the spinal canal owing to the normally mild thoracic kyphosis (see **Fig. 12**). CSF often has patchy areas of low signal because of turbulence of flow and/or other flow artifacts related to pulsation effects; these can be particularly troublesome in images with longer echo delays and in those acquired using high magnetic field strength systems (see **Fig. 14**).

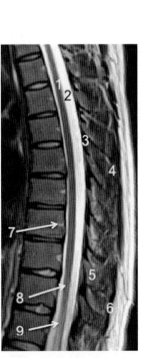

Fig. 12. Sagittal T2-weighted image, thoracic spine. 1, Thoracic spinal cord; 2, Subarachnoid space; 3, Ligamentum flavum; 4, Transversospinalis (multifidus) muscle; 5, Spinous process; 6, Supraspinous ligament; 7, Basivertebral vein; 8, Conus medullaris; 9, Cauda equina.

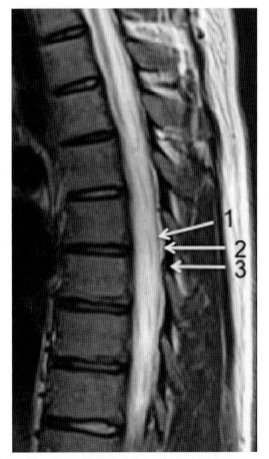

Fig. 13. Parasagittal T2-weighted image, thoracic spine. 1, Posterior thecal sac dura; 2, Posterior epidural fat; 3, Ligamentum flavum.

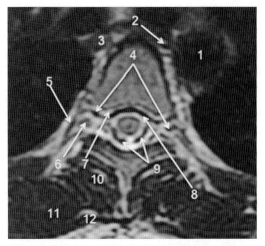

Fig. 14. Axial T2-weighted image, thoracic spine. 1, Aorta; 2, Hemiazygous vein; 3, Azygous vein; 4, Foraminal veins; 5, Thoracic intercostal vein; 6, Dorsal root ganglion; 7, Basivertebral veins, slow flow; 8, Posterior longitudinal ligament; 9, CSF flow artifacts; 10, Transversospinalis (multifidis) muscle; 11, Longissimus dorsi muscle; 12, Trapezius muscle.

T2* images intensify structures with long T2 relaxation times such as CSF, the nucleus pulposis, and facet joint cartilage. On T2* images, the high signal intensity of the venous plexus posterior

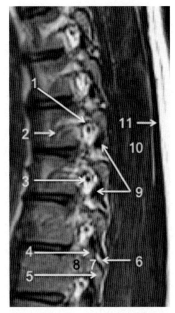

Fig. 15. Parasagittal T2: thoracic neural foramen. 1, Foraminal vein; 2, Thoracic paravertebral intercostal vein and artery; 3, Foraminal nerve root; 4, Superior articular process; 5, Inferior articular process; 6, Facet joint; 7, Pars interarticularis; 8, Pedicle; 9, Ligamentum flavum; 10, Erector spinae muscle group; 11, Trapezius muscle.

to the vertebral body separates the posterior longitudinal ligament and cortical bone of the vertebral body. T2* imaging also allows differentiation of the gray and white matter of the spinal cord. Gray matter appears as a butterfly-shaped region of high signal intensity centrally within the spinal cord when using this technique.[23]

NORMAL SPINAL BONE MARROW MR IMAGING

The axial skeleton contains red marrow, a major site of hematopoiesis throughout life. There is normally a gradual conversion of red marrow to fatty marrow in the appendicular skeleton, which is completed by approximately 25 years of life. The red marrow in the vertebrae also normally undergoes conversion of fatty marrow, although more subtly than in the appendicular skeleton. The fat content of the vertebral body varies with age, degeneration of adjacent discs, therapy, such as radiation, and increased hematopoiesis in processes such as sickle cell disease or other diseases affecting the bone marrow.[20] In younger patients, high-signal fatty marrow can be seen as linear areas adjacent to the basivertebral vein. With advancing age, fatty marrow may appear bandlike, triangular, or multifocal and may take up relatively large areas of the vertebral body in patients older than 40.[20] There is significant variability in the marrow pattern among adults and even within an individual.[20,24]

Ricci and colleagues[25] identified several patterns of marrow distribution in the spine. In pattern 1, the vertebral body demonstrates uniformly low signal on T1-weighted images except for linear areas of high, fatty signal surrounding the basivertebral vein. In pattern 2, bandlike and triangular areas of high signal are found near the end plates and corners of the vertebral body, possibly related to mechanical stress near the end plates. In pattern 3, there are diffusely distributed areas of high signal from fat measuring a few millimeters (pattern 3a) or relatively well-marginated areas on the range of 1 cm (pattern 3b).

In the cervical spine, pattern 1 is found predominantly in patients younger than 40 with patterns 2 and 3 in those who are older than 40. Patterns 2 and 3 generally develop earliest in the lumbar spine, followed by the thoracic spine, and lastly in the cervical spine.[25] Overall, there is continued gradual replacement of hematopoietic marrow with fatty marrow that continues until death. Healthy elderly patients have marked high signal throughout the vertebral body, reflecting the predominance of fatty marrow. Large variations exist, however, secondary to differences among individuals and responses to mechanical stress.[25]

Chemical shift artifact, used extensively in imaging of the adrenal glands and the liver, can be used to assess the bone marrow of the spine in certain instances. In-phase/opposed-phase imaging assesses for the presence of fat and water in a voxel of tissue. The technique takes advantage of the fact that water and fat protons precess at different frequencies and without a refocusing pulse, when there are both fat and water protons in a given voxel, there will be some signal intensity loss on images that are obtained when the protons are in their opposed phase. The utility of chemical shift imaging lies in the fact that in cases of spinal neoplastic disease, normal fat-containing marrow is replaced with tumor, which can result in lack of signal suppression on the opposed phase images. There have been a few reports that have described in-phase/opposed-phase imaging of the spinal bone marrow.[26–28]

MR IMAGING FINDINGS OF VERTEBRAL HEMANGIOMAS

Hemangiomas, composed of angiomatoid fibroadipose tissue interspersed among tortuous thin-walled sinuses, are the most common benign tumors of the spine, seen in 10% or more of healthy adults.[29] They are most common in the thoracic spine followed by the lumbar spine and are relatively rare in the cervical spine.[29] They tend to be well-circumscribed tumors within the vertebral bodies demonstrating high signal intensity on both T1-weighted and T2-weighted images. The T1 shortening is produced by the fatty component, whereas the T2 prolongation is produced by the angiomatous component. The very low signal of the bony trabeculae, which can classically be seen on CT, is overshadowed on MR imaging by the signals from the internal elements described previously. Focal fatty infiltration, a common marrow variant, may be confused with hemangiomas on T1-weighted images; however, the expected corresponding decrease in signal intensity on T2-weighted images serves to distinguish focal fat from the normally high T2-weighted signal of hemangiomas.[30] Hemangiomas may sometimes have a paucity of fatty elements, which may render these lesions isointense or hypointense on T1-weighted images.[30]

NORMAL MR IMAGING OF INTERVERTEBRAL DISCS

In the neonate, the nucleus pulposis is a highly gelantinous, translucent, relatively large, ovoid structure. The anulus fibrosus consists of dense fibers organized as concentric lamellae similar to tree rings. In the second decade of life, the outer portion of the disc is replaced by solid tissue and the anulus becomes more dense. In adults, the nucleus pulposis consists of amorphous fibrocartilage and the anulus becomes even more dense. The demarcation between the nucleus and anulus becomes less distinct with age. In adults, a transversely oriented band of low signal intensity in the midportion of the disc represents a fibrous plate visible on MR imaging. Concentric tears of the annulus are seen in normal discs, and transverse tears, although a manifestation of degenerative disease, are not infrequently seen in asymptomatic adults.[17,19]

Intervertebral herniation of disc material may remodel the vertebral end plate or may extend into the vertebral body. Such herniations are typically referred to as Schmorl nodes.[29] This type of herniation is presumed to have little clinical significance, and it has been observed as early as the second decade of life.

There are abnormalities and normal variants that may mimic the appearance of an extruded or sequestered disk on MR imaging. These include synovial cysts, dilated nerve root sleeves (arachnoid diverticulae), perineural cysts, conjoined nerve roots, nerve sheath tumors, and foreign material such as bullet fragments, metallic hardware, and cement from vertebroplasties. Dilated nerve root sleeves demonstrate signal characteristics identical to CSF, which should allow for differentiation of these from disk material.[4]

COMMON NORMAL SPINAL MR IMAGING ARTIFACTS

The most common source of artifact in MR imaging occurs secondary to patient motion. Whereas random movement leads to blurring, periodic motion, such as with CSF pulsation, cardiac motion, and respiratory motion, leads to ghosting artifacts in the form of image harmonics along the phase-encoding direction because phase information is acquired over an entire scan (minutes), whereas frequency information is acquired over a single frequency readout (milliseconds).[21]

CSF flow-related phenomena can be divided into time-of-flight (TOF) effects and turbulent flow, which produces dark signal. TOF effects are divided into TOF signal loss resulting in dark CSF signal and flow-related enhancement producing bright CSF signal. TOF loss typically occurs in spin-echo or fast spin-echo imaging when protons do not experience both the initial radiofrequency pulse and the subsequent radiofrequency refocusing pulse. TOF loss effects are more pronounced (darker signal) with faster proton velocity, thinner slices, longer TE, and an imaging plane perpendicular to flow. Gradient-recalled echo techniques are less susceptible to TOF loss because of the short TE.

Typical locations for TOF losses include the lateral ventricles just superior to the foramen of Monro, the third ventricle, the fourth ventricle, and within the cervical and thoracic spinal canal. Given the positive relationship between CSF velocity and TOF losses, this effect is magnified in individuals with an underlying abnormally hyperdynamic state, such as hydrocephalus. In addition, laminar flow results in peripherally located protons moving at a slower velocity and leads to a reduction in TOF losses. Turbulent flow results in a broader spectrum of proton velocities and a wide range of flow directions that are not seen in typical laminar flow. This results in more rapid dephasing and signal loss termed "intravoxel dephasing." A commonly encountered CSF flow artifact is the signal void in the dorsal subarachnoid space on sagittal T2-weighted images of the thoracic spine owing to a combination of the respiratory-related and cardiac-related pulsatile CSF flow superimposed on cranially directed bulk CSF flow and turbulent flow from CSF moving from the ventral subarachnoid space to the dorsal subarachnoid space (see **Fig. 14**; **Fig. 16**).

Another common artifact that occurs normally on MR imaging relates to chemical shift and occurs because water and fat protons resonate at slightly different frequencies because of the effects of their local magnetic environment. The most common type of chemical shift artifact occurs along the frequency-encoding axis and results in a spatial misregistration.[31] In the spine, this artifact is manifested as artifactual black lines along the frequency-encoding axis and are most evident in the sagittal T1-weighted images where they produce asymmetric thicknesses of the vertebral end plates. The hyaline cartilage end plate is usually difficult to visualize on MR imaging owing to overlap from chemical shift artifact.[32] Phase-encoding and frequency-encoding gradients may be reversed for imaging the spine in the sagittal plane to avoid chemical shift artifacts in the end plates and disks from the discovertebral interfaces.[32] Chemical shift is proportional to the magnetic field strength.

Truncation artifact, known as Gibb phenomenon, is seen as bands parallel to the spinal cord. This occurs at the interface of CSF and spinal cord because of high-contrast boundaries and is related to acquisition parameters, such as FOV and voxel size (**Fig. 17**).[33,34]

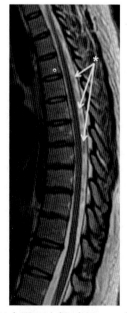

Fig. 16. Sagittal T2-weighted image demonstrating CSF pulsation artifact within the posterior aspect of the thecal sac (*asterisk*).

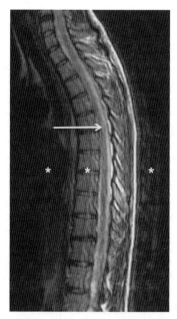

Fig. 17. Artifact degraded sagittal T2-weighted image, thoracic spine. Trucation artifacts (*asterisk*). Trucation artifact simulating spinal cord syrinx (*solid white arrow*).

SUMMARY

Spinal MR imaging is an excellent tool for identifying details of spinal anatomy, including the intraspinal contents, neural foramina, joints, ligaments, intervertebral discs, and bone marrow. The cortical bony structures of the spine, as elsewhere in the body, are generally better imaged using CT. Motion-related and flow-related artifacts may occur during spinal MR imaging and should not be mistaken for pathology. As advancements continue to be made in both MR imaging hardware and software, spinal MR imaging can continue to expand its role in the delineation of both normal and abnormal spinal anatomy.

REFERENCES

1. Brown BM, Schwartz HR, Frank E, et al. Preoperative evaluation of cervical radiculopathy and myelopathy by surface-coil MR imaging. AJNR Am J Neuroradiol 1988;9:859–66.

2. Norman D, Mills CM, Grant-Zawadzki M, et al. Magnetic resonance imaging of the spinal cord and canal: potentials and limitations. AJR Am J Roentgenol 1983;141:1147–52.

3. Chan WP, Lang P, Genant HK, et al. MRI of the musculoskeletal system. Philadelphia: W.B. Saunders Company; 1994.

4. Kaplan PA, Helms CA, Dussault R, et al. Musculoskeletal MRI. Philadelphia: W.B. Saunders Company; 2001.

5. Demaerel P, Sunaert S, Wilms G. Sequences and techniques in spinal MR imaging. JBR-BTR 2003; 86:221–2.

6. Dagirmanjian A, Schils J, McHenry MC. MR imaging of spinal infections. Magn Reson Imaging Clint N Am 1999;7:525–38.

7. Maksymowych WP, Crowther SM, Dhillon SS, et al. Systematic assessment of inflammation by magnetic resonance imaging in the posterio elements of the spine in ankylosing spondylitis. Arthritis Care Res 2010;62:4–10.

8. Myslivecek M, Nekula J, Bacovsky J, et al. Multiple myeloma: predictive value of tc-99m mibi scintigraphy and MRI in its diagnosis and therapy. Nucl Med Rev Cent East Eur 2008;11:12–6.

9. Williams RL, Hardman JA, Lyons K. MR imaging of suspected acute spinal instability. Injury 1998;29: 109–13.

10. Breger RK, Williams AL, Daniels DL, et al. Contrast enhancement in spinal MR imaging. AJNR Am J Neuroradiol 1989;10:633–7.

11. Hedberg MC, Drayer BP, Flom RA, et al. Gradient echo (GRASS) MR imaging in cervical radiculopathy. AJNR Am J Neuroradiol 1988;9:145–51.

12. Wang M, Dai Y, Han Y, et al. Susceptibility weighted imaging in detecting hemorrhage in acute cervical spinal cord injury. Magn Reson Imaging 2011;29: 365–73.

13. Parke WW, Sherk HH. Normal adult anatomy. In: Sherk HH, editor. The cervical spine. Philadelphia: JB Lippincott; 1989. p. 11.

14. Yenerich DO, Haughton VM. Oblique plane MR imaging of the cervical spine. J Comput Assist Tomogr 1986;10:823.

15. Modic MT, Masaryk TJ, Ross JS, et al. Cervical radiculopathy: value of oblique MR imaging. Radiology 1987;163:227.

16. Drake RL, Vogl AW, Mitchell AW, et al. Gray's atlas of anatomy. Philadelphia: Churchill Livingstone; 2007.

17. Boden S, Davis D, Dina T, et al. Abnormal magnetic resonance scans of the lumbar spine in asymptomatic subjects: a prospective investigation. J Bone Joint Surg Am 1990;72:403–8.

18. Yu S, Haughton V, Sether LA. Anulus fibrosus in bulging intervertebral disks. Radiology 1988;169: 761–3.

19. Jensen M, Brant-Zawadski M, Obuchowski N, et al. Magnetic resonance imaging of the lumbar spine in people without back pain. N Engl J Med 1995;331: 69–73.

20. Dooms GC, Fisher MR, Hricack H, et al. Bone marrow imaging: magnetic resonance studies related to age and sex. Radiology 1985;155: 429–32.

21. Reicher MA, Gold RH, Halbach VV, et al. MR imaging of the lumbar spine: anatomic correlations and the effects of technical variations. Am J Roentgenol 1986;147:891–8.

22. Czervionke LF, Daniels DL, Ho PSP, et al. Cervical neural foramina: correlative anatomic and MR imaging study. Radiology 1988;169:753.

23. Czervionke LF, Daniels DL, Ho PSP, et al. The MR appearance of gray and white matter in the cervical spinal cord. AJNR Am J Neuroradiol 1988;9:557–62.

24. Loevner L, Tobey JD, Yousem DM. MR imaging characteristics of cranial bone marrow in adult patients with underlying systemic disorders compared with healthy control subjects. AJNR Am J Neuroradiol 2002;23(2):248–54.

25. Ricci C, Cova M, Kang YS, et al. Normal age-related patterns of cellular and fatty bone marrow distribution in the axial skeleton: MR imaging study. Radiology 1990;177:83–8.

26. Eito K, Waka S, Naoko N, et al. Vertebral neoplastic compression fractures: assessment by dual-phase chemical shift imaging. J Magn Reson Imaging 2004;20:1020–4.

27. Baker LL, Goodman SB, Perkash I, et al. Benign versus pathologic compression fractures of vertebral bodies: assessment with conventional spin-echo,

chemical-shift, and STIR MR imaging. Radiology 1990;174:495–502.

28. Erly WK, Oh ES, Outwater EK. The utility of in-phase/opposed-phase imaging in differentiating malignancy from acute benign compression fractures of the spine. AJNR Am J Neuroradiol 2006;27:1183–8.

29. Schmorl G, Junghanns H. The human spine in health and disease. New York: Grune and Stratton; 1959. p. 12.

30. Laredo JD, Reizine D, Bard M, et al. Vertebral hemangiomas: radiologic evaluation. Radiology 1986;161:183.

31. Bronskill MJ, McVeigh ER, Kucharazyk W, et al. Syrinx-like artifacts on MR images of the spinal cord. Radiology 1988;166:485–8.

32. Bellon EM, Haacke EM, Coleman PE, et al. MR artifacts: a review. Am J Roentgenol 1986;147:1271–81.

33. Pusey E, Lufkin R, Brown R, et al. Magnetic resonance imaging artifacts: mechanisms and clinical significance. Radiographics 1986;6:891–911.

34. Czervionke LF, Czervionke JM, Daniels DL, et al. Characteristic features of MR truncation artifacts. AJNR Am J Neuroradiol 1988;9:815–24.

Normal Magnetic Resonance Imaging of the Thorax

Vikram Venkatesh, MD, Daniel Verdini, MD,
Brian Ghoshhajra, MD, MBA*

KEYWORDS

- Magnetic resonance imaging • Thorax
- MR pulse sequences • Intrathoracic structures

Functionally, the human chest is composed of the cardiorespiratory system, the main purpose of which is to facilitate gas exchange and deliver oxygenated blood to the remainder of the body.

Anatomically, the chest contains the lungs, which comprise airspace, interstitial spaces and airways; the mediastinum, including the aorta and great vessels as well as the trachea, esophagus, fat and lymph nodes; and the heart and pericardium as well as the pulmonary vasculature. The pleura cover the lungs, the chest wall provides the basic skeleton for the thoracic cage, and the diaphragm provides the muscular support for passage of air through the lungs.

LUNG

The normal lung arises embryologically from the primitive foregut.[1] The right lung has 3 lobes, divided by horizontal and oblique fissures, whereas the left lung has 2 lobes, divided by a single oblique fissure.[2] Although the lung fissures are important landmarks on chest radiography and on computed tomography (CT) scans, the paramagnetic properties of air do not allow for good delineation of these anatomic landmarks on magnetic resonance (MR) imaging.[3] Furthermore, for diagnostic purposes, the secondary pulmonary lobule, the basic unit of lung anatomy and basis for high-resolution chest CT, cannot be delineated on MR imaging. These factors make anatomic delineation of disease process of the lungs with MR imaging suboptimal. However, there does remain an important role for disorders that require tissue characterization, such as cystic lesions.

PLEURA

The lungs are invested in a 2-layered pleural covering. The visceral pleura envelopes the lung, whereas the parietal pleura forms an exterior membrane. The space between these layers is known as the pleural space. The visceral pleural layer invaginates to form the fissures.[4] The pleural space becomes distended with pleural fluid in several disease processes and can then be seen; however, the pleura are not routinely visualized on MR scanning of the thorax. The role of MR scanning for pleural diseases is important, but largely confined to disorders in which it is important to achieve tissue characterization instead of anatomic delineation.[5]

DIAPHRAGM

The diaphragms are dome-shaped muscles that descend on normal inspiration, and ascend on expiration. The normal position of the diaphragms is at the fifth to sixth rib anteriorly and the 10th rib posteriorly.[6] The right diaphragm is usually higher than the left. The diaphragmatic position can be depicted using several modalities including plain radiography, CT, and MR imaging.[7] MR imaging has the added benefit of being able to show diaphragmatic motion using cine sequences.[8]

This article includes a discussion of off label usage of contrast material, which has not received FDA approval.
Cardiac MR PET CT Program, Department of Radiology, Massachusetts General Hospital, 55 Fruit Street, Boston, MA 02114, USA
* Corresponding author.
E-mail address: bghoshhajra@partners.org

Magn Reson Imaging Clin N Am 19 (2011) 489–506
doi:10.1016/j.mric.2011.05.014

CHEST WALL

The chest wall forms the structure for the thoracic cage. It comprises bones including the ribs and thoracic vertebral bodies, as well as the intercostal muscles (**Fig. 1**). The intercostal nerves, arteries, and veins course just inferior to the ribs but cannot be readily resolved on routine imaging sequences, except in pathologic processes.[9] The thoracic musculature can also be depicted on MR imaging including the muscles of the anterior chest (such as the pectoralis muscles) and of the back (such as the latissimus dorsi, and trapezius). The reader is referred to any standard anatomy textbook for further elucidation on musculoskeletal anatomy.[2] The superior contrast resolution of MR imaging makes it well suited for depicting these normal structures. The distinction between fat and muscle planes is well seen on MR imaging (**Fig. 2**). Knowledge of the MR anatomy of the chest wall is important for determination of disorders, particularly related to the musculoskeletal system.

NONVASCULAR MEDIASTINUM

MR imaging can identify several normal nonvascular structures in the mediastinum including the thymus, the trachea, the esophagus, and occasional lymph nodes.

Thymus

The thymus is an arrowhead-shaped structure that occupies the anterior mediastinum.[10] It is usually visible in childhood (**Fig. 3**), after which it gradually involutes, but may be visible as a normal structure up to approximately 40 years of age.[11] After this point, the thymus is typically completely replaced by fat. The thymus has a right and left lobe that are typically not distinguished by imaging. The MR appearance of thymus mimics the fatty replacement that is seen with progressive T1 shortening with age, whereas the T2 properties remain constant regardless of patient age.[11] Notably, the thymic signal often parallels that of lymph nodes, particularly in those less than 40 years of age, and therefore distinguishing these 2 entities can often prove challenging.[11]

Esophagus

The esophagus is a tubular structure seen in the middle or posterior mediastinum (depending on classification scheme), coursing through the diaphragm and entering the stomach.[12] It is often collapsed in normal thoracic MR imaging and typically has a small amount of air within it. Although MR imaging of the esophagus is not considered a first-line diagnostic modality, there is increasing

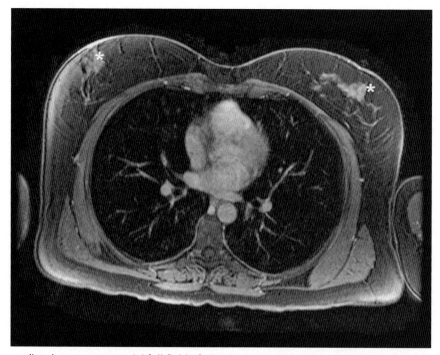

Fig. 1. Extracardiac chest anatomy. Axial full field of view postcontrast image, with fat saturation, shows normal vascular, soft tissue, and breast (*asterisk*) enhancement.

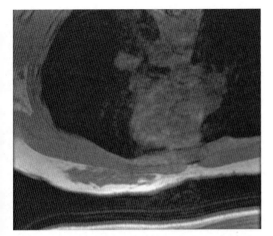

Fig. 2. Extracardiac chest anatomy. Prone noncontrast T1 image obtained for evaluation of the anterior chest wall shows normal musculature, subcutaneous fat, and breast tissue. Note the cardiac pulsation artifact seen on this image performed without cardiac gating.

evidence for use of MR to examine disorders of the gastroesophageal junction such as reflux using cine-MR techniques.[13–15] The esophagus passes in close proximity to the inferior pulmonary veins,

and, because of its close proximity, can be injured during pulmonary vein ablation/isolation procedures, in which case late gadolinium enhancement in that area may be observed.[16]

Trachea and Bronchi

The thoracic portion of the trachea courses from the thoracic inlet and terminates at the carina in the middle mediastinum. The trachea consists of cartilaginous rings anteriorly with a membranous posterior portion. On MR examination, the signal void associated with the tracheal air column can be appreciated, as can the walls of the trachea. The mainstem bronchi and large segmental bronchi can be visualized; however, the smaller subsegmental bronchi, visualized easily on CT, are not readily visualized by MR imaging. The left mainstem bronchus is the hyparterial bronchus, whereas the right mainstem bronchus is the eparterial bronchus, which allows for morphologic delineation of the respective lungs. The tracheal wall can be assessed in pediatric patients to evaluate collapsibility, as well as for stenoses and its relation to vascular structures, using various MR pulse sequences.[17–19]

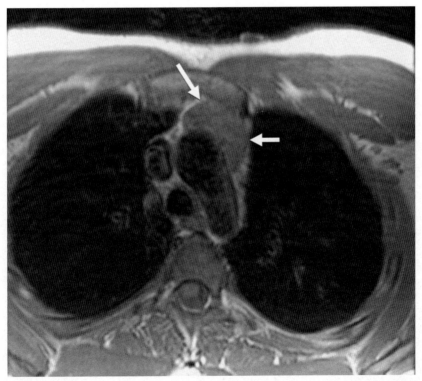

Fig. 3. Extracardiac chest anatomy. Axial T1-weighted black blood image in a young patient (28 years old) shows asymmetric residual thymic tissue (*white arrows*), within the spectrum of normal. Normal thymic tissue is present at birth, and gradual involution occurs, with complete replacement by normal fat usually seen by the fourth decade.

Lymph Nodes

MR imaging is not currently the preferred method to assess for lymph node enlargement; however, knowledge of lymph node stations in the thorax is key to avoiding confusion with other processes and other mediastinal structures. A complete review of the most recent American Joint Committee on Cancer (AJCC) lymph node staging system is beyond the scope of this article, and the reader is referred to the official publication for more information.[20] The characterization of lymph nodes on MR is variable on both T1 and T2 imaging. As per CT, size criteria determine the likelihood of malignancy, although work with diffusion-weighted MR imaging may hold promise for increasing specificity for pathologic involvement.[21,22]

AORTA AND GREAT VESSELS

MR of the aorta (**Fig. 4**) is a commonly performed examination. MR acquisition can be performed in true planes using double-oblique localizers, and cardiac gating can eliminate motion artifacts (**Fig. 5**). There are several techniques that are used to image the aorta, including black blood imaging by means of conventional spin-echo and fast spin-echo sequences, bright blood imaging, such as balanced steady-state free precession, time of flight, and phase contrast sequences, as well as gadolinium-enhanced MR angiography sequences (**Fig. 6**).

The thoracic aorta arises centrally from the left ventricle (LV) and is the main conduit for systemic blood flow, extending to the crus of the diaphragm inferiorly. Initially, the aorta follows a superior course, known as the ascending aorta, followed by a transversely oriented arch, and subsequently a descending portion. From the left ventricular outflow tract (LVOT) and its junction with the aortic annulus, the ascending aorta is divided into the aortic root and the tubular ascending aorta, which is divided by the sinotubular junction (**Fig. 7**). The proximal 3 cm of the aorta ascends within the pericardium; this portion is most susceptible to pulsatile cardiac motion. The sinuses of Valsalva give rise to the coronary arteries (discussed later). Normal branching occurs at the arch and consists of 3 vessels: a brachiocephalic trunk that subsequently divides into the right common carotid artery and subclavian artery, a left common carotid artery, and a left subclavian artery. Variations in the branching pattern of the aortic vessels are also common. The most common variation is known

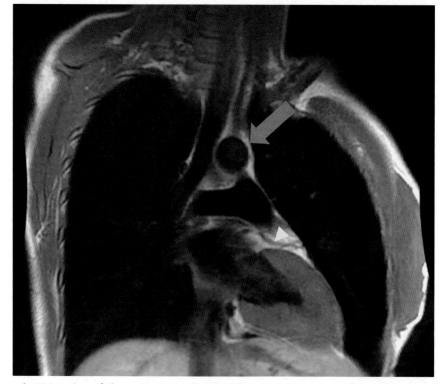

Fig. 4. Normal MR imaging of the aorta. Fast spin-echo black blood image obtained through the aortic arch (*orange arrow*) shows no evidence for aneurysm of dissection. Incidental normal flow void is also seen in the left anterior descending coronary artery (*yellow arrowhead*).

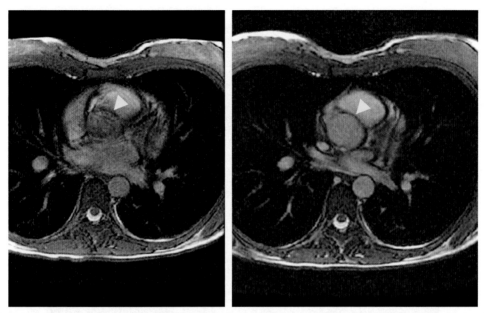

Fig. 5. Normal MR imaging of the aorta. Nongated, breath-hold-balanced, steady-state free precession (SSFP) image at the axial level of the aorta (*left image*) shows cardiac motion artifact (*yellow arrowhead*) that precludes detailed anatomic assessment. Axial, segmented, balanced SSFP image at the same level (*right image*) allows motion-free imaging of the aortic root (*yellow arrowhead*).

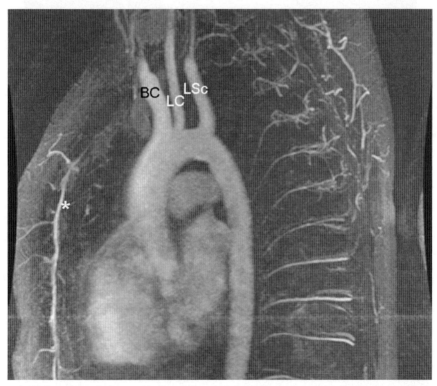

Fig. 6. Normal MR imaging of the aorta. Contrast-enhanced MR angiography (nonsegmented, time-resolved, dynamic, bolus-enhanced, gradient-recalled acquisition, obtained with parallel imaging techniques) oblique maximum intensity projection (MIP) reconstruction in the candy cane view shows the benefits of T1 shortening with gadolinium, such as rapid acquisition times, and visualization of small structures (eg, the chest wall small vessels such as the left internal mammary artery [*asterisk*] seen in this image). The right brachiocephalic trunk (BC), left common carotid (LC), and left subclavian (LSc) arteries, representing the normal aortic branching pattern, are marked. Note the lack of definition of the aortic root on this nongated acquisition.

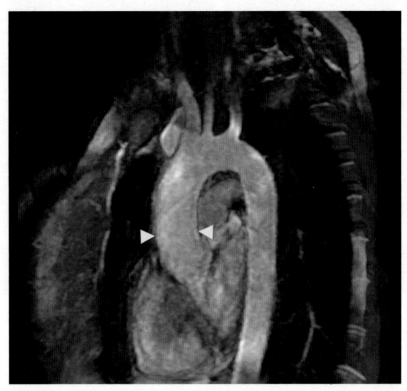

Fig. 7. Normal MR imaging of the aorta. Candy cane view, noncontrast oblique, segmented, balanced SSFP image through the long axis of the aortic arch allows visualization of the course of the normal arch in a single image. Assessment of the aorta does not require contrast. The sinotubular junction (*yellow arrowheads*) is preserved in this healthy, normal patient.

as a bovine arch, in which case the brachioce-phalic trunk and left common carotid share an ostium, and the left subclavian artery has its own branch. The next most common branching pattern involves a left vertebral artery that has a separate origin from the arch, rather than an origin from the left subclavian artery. Bicarotid trunks are a normal variant whereby both carotid arteries originate from a common trunk. An aberrant right subclavian artery is within the spectrum of normal variation, whereby the right subclavian artery is the last branch from the aortic arch, coursing posterior to the esophagus before resuming its normal course. A myriad of other arch variants exist, but a complete review is beyond the scope of this article.[23]

The normal aortic measurements vary with age and body size. There is normal systolic distension of the aorta, which differs significantly from the diastolic. Normative measurement of the aorta is lacking on MR imaging, but has been extensively validated by two-dimensional (2D) echocardiog-raphy and, more recently, CT.[24] In general, there is close correlation with 2D-echo results.[25,26] Consensus data on normal MR measurements of the ascending, arch, and descending thoracic

aorta are scarce. At our institution, we use a general rule of 4.0 cm as a top normal size of the aortic sinuses, and 3.8 cm as a top normal for the ascending aorta (specifically at the level of the right pulmonary artery). However, care should be taken when reporting aortic sizes; more accurate correlation with outcomes has been shown when indexing values to body size.[27]

PULMONARY ARTERIAL ANATOMY

The pulmonary arteries function to deliver deoxy-genated blood from the right ventricle (RV) to the lungs. The pulmonary arteries arise from the muscular infundibulum of the RV at the pulmonic valve. The main pulmonary artery is an intraperi-cardial structure that courses superiorly from the right ventricular outflow tract (RVOT). The main pulmonary artery subsequently bifurcates into a longer right pulmonary artery that crosses the midline to supply the right lung, and a shorter left pulmonary artery.[28]

The right pulmonary artery courses posterior to the superior vena cava (SVC) and anterior to the right mainstem bronchus. It then divides into a truncus anterior, supplying the right upper lobe, and an interlobar artery, which supplies the right middle lobe and lower lobe. The pulmonary arteries course with their respective bronchi.[2]

The left pulmonary artery passes anterior and lateral to the left mainstem bronchus and is located higher than the right main pulmonary artery in normal individuals. The left main pulmonary artery divides into a left upper lobe artery and an interlobar artery that supplies the lingula and lower lobe. The blood supply generally follows the adjacent bronchi.[2]

Normative measurements have not been widely reported by MR imaging. One publication measured pulmonary artery diameters in true double-oblique, short-axis measurements. This study by Lyn and colleagues,[29] reported normal main pulmonary arteries between 1.89 and 3.03 cm (fifth to 95th percentiles). This result varied significantly with height and body weight. The pulmonary artery/aorta ratio varied between 0.66 and 1.13.[29]

PULMONARY VENOUS ANATOMY

Dedicated MR of the pulmonary veins is a commonly performed procedure, owing to pulmonary vein ablation/isolation procedures. Techniques used to image the pulmonary veins include dark blood spin-echo sequences, bright blood sequences, as well as gadolinium-enhanced MR angiography techniques.

The pulmonary veins deliver oxygen-rich blood from the pulmonary capillaries to the left atrium (**Fig. 8**). Variation in pulmonary anatomy is the rule rather than the exception. Clinically, delineation of the pulmonary vein ostia with the left atrium is most important (**Fig. 9**). The branching of the pulmonary veins more distally is variable.[30] The most common pulmonary venous anatomy is 2 right-sided pulmonary veins, the superior supplying the right upper lobe, and the inferior supplying the lower and middle lobes, and 2 left-sided pulmonary veins, the superior supplying the left upper lobe (**Fig. 10**) and the inferior supplying the left lower lobe. The superior pulmonary veins course anterosuperiorly, whereas the inferior pulmonary veins course posteroinferiorly. Normal variants are plentiful in the pulmonary venous system; the most common is a third right-sided pulmonary vein (**Fig. 11**) that courses anteriorly to supply the right middle lobe, or, less frequently, courses posteriorly to supply the superior segment of the right lower lobe. On the left side, the most common variant is a common trunk arising from the left atrium that subsequently branches to drain the entire left lung. Only rarely is a fifth pulmonary vein seen arising from the left

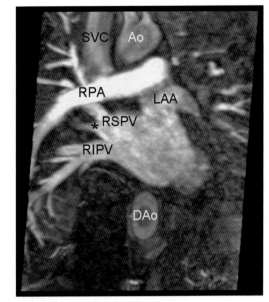

Fig. 8. Pulmonary vein anatomy. An oblique radial multiplanar reformation, reconstructed from a gadolinium-enhanced MR venography, through the long axis of the right superior pulmonary vein (RSPV) shows a wide ostium, no evidence of stenosis, and a normal variant branching pattern with a wide common ostium of the right upper (RSPV) and middle (*asterisk*) pulmonary vein. Note the positions of the superior vena cava (SVC), aortic arch (Ao), descending aorta (DAo), and overlying right pulmonary artery (RPA). The left atrial appendage (LAA) is evident in this plane, and should be distinguished from the left-sided pulmonary veins. RIPV, right inferior pulmonary vein.

side.[30–34] Rarer still is the presence of a right top pulmonary vein that arises from the roof of the left atrium and drains an apical portion of the right upper lobe.[32]

Normal pulmonary vein ostia are similar in both right-sided and left-sided pulmonary veins, and similar in both the right and left inferior pulmonary veins. The superior pulmonary veins are typically larger than the inferior pulmonary veins. The proximal pulmonary vein trunks can be either straight or funnel shaped.[30] The branching pattern is also variable, with early branching occurring frequently and of particular importance in planning electrophysiologic interventions.

HEART AND PERICARDIUM
Imaging Technique

The heart can be imaged using both spin-echo and gradient-echo techniques. Spin-echo acquisitions are black blood sequences (**Fig. 12**) and can provide important morphologic information. Rapid

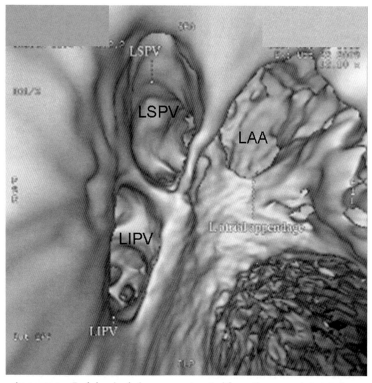

Fig. 9. Pulmonary vein anatomy. Endoluminal view, reconstructed from the same dataset, shows the relationship of the ostia of the left superior pulmonary vein (LSPV) and left lower pulmonary vein (LIPV), and the left atrial appendage (LAA). This view is helpful for planning of pulmonary vein isolation procedures in patients with atrial arrhythmias.

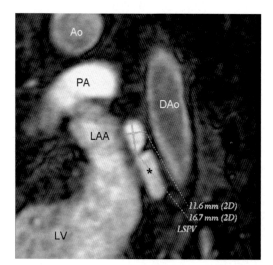

Fig. 10. Pulmonary vein anatomy. Oblique MIP image in the short axis of the left superior pulmonary vein (LSPV) (*crosshairs*) shows normal size, and no evidence for stenosis at this level. The minimally opacified aortic arch (Ao) and descending aorta (DAo), brightly enhanced main pulmonary artery (PA), left inferior pulmonary vein (*asterisk*), and left ventricular blood pool (LV) are marked. By acquiring the center of k-space early during bolus contrast delivery, the pulmonary circulation is more opacified relative to the systemic arterial circulation.

repetition sequences are used to generate bright blood images and are now predominantly used to generate functional information. Perfusion and delayed enhancement (**Fig. 13**) images can be generated using separate imaging sequences that are tailored for speed in the former, and more for detail in the latter.

Normal cardiac MR imaging requires both cardiac and respiratory gating to suppress motion-related artifacts. This suppression is achieved by synchronizing electrocardiographic tracings with cardiac MR image acquisitions. Images can be gated prospectively or retrospectively depending on the type of sequence being performed.[35] Respiratory gating can also be performed to minimize motion, which is typically performed by acquiring breath-hold sequences, although other strategies exist to minimize respiratory motion. These strategies include increasing the number of signal averages (also called number of excitations [NEX]) per image to average motion, as well as navigator sequences whereby electrocardiograph and respiratory gating information is synchronized for acquisition at a specific time point in both the cardiac and respiratory cycle. These techniques are associated with significantly increased imaging times.

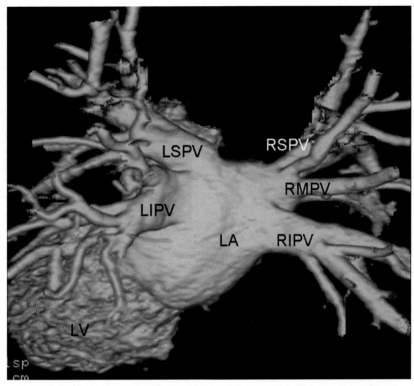

Fig. 11. Pulmonary vein anatomy. Three-dimensional (3D) volume-rendered image, viewed from posterior, reconstructed from the same dataset shows normal branching, with 3 right-sided pulmonary veins (RSPV, right superior pulmonary vein; RMPV, right middle pulmonary vein; RIPV, right inferior pulmonary vein), and 2 left-sided pulmonary veins (LSPV, left superior pulmonary vein; LIPV, left inferior pulmonary vein), each draining the corresponding lobe of the lung in the same patient. The posterior wall of the left atrium (LA) faces the viewer, draining to the LV. The pulmonary arteries, aorta, and thoracic cage have been subtracted during postprocessing.

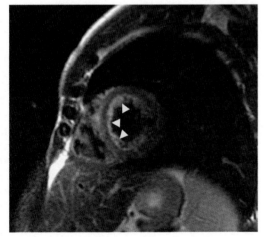

Fig. 12. Basic imaging options for the LV. Using fast spin-echo techniques with inversion recovery, a T2-weighted black blood image is obtained. The blood pool is dark because of entry refreshed spins in the blood pool from protons that were saturated by the initial blood suppression pulse. Signal from in-plane slow flow along the LV wall (*yellow arrowheads*) should not be confused with evidence of disease.

Imaging Planes

The axis of the heart is oblique within the thorax, with the normal axis of rotation lying roughly 45 degrees to the sagittal and coronal planes. It lies between the lungs, above the diaphragm, and below the carina. In the conventionally positioned heart, the apex is in the left side of the chest, with the RV lying anterior to the LV on axial images. Although this is the conventional positioning of the heart, any combination is possible, and therefore imagers should know the morphologic characteristics that distinguish the cardiac chambers.

True cardiac planes are always double oblique to the body (**Fig. 14**). When imaging the LV, all long-axis views must bisect the mitral valve plane and the left ventricular apex, whereas the short-axis view is perpendicular to long-axis views (**Figs. 15** and **16**). Several methods can be used to create these double-oblique planes, which are slightly different in each patient, and dependent on a consistent respiratory excursion (ie, end inspiration or end expiration). At our institution, this begins with the acquisition of sagittal and axial

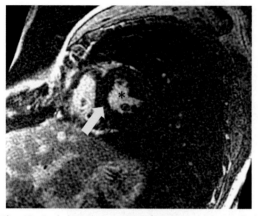

Fig. 13. Basic imaging options for the LV. Myocardial delayed enhancement images are obtained by using a double-inversion recovery technique that allows nulling of the enhanced, normal myocardium (*yellow arrow*). This image was timed for nulling of signal with a T1 relaxation time of 180 milliseconds. This inversion time was tailored to the patient's unique nulling time for normal myocardium. Note that the blood pool (*black asterisk*) and peripheral anatomy show bright signal and contrast enhancement, caused by the different T1 relaxation times, and therefore lack of nulling, of these tissues.

localizers. From the axial localizer, a paraseptal long-axis view is obtained by prescribing a long-axis image parallel to the interventricular septum, transecting the mitral valve and the cardiac apex (*yellow line* in **Fig. 14**). Using this view, we then prescribe a perpendicular short-axis view (*yellow line* in **Fig. 15**). From the short-axis view, a 3-chamber long axis can be defined through the LVOT, whereas a 4-chamber long-axis view (**Fig. 17**, defined by the *yellow line* in **Fig. 16**) can be defined through the margin of the RV. These 4 standard left ventricular planes are most commonly used in cardiac MR. In addition, MR offers the possibility acquiring images in any desired plane, and less commonly used views include radial long-axis views (in any desired long-axis view), or right ventricular views such as RV inflow and outflow views (**Fig. 18**). Right ventricular inflow views are prescribed from the 4-chamber view, parallel to the septum, centered on the RV; right ventricular outflow views are prescribed from the axial localizer, in a near-sagittal plane centered on the tricuspid valve and the pulmonary artery.

SVC/IVC and Right Atrium

The atria can be divided into several components based largely on their embryologic origin. Embryologically, the right atrium (RA) is formed from the sinus venosus and the primitive auricle. These 2

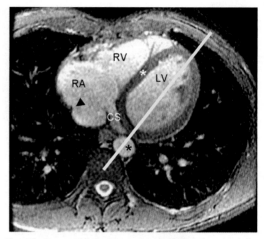

Fig. 14. True cardiac planes. An algorithm for obtaining true cardiac planes is shown. All true cardiac planes are double oblique to the body. Nonsegmented, breath-hold-balanced SSFP localizer is obtained. Although all 4 chambers can be identified in some slices of this plane, the axial view is not a true 4-chamber view. On this image, the right atrium (RA), right ventricle (RV), LV, interventricular septum (*white asterisk*), coronary sinus (CS), and descending aorta (*black asterisk*) are readily identified. Note the small irregularity in the posterior wall of the RA (*arrowhead*), which represents the crista terminalis, seen in cross section. This is a normal structure with a slightly variable appearance, which should not be confused with masses or thrombi.

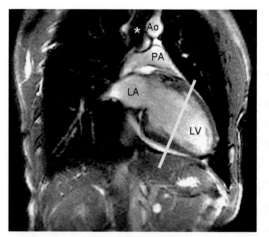

Fig. 15. True cardiac planes. An algorithm for obtaining true cardiac planes is shown. All true cardiac planes are double oblique to the body. From the axial localizer, a segmented, cine-balanced SSFP parasternal long-axis (2-chamber) view is obtained, which was planned via the yellow line drawn in **Fig. 14**. The left atrium (LA), LV, pulmonary artery (PA), and aorta (Ao) are easily identified on this bright blood sequence. The signal void in the lung parenchyma is difficult to distinguish from the lack of signal in the trachea (*white asterisk*). The azygous arch (bright signal) lies immediately to the right of the asterisk.

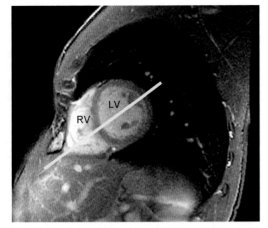

Fig. 16. An algorithm for obtaining true cardiac planes is shown. All true cardiac planes are double oblique to the body. Using the parasternal long-axis view, a perpendicular line that is parallel to the mitral valve plane, and perpendicular to the long axis of the LV, is prescribed (*yellow line* in **Fig. 15**), yielding this short-axis view imaged with segmented cine-balanced SSFP. The right ventricle is marked (RV).

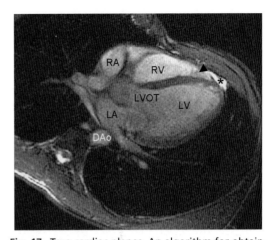

Fig. 17. True cardiac planes. An algorithm for obtaining true cardiac planes is shown. All true cardiac planes are double oblique to the body. The short-axis view allows prescription of a true 4-chamber view, by drawing a plane through the center of the mitral valve, the apex of the heart, and the angle of the right ventricle (RV) margin (*yellow line* in **Fig. 16**). This 4-chamber plane (again imaged with cine-segmented balanced SSFP) allows visualization of the right atrium (RA), RV (with the moderator band identified by an arrowhead), left ventricle (LV), left ventricular outflow tract (LVOT), and left atrium (LA). The descending aorta (DAo) is identified immediately posterior to the left atrium. Note a trace amount of normal pericardial fat seen near the LV apex (*black asterisk*). The distinction between pericardial fluid and epicardial and pericardial fat can be difficult using balanced SSFP sequences, which exhibit both T1 and T2 properties. Often, additional sequences are necessary to evaluate the pericardium.

parts are separated by the crista terminalis on the inside and the sulcus terminalis on the outside. Owing to its venous origin, the posterior aspect of the right heart is smooth walled. The wall is also thin, and should measure no more than 3 mm. The primitive auricle is highly trabeculated and also gives rise to the trabeculated atrial appendage. The appendage itself drapes along the lateral margin of the RA. The right atrial appendage is a broad and triangular structure, with pectinate muscles running through it.[28,36,37]

The SVC, IVC, and coronary sinus drain into the smooth portion of the RA, which is venous in origin. The coronary sinus receives its supply from the great, small, and middle cardiac veins and drains directly into the RA via the thebesian valve and follows a course along the posteroinferior heart. The crista terminalis is visible on several views and familiarity with its location is important to avoid confusion of this normal structure with mass lesions or thrombi.[28,36,37]

RV

The role of the RV is to pump desaturated blood to the lungs for oxygenation. In the normally oriented heart, the RV is the more anterior ventricle, directly posterior to the sternum **Fig. 19**. In conditions of hypertrophy, it contacts the sternum anteriorly, producing a typical appearance on chest radiographs. In the normal heart, the RV wall is thin, measuring approximately 2 to 3 mm, and usually no more than 5 mm. It assumes a pyramidal

configuration, with the posterior and base being larger than the apex.[38] The ventricles can be thought of as a system with an inflow, a contractile portion, and an outflow.[39]

The tricuspid valve is markedly different than the mitral valve, possessing 3 leaflets (inferior, septal, and anterosuperior). One of the most characteristic features distinguishing it from the mitral valve is the connection of tendinous chords from the septal leaflet to the interventricular septum.[28,40] There are both medial and anterior papillary muscles supporting the tricuspid valve apparatus. The smaller, medial papillary muscle originates from the crista supraventricularis and the septomarginal trabeculations and is known as the muscle of Lancisi.[38] The anterior papillary muscle arises from the lateral third of the septomarginal trabeculations.

Morphologically, the RV apex is more trabeculated than the LV (**Table 1**). Furthermore, on pathologic specimens, the trabeculated crista supraventricularis extends from the tricuspid valve

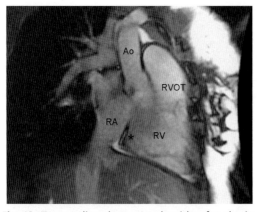

Fig. 18. True cardiac planes. An algorithm for obtaining true cardiac planes is shown. All true cardiac planes are double oblique to the body. Cine-segmented balanced SSFP RV inflow view is obtained perpendicular to the tricuspid valve prescription (not shown). Although less frequently performed, RV inflow or outflow views can be useful in assessing right ventricular or right heart valvular disorders. The right atrium (RA) is separated from the RV by the tricuspid valve, which can be difficult to visualize in normal cases. The tricuspid valve plane contains a normal amount of epicardial fat, which on this image causes India ink artifact, which allows tissue differentiation. This view is not optimized for the right ventricular outflow tract (RVOT), which requires a separate, in most cases parasagittal, view. Note the trabeculations of the RV, which distinguish the RV from the LV. Oblique view through the aortic root and ascending aorta (Ao) is noted.

apparatus to the level of the pulmonic valve.[28,36,40] The septal aspect of the crista supraventricularis breaks up to form the septomarginal trabeculations, which comprise the moderator band at the RV apex and the septal trabeculations. Functionally, the RV relies more heavily on longitudinal shortening than the LV (believed to be related to differences in the muscular composition of the ventricles), which can be assessed by the degree of excursion of the tricuspid valve.[40]

The RV outflow tract is also known as the infundibulum. It is supported by the crista supraventricularis, which extends from tricuspid valve to pulmonic valve, giving muscular separation between the 2 valves (unlike the aortic and mitral valves, which have fibrous continuity). The crista supraventricularis forms the posterior portion of the RVOT, whereas only a small portion of the anterior RVOT is truly muscular. Septoparietal trabeculations run along the anterior RVOT as well.[28,38,40,41]

Left Atrium

The function of the left atrium is to receive oxygenated blood from the lungs via the pulmonary veins and subsequently deliver it to the LV. The left atrium lies inferior to the carina, which can be displaced anterior to the esophagus and descending aorta in cases of left atrial enlargement.[2,28,36,37]

Embryologically, the left atrium is also derived from the sinus venosus and a primitive auricle.[28]

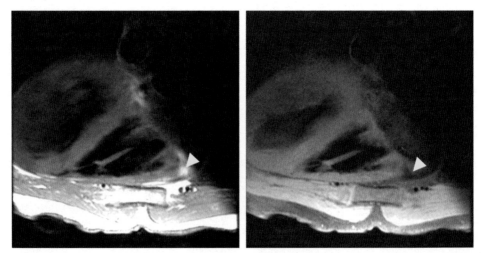

Fig. 19. Normal RV. Prone high-resolution (NEX = 4) T1 images obtained without (left) and with (right) fat suppression show normal tissue characteristics in the free wall of the right ventricle. There is normal fat in the right AV groove (arrowheads), confirmed by decreased signal on fat suppression. These images were obtained to evaluate for fibrofatty metaplasia, a finding which can indicate changes of arrhythmogenic right ventricular dysplasia (ARVD). Prone imaging is believed to lead to decreased respiratory variation, which is necessary when obtaining free breathing images to allow multiple excitations, as in these images. The diagnosis of ARVD cannot be made by MR imaging alone, and fatty infiltration of the free wall of the RV can also be seen in normal patients, or from other common causes such as prior myocardial infarction.

Table 1 Morphologic distinguishing features between LV and RV	
RV	**LV**
No fibrous continuity between tricuspid valve and pulmonic valve	Fibrous continuity between mitral and aortic valve
Trabeculated septum	No trabeculation along septum
Moderator band	No moderator band
Trabeculated and muscular outflow tract	Smooth outflow tract

Similar to the RA, the sinus venosus provides a smooth back wall to the atrium, but, unlike the RA, almost the entire atrial wall is baldly smooth.[36]

The left atrial appendage is derived from the primitive auricle. Although there is variability in its shape and position, it is a blind-ending structure that is often located superior to the left superior pulmonary vein.[42] It has a thin, pectinate muscle architecture, not as thick as the right atrial appendage, and is distinguished from the typically smooth left atrium. Unlike the right atrial appendage, the left atrial appendage does not usually drape over the atrium. The left atrial appendage typically lies above the atrioventricular groove and covers the proximal left circumflex coronary artery.

LV

In the normal heart, the function of the LV is to pump blood into the systemic circulation, and is typically a thick-walled chamber owing to this demand. In conventional anatomy, it is oriented posterior to the RV. The inferior margin of the LV is adjacent to the diaphragm. The lateral wall is located laterally on short-axis images but obliquely on conventional axial images. The medial wall shares its wall with the RV as part of the interventricular septum, and is therefore known as the septal wall. The anterior wall is opposite the inferior wall and forms the superior margin of the LV.[2,28,36,43]

The interventricular septum in the LV is smooth and free of any muscular or chordal attachments. The apex can contain fine trabeculations, but is distinguished in appearance by the coarse trabeculations seen in the RV.[40] Occasional thin intraventricular strands known as false tendons are seen in the apical LV, which are defined as

structures that traverse the LV without any connection to the valve leaflets.[44] There is no moderator band or septomarginal trabeculations in the LV.

The mitral valve has anterior and posterior leaflets that are positioned obliquely. The anterior valve leaflet shows fibrous continuity with the aortic valve, whereas the posterior valve leaflet is contiguous with the LV wall (**Fig. 20**). There are 2 papillary muscles that support the mitral valve apparatus: the anterolateral and the posteromedial (**Fig. 21**).[28] These can be thought of more as one being anterosuperior, and the other being inferomedial or inferoseptal. They attach to the left ventricular free wall, and do not attach to the ventricular septum. The papillary muscles subsequently spread into tendinous chords that attach to both mitral valve leaflets; therefore, each papillary muscle contributes function to both mitral valve leaflets. Owing to the obliquity of the mitral valve apparatus, the orifice-covering area is asymmetric with the posterior leaflet, contributing approximately two-thirds of the mitral valve area, whereas the anterior cusp provides continuity to one-third. There is a solitary zone of coaptation of the valves. It is important for the tendinous chords to support the valve leaflets equally to avoid prolapse of the valve leaflets.[40] The LVOT is much smaller than the RVOT, and located centrally within the heart. This difference is caused by the fibrous continuity of the mitral valve with the aortic valve. Portions of 2 of the 3 aortic valve

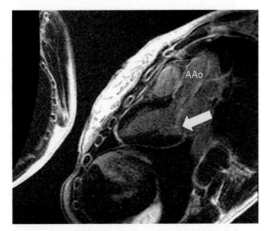

Fig. 20. Basic imaging options for the LV. Radial view of the LV double-inversion recovery with tailored inversion time (in a roughly 3-chamber or LV outflow tract view), show nulling of the healthy normal myocardium. Note late gadolinium enhancement of the fibrous mitral (*yellow arrow*) and aortic valves, which is a normal phenomenon. Note also that all long-axis views must bisect the LV apex and the mitral valve. AAo, ascending aorta.

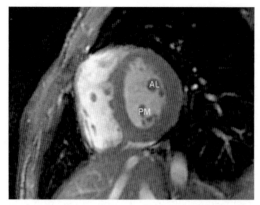

Fig. 21. Basic imaging options for the LV. Using segmented cine-balanced SSFP images, bright signal in the blood pool is obtained. Although fast, robust images can be easily obtained with or without cine functional imaging, the sequence is not normally used for tissue characterization because of the combined T1 and T2 properties of the images and resulting myocardial signal. In this short-axis view of the mid–left ventricular level, the anterolateral (AL) and posteromedial papillary muscles (PM) are readily identified.

leaflets have muscular attachments, whereas 2 of the 3 aortic valve leaflets have fibrous attachments.[28,40] The morphology of the LVOT creates a situation in which there can be dynamic obstruction at this level, as seen in cases such as hypertrophic cardiomyopathy. The ability of MR imaging to achieve true imaging planes can be clinically relevant in discerning the severity of dynamic outflow obstruction through the use of phase contrast imaging as well as planimetric imaging.

Interatrial Septum

The interatrial septum can be thought of as an invagination of the walls of the atria.[41] This is true of the superior and posterior rims as well as of much of the anterior rim. Therefore, the septum secundum is a meeting of the 2 atrial walls formed predominantly by the SVC entering the RA and the right pulmonary veins entering the left atrium. The fossa ovalis is a flap valve (remnant of the septum primum) that, along with the anteroinferior septum, forms the true atrial septum.[41] Typically, the high pressure in the left atrium after birth causes fusion of the interatrial septum, but, in approximately 20% to 30% of the population, the fusion is imperfect, resulting in a patent foramen

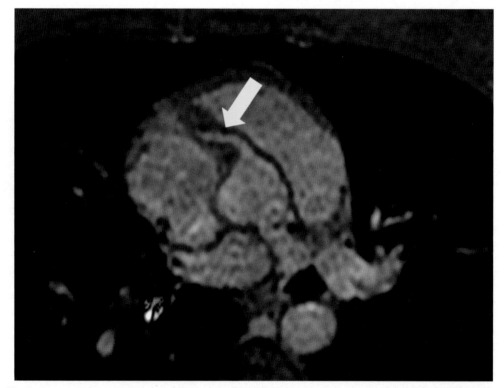

Fig. 22. Coronary artery anatomy. An oblique, breath-held, noncontrast, segmented, balanced SSFP obtained at high resolution shows normal ostium of the proximal RCA (*yellow arrow*). By obtaining an overlapping stack of images in a 3D acquisition, the tortuous coronary arteries can be visualized.

ovale.[45,46] The septum primum typically fuses with the endocardial cushions in fetal life, thus closing the fetal ostium primum. The ostium secundum is located superior to the septum primum and is typically sealed by growth of the septum secundum during fetal life.[47] Typically, a full interatrial septum can be seen on MR imaging; however, the thin fossa ovalis can occasionally appear as a communication between the atria, and this should not be interpreted incorrectly as a pathologic process.

There are muscular connections between the atrial walls, which allow conduction between them; however, these are not well visualized by MR. The most important of these is the Bachmann bundle, which originates at the crista terminalis.[48]

Coronary Arteries

The assessment of coronary arteries by MR has yet to gain widespread acceptance, although,

with advances in MR technology and sequences, this may become a reality in the foreseeable future.

The right coronary artery (RCA) arises from the right coronary cusp of the aorta (**Fig. 22**). It follows the right atrioventricular groove and typically gives off a conus branch and the sinoatrial nodal branch. The RCA gives off a variable number of acute marginal branches. In most individuals, the RCA gives rise to the posterior descending artery and posterior left ventricular branch, and is therefore the dominant coronary artery, supplying the inferior heart. The left coronary artery arises from the left coronary cusp and divides into the left anterior descending (LAD) coronary artery and the left circumflex (LCx) coronary artery. The LAD runs along the anterior interventricular septum and gives rise to multiple septal perforator branches as well as numerous diagonal branches. The LCx follows a course along the left atrioventricular groove and then a more posterior course, and gives off multiple obtuse marginal branches. It is

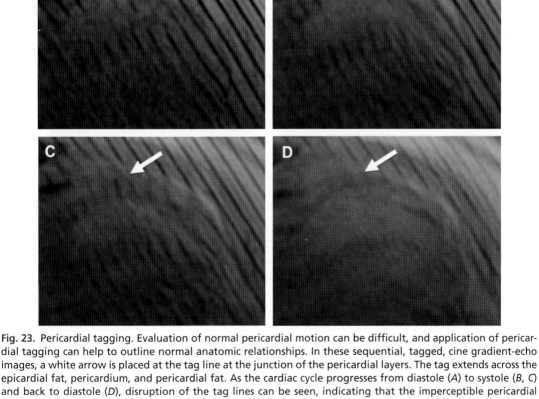

Fig. 23. Pericardial tagging. Evaluation of normal pericardial motion can be difficult, and application of pericardial tagging can help to outline normal anatomic relationships. In these sequential, tagged, cine gradient-echo images, a white arrow is placed at the tag line at the junction of the pericardial layers. The tag extends across the epicardial fat, pericardium, and pericardial fat. As the cardiac cycle progresses from diastole (A) to systole (B, C) and back to diastole (D), disruption of the tag lines can be seen, indicating that the imperceptible pericardial layers are sliding across one another. In cases of pericardial adhesions, the visceral and parietal layers do not slide past one another, and the tag lines maintain their form throughout the cardiac cycle. The layers of the pericardium are often difficult to identify unless they are pathologically thickened.

the dominant circulation in a small number of individuals.

According to the American Heart Association 17-segment model, the segments are given numbers in a counter-clockwise direction starting at the base (6 segments), the midmyocardium (6 segments), and the apex (4 segments), with segment 17 representing the apical tip.[49] Traditionally, it has been believed that segments 1, 2, 7, 8, 13, 14, and 17 are in the LAD territory; segments 3, 4, 9, 10, and 15 are in the RCA territory; and the remainder are in the LCx territory (segments 5, 6, 11, 12, and 16). Recent MR studies have shown that the coronary artery supply based on segments is variable.[50]

PERICARDIUM

The pericardium provides a sac in which the heart is contained. The heart in nondiseased states should be freely mobile within the pericardium.[37,51] The pericardium is typically imaged in the standard cardiac imaging planes already described. In disease states, the use of pericardial tag lines can be of value to delineate the restriction of motion of the heart within the pericardial sac (**Fig. 23**). Phase contrast imaging can also be of value to determine the present of mobile fluid versus stationary mass lesions of the pericardium in appropriate clinical settings.[37]

The pericardium consists of 2 layers, a serous or visceral pericardium, which is directly and inseparably attached to the epicardium, and a fibrous or parietal pericardium on the exterior.[52,53] The pericardial space is located between the 2 layers of pericardium and can contain a small amount of physiologic fluid. It can be difficult to distinguish adjacent epicardial fat and fluid within the pericardial space, and the tissue characterization abilities of MR can be useful in making this distinction.[53] The layer outside the fibrous pericardium contains the pericardial fat. The normal pericardium is typically less than 2 mm and has been found to be abnormal when greater than 4 mm.[37,54,55]

The pericardium contains the heart as well as the origin of the great vessels. It extends superiorly from the heart to form 2 tubelike structures, 1 of which invests the origin of the aorta and the pulmonary trunk, whereas the other invests the superior and inferior vena cava.[56] Superiorly, a transverse sinus connects these 2 tubes, into which there are several recesses that are normally filled with small amounts of pericardial fluid (**Fig. 24**). The superior pericardial recess forms a sleeve around the aorta (aortic recesses) and pulmonary (pulmonic recesses) trunks, but is typically best seen posterior to the ascending aorta.

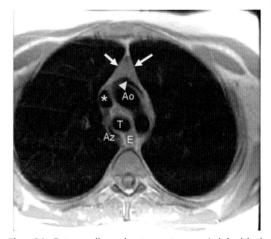

Fig. 24. Extracardiac chest anatomy. Axial, black blood, T1 image obtained in a young female patient shows normal pericardial recesses (*yellow arrowhead*), and a symmetric, sliplike normal thymus (*white arrows*). The aortic arch (Ao), SVC (*white asterisk*), azygous arch (Az), trachea (T), and esophagus (E) are labeled. Note that on spin-echo sequences, moving blood, moving fluid, and air all show signal voids, making knowledge of normal anatomy essential, especially on oblique images.

There is a smaller oblique recess within the pericardium, located adjacent to the left atrium, which gives rise to potential pulmonary vein recesses and caval recesses.[56] Knowledge of these recesses is helpful to avoid confusion with other pericardial space structures such as lymph nodes. The pericardium also contains nerves as well as veins, in addition to the coronary arteries that course in the epicardial fat.

SUMMARY

The soft tissue contrast properties of MR allow excellent discrimination of most intrathoracic structures other than the lungs, and allow good insight into normal anatomy. Using MR imaging, the normal cardiorespiratory system, including portions of the lungs and pleural spaces, as well as the mediastinal, chest wall, and cardiac structures in particular, can be well depicted. In addition, using newer MR pulse sequences, cinematic imaging can also be achieved, which allows a window into the normal functional processes of these organs.

REFERENCES

1. Kasprian G, Balassy C, Brugger PC, et al. MRI of normal and pathological fetal lung development. Eur J Radiol 2006;57:261–70.

2. Moore KL, Dalley AF. Clinically oriented anatomy. 5th edition. Baltimore (MD): Lippincott; 2005.

3. Kauczor HU, Kreitner KF. Contrast-enhanced MRI of the lung. Eur J Radiol 2000;34:196–207.

4. McLoud TC, Flower CD. Imaging the pleura: sonography, CT, and MR imaging. AJR Am J Roentgenol 1991;156:1145–53.

5. McLoud TC. CT and MR in pleural disease. Clin Chest Med 1998;19:261–76.

6. Lennon EA, Simon G. The height of the diaphragm in the chest radiograph of normal adults. Br J Radiol 1965;38:937–43.

7. Roberts HC. Imaging the diaphragm. Thorac Surg Clin 2009;19:431–50, v.

8. Taylor AM, Jhooti P, Wiesmann F, et al. MR navigator-echo monitoring of temporal changes in diaphragm position: implications for MR coronary angiography. J Magn Reson Imaging 1997;7:629–36.

9. Fortier M, Mayo JR, Swensen SJ, et al. MR imaging of chest wall lesions. Radiographics 1994;14:597–606.

10. Moore AV, Korobkin M, Olanow W, et al. Age-related changes in the thymus gland: CT-pathologic correlation. AJR Am J Roentgenol 1983;141:241–6.

11. de Geer G, Webb WR, Gamsu G. Normal thymus: assessment with MR and CT. Radiology 1986;158:313–7.

12. Felson B. The mediastinum. Semin Roentgenol 1969;4:41–58.

13. Curcic J, Fox M, Kaufman E, et al. Gastroesophageal junction: structure and function as assessed by using MR imaging. Radiology 2010;257:115–24.

14. Manabe T, Kawamitsu H, Higashino T, et al. Observation of gastro-esophageal reflux by MRI: a feasibility study. Abdom Imaging 2009;34:419–23.

15. Kulinna-Cosentini C, Schima W, Cosentini EP. Dynamic MR imaging of the gastroesophageal junction in healthy volunteers during bolus passage. J Magn Reson Imaging 2007;25:749–54.

16. Meng J, Peters DC, Hsing JM, et al. Late gadolinium enhancement of the esophagus is common on cardiac MR several months after pulmonary vein isolation: preliminary observations. Pacing Clin Electrophysiol 2010;33:661–6.

17. Faust RA, Remley KB, Rimell FL. Real-time, cine magnetic resonance imaging for evaluation of the pediatric airway. Laryngoscope 2001;111:2187–90.

18. Faust RA, Rimell FL, Remley KB. Cine magnetic resonance imaging for evaluation of focal tracheomalacia: innominate artery compression syndrome. Int J Pediatr Otorhinolaryngol 2002;65:27–33.

19. Hofmann U, Hofmann D, Vogl T, et al. Magnetic resonance imaging as a new diagnostic criterion in paediatric airway obstruction. Prog Pediatr Surg 1991;27:221–30.

20. Mountain CF, Dresler CM. Regional lymph node classification for lung cancer staging. Chest 1997; 111:1718–23.

21. Hasegawa I, Boiselle PM, Kuwabara K, et al. Mediastinal lymph nodes in patients with non-small cell lung cancer: preliminary experience with diffusion-weighted MR imaging. J Thorac Imaging 2008;23: 157–61.

22. Nakayama J, Miyasaka K, Omatsu T, et al. Metastases in mediastinal and hilar lymph nodes in patients with non-small cell lung cancer: quantitative assessment with diffusion-weighted magnetic resonance imaging and apparent diffusion coefficient. J Comput Assist Tomogr 2010;34:1–8.

23. Natsis KI, Tsitouridis IA, Didagelos MV, et al. Anatomical variations in the branches of the human aortic arch in 633 angiographies: clinical significance and literature review. Surg Radiol Anat 2009;31:319–23.

24. Lin FY, Devereux RB, Roman MJ, et al. Assessment of the thoracic aorta by multidetector computed tomography: age- and sex-specific reference values in adults without evident cardiovascular disease. J Cardiovasc Comput Tomogr 2008;2:298–308.

25. Burman ED, Keegan J, Kilner PJ. Aortic root measurement by cardiovascular magnetic resonance: specification of planes and lines of measurement and corresponding normal values. Circ Cardiovasc Imaging 2008;1:104–13.

26. Vasan RS, Larson MG, Benjamin EJ, et al. Echocardiographic reference values for aortic root size: the Framingham Heart Study. J Am Soc Echocardiogr 1995;8:793–800.

27. Davies RR, Gallo A, Coady MA, et al. Novel measurement of relative aortic size predicts rupture of thoracic aortic aneurysms. Ann Thorac Surg 2006;81:169–77.

28. Bogaert J, Dymarkowski S, Taylor AM. Clinical cardiac MR. Medform (MA): Springer; 2005.

29. Lin FY, Devereux RB, Roman MJ, et al. The right sided great vessels by cardiac multidetector computed tomography: normative reference values among healthy adults free of cardiopulmonary disease, hypertension, and obesity. Acad Radiol 2009;16:981–7.

30. Mansour M, Holmvang G, Sosnovik D, et al. Assessment of pulmonary vein anatomic variability by magnetic resonance imaging: implications for catheter ablation techniques for atrial fibrillation. J Cardiovasc Electrophysiol 2004;15:387–93.

31. Scharf C, Sneider M, Case I, et al. Anatomy of the pulmonary veins in patients with atrial fibrillation and effects of segmental ostial ablation analyzed by computed tomography. J Cardiovasc Electrophysiol 2003;14:150–5.

32. Lickfett L, Kato R, Tandri H, et al. Characterization of a new pulmonary vein variant using magnetic resonance angiography: incidence, imaging, and interventional implications of the "right top pulmonary vein". J Cardiovasc Electrophysiol 2004;15:538–43.

33. Kato R, Lickfett L, Meininger G, et al. Pulmonary vein anatomy in patients undergoing catheter ablation of atrial fibrillation: lessons learned by use of magnetic resonance imaging. Circulation 2003;107:2004–10.

34. Kaseno K, Tada H, Koyama K, et al. Prevalence and characterization of pulmonary vein variants in patients with atrial fibrillation determined using 3-dimensional computed tomography. Am J Cardiol 2008;101:1638–42.

35. Lee V. Cardiovascular MRI: physical principles to practical protocols. Baltimore (MD): Lippincott; 2005.

36. Kwong R. Cardiovascular magnetic resonance imaging. Totowa (NJ): Humana Press; 2007.

37. Miller S. Cardiac imaging: the requisites. Maryland Heights (MO): Mosby; 2004.

38. Boxt LM. Radiology of the right ventricle. Radiol Clin North Am 1999;37:379–400.

39. Anderson RH, Ho SY. What is a ventricle? Ann Thorac Surg 1998;66:616–20.

40. Anderson RH, Razavi R, Taylor AM. Cardiac anatomy revisited. J Anat 2004;205:159–77.

41. Anderson RH, Cook AC. The structure and components of the atrial chambers. Europace 2007; 9(Suppl 6):vi3–9.

42. Ramaswamy P, Lytrivi ID, Srivastava S, et al. Left atrial appendage: variations in morphology and position causing pitfalls in pediatric echocardiographic diagnosis. J Am Soc Echocardiogr 2007; 20:1011–6.

43. Partridge JB, Anderson RH. Left ventricular anatomy: its nomenclature, segmentation, and planes of imaging. Clin Anat 2009;22:77–84.

44. Bhatt MR, Alfonso CE, Bhatt AM, et al. Effects and mechanisms of left ventricular false tendons on functional mitral regurgitation in patients with severe cardiomyopathy. J Thorac Cardiovasc Surg 2009; 138:1123–8.

45. Hagen PT, Scholz DG, Edwards WD. Incidence and size of patent foramen ovale during the first 10 decades of life: an autopsy study of 965 normal hearts. Mayo Clin Proc 1984;59:17–20.

46. Krasuski RA, Hart SA, Allen D, et al. Prevalence and repair of intraoperatively diagnosed patent foramen ovale and association with perioperative outcomes and long-term survival. JAMA 2009;302: 290–7.

47. Anderson RH, Brown NA, Webb S. Development and structure of the atrial septum. Heart 2002;88: 104–10.

48. Khaja A, Flaker G. Bachmann's bundle: does it play a role in atrial fibrillation? Pacing Clin Electrophysiol 2005;28:855–63.

49. Cerqueira MD, Weissman NJ, Dilsizian V, et al. Standardized myocardial segmentation and nomenclature for tomographic imaging of the heart: a statement for healthcare professionals from the Cardiac Imaging Committee of the Council on Clinical Cardiology of the American Heart Association. Circulation 2002;105:539–42.

50. Ortiz-Pérez JT, Rodríguez J, Meyers SN, et al. Correspondence between the 17-segment model and coronary arterial anatomy using contrast-enhanced cardiac magnetic resonance imaging. JACC Cardiovasc Imaging 2008;1:282–93.

51. Masui T, Finck S, Higgins CB. Constrictive pericarditis and restrictive cardiomyopathy: evaluation with MR imaging. Radiology 1992;182:369–73.

52. Misselt AJ, Harris SR, Glockner J, et al. MR imaging of the pericardium. Magn Reson Imaging Clin N Am 2008;16:185–99, vii.

53. Sechtem U, Tscholakoff D, Higgins CB. MRI of the abnormal pericardium. AJR Am J Roentgenol 1986;147:245–52.

54. Soulen RL, Stark DD, Higgins CB. Magnetic resonance imaging of constrictive pericardial disease. Am J Cardiol 1985;55:480–4.

55. Smith WH, Beacock DJ, Goddard AJ, et al. Magnetic resonance evaluation of the pericardium. Br J Radiol 2001;74:384–92.

56. Rienmüller R, Gröll R, Lipton MJ. CT and MR imaging of pericardial disease. Radiol Clin North Am 2004; 42:587–601, vi.

Breast MR Imaging: Normal Anatomy

Sara C. Gavenonis, MD

KEYWORDS

- Breast MR imaging • Normal anatomy
- Structural anatomy • Functional anatomy

Breast cancer is one of the most common cancers in American women, with the American Cancer Society estimating more than 200,000 women being newly diagnosed with breast cancer in 2010.[1] As an adjunct to mammography, breast magnetic resonance (MR) imaging has emerged as a powerful and useful tool in the detection and evaluation of breast cancer. Dynamic contrast-enhanced breast MR has sensitivities reported as approaching 100% for invasive breast cancer.[2–4] Given this sensitivity, breast MR imaging is increasingly being used in both screening and diagnostic breast imaging applications. In 2007, the American Cancer Society published guidelines for the application of screening breast MR imaging in women with an elevated risk of breast cancer, either by family history–based calculation or because of prior medical history.[5] The use of breast MR imaging in specific diagnostic scenarios such as evaluating the extent of disease in a patient with breast cancer has also been studied.[6–11] As the applications of breast MR imaging increase and are refined, an understanding of the normal anatomy of the breast on MR imaging and the basic rationale behind the imaging of this structure is invaluable. Only with a strong foundation of knowledge of the "normal" can pathology be recognized appropriately.

The goals of this article are as follows:

1. Review a basic protocol for breast MR imaging
2. Review normal structural anatomy of the breast
3. Review expected range of normal functional anatomy of the breast, as seen on dynamic contrast-enhanced images of the breast.

PROTOCOL: TECHNICAL CONSIDERATIONS

Breast MR imaging has the ability to depict both structural and functional anatomy of the breast. Breast MR imaging protocol uses a multiplanar imaging approach as well as the use of intravenous gadolinium to achieve the goals of anatomic depiction. This discussion focuses on the protocol currently used at the Hospital of the University of Pennsylvania (HUP), with reference to general principles of breast MR imaging techniques.

At present, the standard clinical protocol for breast MR imaging at this institution is acquired with a 1.5-T magnet with a dedicated bilateral breast coil. A minimum field strength of 1.5 T is recommended for optimal breast MR imaging. It is important that there is good magnetic field homogeneity across both breasts, to allow for optimal in-plane image resolution and signal to noise ratio per pixel. Also, this allows for optimal fat suppression across both breasts.

The importance of patient positioning should be emphasized. For breast MR imaging, the patient is positioned prone with the breasts pendant. It is essential that the technologist positioning the patient is aware of the pitfalls sometimes associated with use of the breast coil and prone positioning. For example, lateral and axillary breast tissue is often excluded from the coil, and this is sometimes only apparent during localizer sequences (**Fig. 1**). This situation can lead to nonvisualization or suboptimal evaluation of the excluded portions of the breast. Such malpositioning may limit the visualization of not only the structural anatomy of those portions of the breast(s). It

Funding: Not applicable.

The author has nothing to disclose.

Breast Imaging, Department of Radiology, Hospital of the University of Pennsylvania, 1 Silverstein, 3400 Spruce Street, Philadelphia, PA 19104, USA

E-mail address: Sara.Gavenonis@uphs.upenn.edu

Magn Reson Imaging Clin N Am 19 (2011) 507–519

doi:10.1016/j.mric.2011.05.009

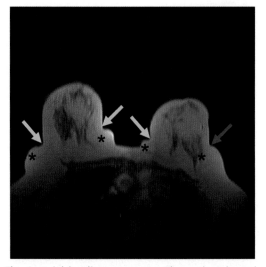

Fig. 1. Axial localizer sequence. The patient is positioned prone, with the breasts pendant in the dedicated breast coil. Asterisks indicate tissue that is not fully within the chambers of the coil. Stepoffs of tissue between breast within and outside of the chamber are seen (*blue arrows*), created by the patient's weight on the breast. On the left side, breast parenchyma is in the region of this stepoff (*red arrow*), and the weight on this portion could theoretically obscure structural anatomy as well as have an effect on the vascular enhancement of this region (thereby affecting the functional anatomy). Ideally, this patient should be repositioned.

must be noted that the pressure from the patient's weight on the portions of the breast excluded from the coil also alters the vascular flow dynamics of those areas. Thus, the functional anatomy of those portions of the breast is also not optimally evaluated, which can lead to false-negative results (**Fig. 2**).

Positioning is also of paramount importance during MR imaging–guided breast interventional procedures. Although this topic is beyond the scope of this article, it is important to be aware of the impact of positioning on the potential success of any MR imaging–guided breast procedure. Consideration should be given to physical access to the target site and to the impact of altering the enhancement dynamics to the target site during such procedures.

The patient's arms are variably positioned either above the head or at the sides, depending on patient mobility, patient comfort, and ability to image or access the target region of the breast. The patient's peripheral intravenous access is connected to the injector before imaging, to minimize any subsequent patient motion.

Localizer sequences are first performed (**Table 1**). In addition, patient positioning can also be assessed

on localizer sequences. If necessary, the patient should be repositioned (see **Fig. 1**; **Fig. 3**).

At the author's institution, sagittal plane imaging is performed for all precontrast series and dynamic enhanced series. A delayed axial postcontrast series is also obtained for multiplanar reference purposes, as well as for delayed enhancement information. The ability to cross-reference between planes is useful in establishing the 3-dimensional characteristics of any finding. Sagittal image acquisition is chosen at HUP to maximize the in-plane spatial resolution of the images, thus optimizing morphologic assessment of any findings. Axial dynamic image acquisition is an alternative option, and can provide excellent temporal resolution (fewer total slices to image both breasts) and also provides the ability to compare symmetry on the same image. There are pros and cons to each approach; one compromise solution is to obtain dynamic enhanced series with isotropic voxels, so that reconstruction in the imaging plane of choice can occur with postprocessing. The essence of any breast MR imaging technique with regard to imaging plane is to ensure there is some capability of multiplanar assessment and cross-referencing, so that any enhancement can be properly assessed in terms of 3-dimensional morphology.

The phase-encoding direction is chosen to minimize artifact from cardiac pulsation. This direction will vary based on the chosen imaging plane. For example, the phase-encoding direction will be craniocaudal in the sagittal imaging plane and transverse in the axial imaging plane. Although in the axial plane this results in some cardiac pulsation artifact in the axillary regions, it is preferable to obscuring the medial portions of the breasts (which is what would occur if the phase-encoding direction were chosen in the orthogonal axis).

After localizer sequences, at HUP a sagittal T2-weighted turbo spin-echo sequence is acquired (see **Table 1**) with fat saturation (**Fig. 4**). The T2 signal intensity of an MR imaging finding has been reported to be useful as an adjunct to morphology and kinetic information.[12] Although there are many benign MR imaging findings that have increased T2 signal, such as cysts and fibroadenomas,[12] it is important to remember that malignant lesions can also have increased T2 signal. One study reported that 30 of 480 cancers displayed increased T2 signal relative to surrounding parenchyma on fat-suppressed T2-weighted imaging.[13] Increased T2 signal intensity of a finding can thus support a benign assessment if morphology and enhancement is otherwise also benign, but the increased T2 signal intensity of a lesion should not trump suspicious morphology or enhancement kinetics.

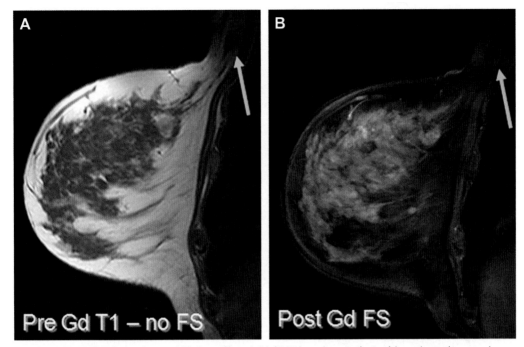

Fig. 2. Altered vascular dynamics: positioning effect. Initial MR imaging study. In this patient, the superior aspect of the breast parenchyma is not fully included in the coil, and the patient's weight is on this excluded tissue. There is a lesion (*blue arrow*) in this excluded tissue, which does not demonstrate enhancement on this MR imaging study. (*A*) Sagittal T1-weighted image, no fat saturation (FS), pre-gadolinium (Gd) contrast. (*B*) Sagittal T1-weighted image, with fat saturation, post contrast (second time point is representatively shown). On a subsequent MR imaging study, obtained with more optimal positioning, the indicated lesion demonstrated suspicious morphology and enhancement. Subsequent biopsy demonstrated invasive ductal carcinoma. In this figure, the positioning of the patient resulted in altered vascular dynamics of the suspicious lesion, as the lesion was excluded from the coil and the patient's weight was on this tissue. This case highlights the importance of positioning of the patient and its effect on vascular dynamics.

Subsequently, a sagittal T1-weighted series without fat saturation is obtained (see **Table 1**) (**Figs. 5** and **6**). This series provides a useful overview of the architecture and fibroglandular tissue distribution of the breast. When used in conjunction with the subsequent fat-suppressed T1-weighted series, this series is also useful in assessing the fat content of any structure, which becomes especially useful in the characterization of fat necrosis or lymph nodes (**Fig. 7**).

A sagittal T1-weighted series with fat saturation is then obtained (see **Table 1**) (**Fig. 8**). This series highlights any areas of intrinsic T1 high intensity that are not fat. For example, material in proteinaceous cysts and areas of hemorrhage are identified. This series also serves as the baseline mask for subtraction after the postcontrast series are obtained. Although theoretically fat saturation is not essential for obtaining information from subtraction series, such an approach also assumes there is no patient motion. If there are areas of intrinsic T1 hyperintensity and there is patient motion during the dynamic series

acquisition, false-positive areas can be seen on the subtraction series. Therefore, to minimize the potential effects of even small amounts of patient motion on the diagnostic quality of the subtraction series, fat saturation is used for this portion of the breast MR imaging examination at the author's institution. In addition, the use of fat saturation optimizes the dynamic range of the image, making any true enhancement more conspicuous on the postcontrast source images.

Intravenous injection of gadolinium contrast agent is then administered with a power injector (2 mL/s), followed by a 20-mL saline flush. At HUP, MultiHance (gadobenate dimeglumine) 529 mg/mL (Bracco Diagnostics, Princeton, NJ, USA) is used, dosed based on the patient's weight, for a dose of 0.1 mmol/kg. Consideration to recent renal function laboratory tests is also given, as patients with impaired renal function may not clear the gadolinium dose optimally and thus be more susceptible to nephrogenic systemic fibrosis. Renal function is assessed by glomerular filtration rate (GFR), with a full dose given for a GFR greater

Table 1
Breast MR imaging protocol at the author's institution (1.5 T)

Parameter	Imaging Series				
	Multiplanar Localizer	Sagittal T2-Weighted	Sagittal T1-Weighted GRE	Sagittal T1-Weighted GRE (pre- and 3 postcontrast series at 90-s intervals)	Axial T1-Weighted GRE
Concatenations	—	2	2	1	1
TR (ms)	20.0	6530	9.76	14.6	8.13
TE (ms)	5.00	86	4.76	3.61	3.83
Fat saturation	No	Yes	No	Yes	Yes
Flip angle	40	180	20	30	15
Field of view (mm)	400	240	240	240	320
Matrix	256	256 × 256	512 × 512	512 × 512	512 × 512
No. of sections	1 each plane	58	88	88	160
Slice thickness (mm)	10.0	3	2.9	2.9	1.5
Voxel size (mm)	3.1 × 1.6 × 10.0	1.3 × 0.9 × 3.0	0.7 × 0.5 × 2.9	0.7 × 0.5 × 2.9	0.9 × 0.6 × 1.5
Bandwidth (Hz/pixel)	180	129	180	280	200
Relative SNR	1.00	1.00	1.00	1.00	1.00
Imaging time (min:s)	0:12	3:57	1:37	1:24 (×4)	1:42

Subtraction images generated using precontrast series as a mask (3 sets of sagittal subtraction series generated).
Abbreviations: GRE, gradient recalled echo; SNR, signal to noise ratio; TE, echo time; TR, repetition time.

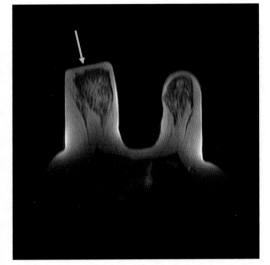

Fig. 3. Axial localizer sequence. The patient is positioned prone, with the breasts pendant in the dedicated breast coil. With larger breast sizes, the anterior portions of the breast may abut the inferior aspect of the coil chamber (*arrow*).

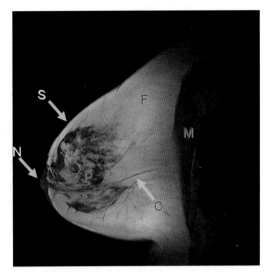

Fig. 5. Sagittal T1-weighted image without fat saturation. Adipose tissue is of high signal intensity, and breast fibroglandular elements appear relatively intermediate to dark. Representative structures are indicated. N, nipple; S, skin; V, vessels; F, fat; P, breast parenchyma (fibroglandular tissue); C, Cooper's ligament; M, pectoralis muscles.

than 45 mL/min/1.73 m^2 and a half dose given for GFR between 30 and 45 mL/min/1.73 m^2. GFR less than 30 mL/min/1.73 m^2 is considered the threshold at HUP as a contraindication for gadolinium administration. Thus, dynamic contrast-enhanced breast MR imaging cannot be performed in patients with GFR in that range. These rules are based on Food and Drug Administration guidelines, which can be viewed at the Web site (http://www.fda.gov).

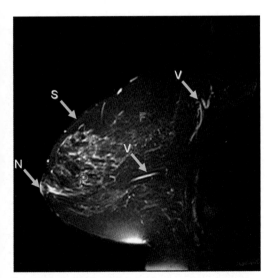

Fig. 4. Sagittal T2-weighted image with fat saturation. Fat appears dark while breast parenchyma appears intermediate to bright. Representative structures are indicated. N, nipple; S, skin; V, vessels; F, fat; P, breast parenchyma (fibroglandular tissue).

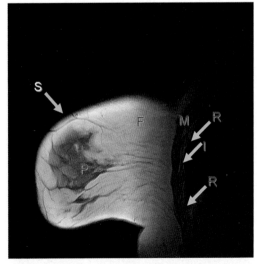

Fig. 6. Sagittal T1-weighted image without fat saturation, in a different case. This representative slice is more medial than the image in Fig. 5 (note the ribs are viewed more in cross section). S, skin; F, fat; P, breast parenchyma (fibroglandular tissue); M, pectoralis muscles; R, ribs; I, intercostal muscles.

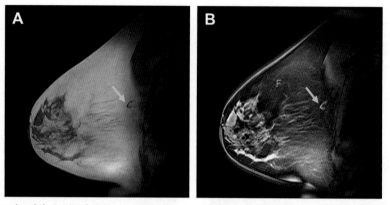

Fig. 7. Lymph node. (*A*) Sagittal T1-weighted image, no fat saturation. A crescentic structure with a T1-hyperintense central hilum is seen (*arrow*). On this image without fat saturation, the fatty hilum of the lymph node is hyperintense, and the relative signal intensity of the cortex is lower. (*B*) Sagittal T1-weighted image, with fat saturation, no contrast. The signal from the fatty hilum of the lymph node is nulled, as is fat elsewhere in the breast. On this image with fat saturation, the relative signal intensity of the cortex to the hilum is higher. Also, the relative signal intensity of fibroglandular elements then becomes intermediate to bright, given that the fat appears dark. F, fat; P, breast parenchyma (fibroglandular tissue).

Dynamic postcontrast T1-weighted series with fat saturation are then obtained in the sagittal plane, with 3 series obtained at 90-second intervals (see **Table 1**) (**Fig. 9**). This timing is based on studies indicating that optimal temporal resolution is achieved when imaging occurs at 60- to 120-second intervals after gadolinium injection.[4,14–16]

An axial delayed T1-weighted series with fat saturation is then obtained (see **Table 1**) (**Fig. 10**). This series permits a larger field of view to visualize

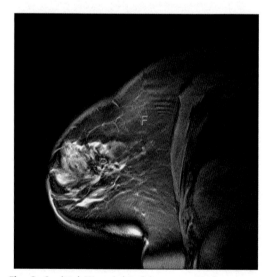

Fig. 8. Sagittal T1-weighted image, with fat saturation. The relative signal intensity of fibroglandular elements is intermediate to bright, given that the fat appears dark (fat signal is nulled). F, fat; P, breast parenchyma (fibroglandular tissue).

the axillary, pectoral, and intramammary regions, which are important in evaluating for lymphadenopathy in cases of breast cancer. However, many extramammary structures are also visualized, though not optimally. It is important to assess these structures as well: for example, the heart, liver, and chest wall musculoskeletal structures, and the anterior lung fields (see **Fig. 10**).

Subtraction images are generated using the combination of the dynamic postcontrast sagittal series and "subtracting" the baseline mask of the precontrast sagittal T1-weighted series with fat saturation (**Figs. 11** and **12**). These images are often viewed as linked series so that the temporal characteristics of the enhancement can be best appreciated.

It can be helpful to use both the source precontrast and postcontrast images in addition to the subtraction images in the interpretation of breast MR imaging, as an important pitfall to avoid is the absence of intravenous (IV) gadolinium. This situation could occur secondary to a failure in the IV line, a leak, or a contrast extravasation not immediately detected. When no gadolinium is actually administered IV but image acquisition continues, there can be the appearance of minimal background enhancement in the breast, but there will also be no enhancement in the great vessels and no contrast in the heart. It is important to avoid this pitfall by assessing the expected locations of contrast in the great vessels and heart, to ensure that contrast has been administered appropriately (see **Fig. 9**C). Otherwise, the study would be deemed nondiagnostic.

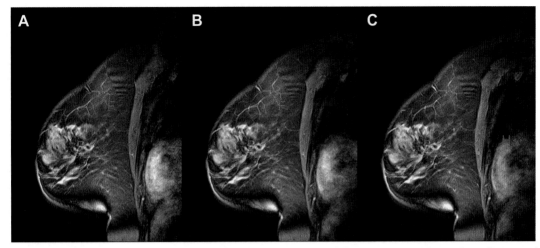

Fig. 9. (A) Sagittal T1-weighted image, with fat saturation, post gadolinium contrast, time point 1 (90 seconds after contrast injection). F, fat; P, breast parenchyma (fibroglandular tissue). (B) Sagittal T1-weighted image, with fat saturation, post gadolinium contrast, time point 2 (180 seconds after contrast injection). F, fat; P, breast parenchyma (fibroglandular tissue). (C) Sagittal T1-weighted image, with fat saturation, post gadolinium contrast, time point 3 (270 seconds after contrast injection). Note the subtle but observable change in contrast in the heart as the time points progress and circulation of contrast agent occurs (H). F, fat; P, breast parenchyma (fibroglandular tissue); H, heart.

NORMAL ANATOMY
Structural Normal Anatomy

In gross anatomic terms, the perimeter of the adult breast is skin at the anterior, medial, and inferior aspects. Posteriorly, the chest wall is the boundary of the breast (pectoralis major and pectoralis minor with associated fascia, ribs, and intercostal muscles) (see **Figs. 4–6**). At the upper outer boundary, breast tissue variably extends into the axilla. Blood vessels are present within the breast and the axilla (see **Figs. 10** and **12**). Lymph nodes are routinely present in the axillary region (see **Figs. 7** and **10B**), and occasionally also within the breast. A normal intramammary lymph node will have the same morphology and MR imaging signal characteristics as lymph nodes elsewhere, generally including an overall crescentic shape and a fatty hilum (see **Fig. 7**).

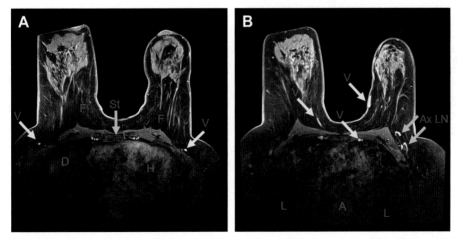

Fig. 10. (A) Axial T1-weighted image, with fat saturation, post gadolinium contrast, delayed time point (approximately 2 minutes after last subtraction image). F, fat; P, breast parenchyma (fibroglandular tissue); M, pectoralis muscles; St, sternum; D, hepatic dome; H, heart; V, vessel, axillary. (B) Axial T1-weighted image, with fat saturation, post gadolinium contrast, delayed time point (approximately 2 minutes after last subtraction image), more superior slice than that shown in a. Ax LN and blue arrows, axillary lymph nodes; V and yellow arrows, vessels, internal mammary; H, heart; L, lung; A, aorta.

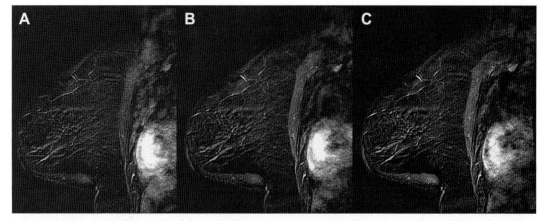

Fig. 11. Sagittal subtraction series. (*A*) Subtraction 1 = Postcontrast time point 1−Precontrast = (9A−8). (*B*) Subtraction 2 = Postcontrast time point 2−Precontrast = (9B−8). (*C*) Subtraction 3 = Postcontrast time point 2−Precontrast = (9C−8).

The mature female breast has glandular components (ducts and lobules), fibrous supporting elements (Cooper's ligaments), and surrounding adipose tissue (see **Figs. 4–6**). The fibroglandular elements of the breast are organized into segments, with approximately 10 to 20 segments

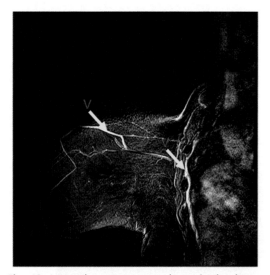

Fig. 12. Internal mammary vessels, sagittal subtraction series. A representative image from a second time-point subtraction series is shown to demonstrate the prominence of the internal mammary vessels on these images (V). Given that branches of the internal mammary vessels can sometimes take a tortuous intramammary course, a pitfall to avoid when viewing a single image in a single plane is mistaking the appearance of a vessel en face (or seen obliquely) as a discrete lesion. Cross-referencing between axial (**Fig. 10B**) and sagittal planes, and scrolling through sequential slices can clarify the finding as vascular, thus avoiding this pitfall.

in each breast. Each segment is arrayed about a major lactiferous duct. The major ducts form from tributaries within each segment called ductules, each of which has associated lobules. A terminal ductule with its associated lobules is termed a terminal ductule-lobular unit or TDLU. The TDLU is the site where many breast cancers arise.[17]

Normal anatomic components of the breast can be visualized and distinguished on MR imaging by assessing signal intensity. On T1-weighted imaging without fat saturation, adipose tissue is of high signal intensity and breast fibroglandular elements appear relatively intermediate to dark (see **Figs. 5** and **6**). The presence of fat can be confirmed by assessing the same region on T1-weighted images with fat saturation, where adipose signal would be expected to be nulled (see **Fig. 7**). In T1-weighted images with fat saturation, the relative signal intensity of fibroglandular elements then becomes intermediate to bright, given that the fat appears dark (see **Fig. 7B**). Similarly, on T2-weighted series with fat saturation, fat appears dark while breast parenchyma appears intermediate to bright (see **Fig. 4**).

On T1-weighted fat saturated images, intrinsically T1-hyperintense material such as proteinaceous fluid in ducts is highlighted. Moreover, on T2-weighted fat saturated images intrinsically T2-hyperintense material or lesions, such as fibroadenomas or simple cysts, are accentuated.

Functional Normal Anatomy

There is wide variation of normality in fibroglandular composition of the breast, and in mammography the breast density percentage is classified and reported as per BI-RADS (Breast Imaging

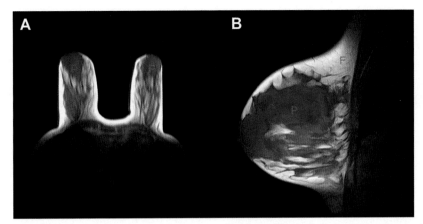

Fig. 13. Minimal background enhancement. Precontrast images without fat saturation demonstrate a large amount of fibroglandular tissue. (*A*) Axial localizer. P, breast parenchyma (fibroglandular tissue). (*B*) Sagittal T1-weighted image, no fat saturation. F, fat; P, breast parenchyma (fibroglandular tissue).

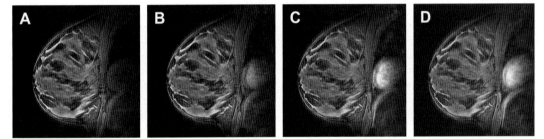

Fig. 14. Minimal background enhancement. Sagittal source images, T1-weighted with fat saturation, demonstrate minimal background enhancement of the breast parenchyma. Fat appears dark, and breast parenchyma (fibroglandular tissue) appears as intermediate to bright signal. (*A*) Precontrast. (*B*) Postcontrast time point 1 (90 seconds after injection). (*C*) Postcontrast time point 2 (180 seconds after injection). (*D*) Postcontrast time point 3 (270 seconds after injection).

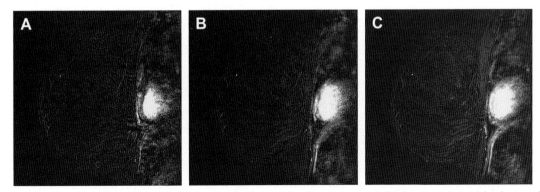

Fig. 15. Minimal background enhancement. Sagittal subtraction images highlight the minimal background enhancement of the breast parenchyma. (*A*) Subtraction 1 = 14B−14A. (*B*) Subtraction 2 = 14C−14A. (*C*) Subtraction 3 = 14D−14A.

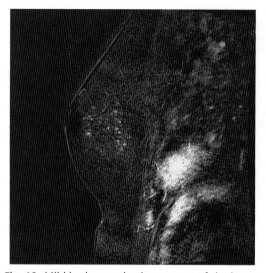

Fig. 16. Mild background enhancement of the breast parenchyma is demonstrated on this representative sagittal subtraction image (representative third time point).

Reporting and Data System).[18] It must be noted that there is also a variable functional anatomy of the fibroglandular tissue, which manifests as enhancement on postcontrast images. This component of the enhancement pattern is termed background enhancement, and has been classified as none/minimal, mild, moderate, and marked.[19]

It is of paramount importance to note the distinction between fibroglandular density and background enhancement. For example, depending on the hormonal status of the patient or other factors such as prior radiation treatment, a breast that appears extremely dense on mammography can theoretically have minimal to mild background enhancement (**Figs. 13–15**). Also, depending on the context, a patient can have marked background enhancement that is normal physiologic enhancement. Correlation with the clinical context and the patient's menstrual cycle is important in the interpretation of these studies.

Examples of background parenchymal enhancement can be seen in **Figs. 16–19**.

Background enhancement varies not only between individuals (see **Figs. 17** and **18**) but can also vary as a function of when a patient is imaged during her menstrual cycle.[20] Having the background enhancement of both breasts is useful for comparison of symmetry. Bilateral studies may raise the theoretical potential for false positives in the breast contralateral to the one of interest, but the potential benefit of being able to compare breast background enhancement is often invaluable. Thus the author prefers to obtain bilateral studies as per routine at HUP, rather than unilateral studies.

Enhancement Kinetics

At HUP, dynamic postcontrast images are obtained at 90-second intervals for 3 time points after injection (see **Fig. 9**). This action permits the evaluation of the enhancement kinetics of any focal findings.

Initial enhancement can be assessed by comparing the precontrast and the first postcontrast series, and is described as rapid, intermediate, or slow.[21–23] Lesions that have relatively higher vascularity (for example, malignant lesions with associated neoangiogenesis) would be expected to have a rapid rate of initial enhancement. The second and third postcontrast series can be used to assess if the pattern of enhancement is gradually increasing (Type 1, persistent), stabilizing (Type 2, plateau), or decreasing (Type 3,

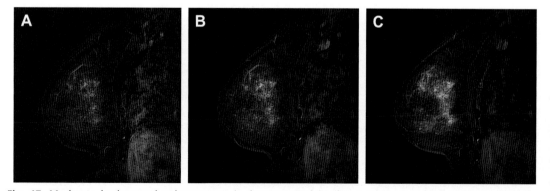

Fig. 17. Moderate background enhancement is demonstrated in this patient, on serial sagittal subtraction images. Note that the enhancement pattern is persistent, and the background enhancement has a relatively confluent appearance globally. (*A*) Subtraction 1. (*B*) Subtraction 2. (*C*) Subtraction 3.

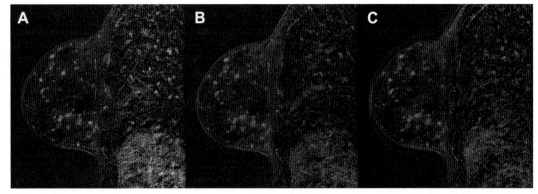

Fig. 18. Moderate background enhancement, in a different patient to the one shown in **Fig. 17**. This patient had multiple prior MR imaging examinations, and this pattern of enhancement had been stable compared with prior studies. Note that while the background enhancement is still classified as "moderate," the morphology of the background enhancement is distinct from the patient in **Fig. 17**. (A) Subtraction 1. (B) Subtraction 2. (C) Subtraction 3.

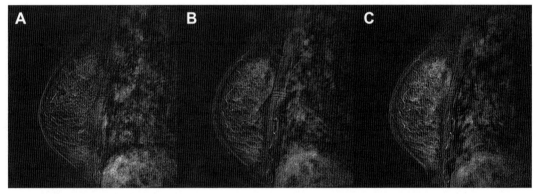

Fig. 19. Marked background enhancement. Note that the enhancement pattern is persistent. (A) Subtraction 1. (B) Subtraction 2. (C) Subtraction 3.

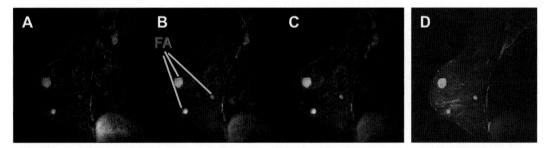

Fig. 20. Multiple fibroadenomas. This patient had a history of prior surgical excision of multiple fibroadenomas. MR imaging examination demonstrated multiple round and oval circumscribed masses, which were T2-hyperintense and which demonstrated persistent enhancement. The findings appeared stable compared with prior MR imaging examinations. The MR characteristics of the findings, in combination with the patient's history and the stability, are all in keeping with benignity. FA, fibroadenomas. (A) Subtraction 1. (B) Subtraction 2. (C) Subtraction 3. (D) Sagittal T2-weighted image with fat saturation.

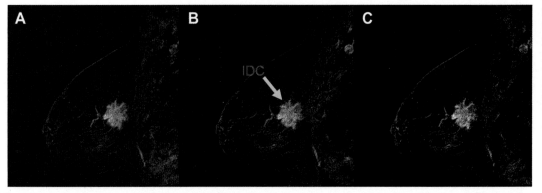

Fig. 21. Invasive ductal carcinoma (IDC). (*A*) Subtraction 1. A representative image from the first sagittal subtraction series demonstrates rapid and heterogeneous enhancement of this irregular mass, which was biopsy-proven malignancy. (*B, C*) Subtraction 2 and subtraction 3. There are components of the mass that demonstrate washout kinetics.

washout). Many benign lesions (such as fibroadenomas) demonstrate persistent enhancement (**Fig. 20**).[22,23] In general, washout enhancement is the most suspicious for malignancy (**Fig. 21**),[22,23] noting that malignant lesion enhancement kinetics can be variable.

It is also important to bear in mind that normal background enhancement is expected to have persistent enhancement (see **Figs. 17** and **19**).

SUMMARY

Dynamic contrast-enhanced breast MR imaging has emerged as a useful tool in different clinical scenarios. Structural and functional anatomy of breast parenchyma and any focal breast findings can be assessed using breast MR imaging, which also has the benefit of being a multiplanar study. It is important to integrate structural anatomy with functional anatomy in the interpretation of breast MR imaging and to interpret breast MR imaging in the clinical context of the patient, as well as in conjunction with other breast imaging modalities such as mammography and ultrasonography.

Dynamic contrast-enhanced MR imaging is a powerful tool in assessing the breast, and a firm understanding of the normal anatomy of the breast provides a foundation on which to detect pathology. The "normal anatomy of the breast" actually encompasses a wide range of normal, both within large patient populations and for an individual patient whose "normal breast anatomy" may vary monthly and across her lifetime. Looking forward, the information breast MR imaging provides about this "normal" anatomy may also be useful in risk assessment and in obtaining imaging biomarkers of functional breast physiology.

REFERENCES

1. Jemal A, Siegel R, Xu J, et al. Cancer statistics, 2010. CA Cancer J Clin 2010;60(5):277–300.
2. Heywang-Kobrunner SH, Bick U, Bradley WG Jr, et al. International investigation of breast MRI: results of a multicentre study (11 sites) concerning diagnostic parameters for contrast-enhanced MRI based on 519 histopathologically correlated lesions. Eur Radiol 2001;11(4):531–46.
3. Orel SG, Schnall MD. MR imaging of the breast for the detection, diagnosis, and staging of breast cancer. Radiology 2001;220(1):13–30.
4. Liu PF, Debatin JF, Caduff RF, et al. Improved diagnostic accuracy in dynamic contrast enhanced MRI of the breast by combined quantitative and qualitative analysis. Br J Radiol 1998;71(845): 501–9.
5. Saslow D, Boetes C, Burke W, et al. American Cancer Society guidelines for breast screening with MRI as an adjunct to mammography. CA Cancer J Clin 2007;57(2):75–89.
6. Orel SG, Schnall MD, Powell CM, et al. Staging of suspected breast cancer: effect of MR imaging and MR-guided biopsy. Radiology 1995;196(1): 115–22.
7. Boetes C, Mus RD, Holland R, et al. Breast tumors: comparative accuracy of MR imaging relative to mammography and US for demonstrating extent. Radiology 1995;197(3):743–7.
8. Esserman L, Hylton N, Yassa L, et al. Utility of magnetic resonance imaging in the management of breast cancer: evidence for improved preoperative staging. J Clin Oncol 1999;17(1):110–9.
9. Fischer U, Kopka L, Grabbe E. Breast carcinoma: effect of preoperative contrast-enhanced MR imaging on the therapeutic approach. Radiology 1999;213(3):881–8.

10. Fischer U, Baum F, Luftner-Nagel S. Preoperative MR imaging in patients with breast cancer: preoperative staging, effects on recurrence rates, and outcome analysis. Magn Reson Imaging Clin N Am 2006; 14(3):351–62, vi.

11. Liberman L. Breast MR imaging in assessing extent of disease. Magn Reson Imaging Clin N Am 2006; 14(3):339–49, vi.

12. Kuhl CK, Klaschik S, Mielcarek P, et al. Do T2-weighted pulse sequences help with the differential diagnosis of enhancing lesions in dynamic breast MRI? J Magn Reson Imaging 1999;9(2): 187–96.

13. Yuen S, Uematsu T, Kasami M, et al. Breast carcinomas with strong high-signal intensity on T2-weighted MR images: pathological characteristics and differential diagnosis. J Magn Reson Imaging 2007;25(3):502–10.

14. Kuhl CK, Schild HH, Morakkabati N. Dynamic bilateral contrast-enhanced MR imaging of the breast: trade-off between spatial and temporal resolution. Radiology 2005;236(3):789–800.

15. Song HK, Dougherty L, Schnall MD. Simultaneous acquisition of multiple resolution images for dynamic contrast enhanced imaging of the breast. Magn Reson Med 2001;46(3):503–9.

16. Szabo BK, Aspelin P, Wiberg MK, et al. Dynamic MR imaging of the breast. Analysis of kinetic and morphologic diagnostic criteria. Acta Radiol 2003; 44(4):379–86.

17. Tot T. The origins of early breast carcinoma. Semin Diagn Pathol 2010;27(1):62–8.

18. American College of Radiology (ACR). BI-RADS—mammography. ACR breast imaging reporting and data system, breast imaging atlas. 4th edition. Reston (VA): American College of Radiology; 2003.

19. Molleran V, Mahoney MC. The BI-RADS breast magnetic resonance imaging lexicon. Magn Reson Imaging Clin N Am 2010;18(2):171–85, vii.

20. Kuhl CK, Bieling HB, Gieseke J, et al. Healthy premenopausal breast parenchyma in dynamic contrast-enhanced MR imaging of the breast: normal contrast medium enhancement and cyclical-phase dependency. Radiology 1997;203(1):137–44.

21. Erguvan-Dogan B, Whitman GJ, Kushwaha AC, et al. BI-RADS-MRI: a primer. AJR Am J Roentgenol 2006;187(2):W152–60.

22. Kuhl CK, Schild HH. Dynamic image interpretation of MRI of the breast. J Magn Reson Imaging 2000; 12(6):965–74.

23. Kuhl CK. MRI of breast tumors. Eur Radiol 2000; 10(1):46–58.

Normal and Variant Abdominal Anatomy on Magnetic Resonance Imaging

Ashish P. Wasnik, MBBS, MD[a], Michael B. Mazza, MD[a],
Usha R. Lalchandani, MBBS[b], Peter S. Liu, MD[a,c,*]

KEYWORDS

- Normal abdominal anatomy • Variant abdominal anatomy
- Magnetic resonance imaging • Organ-specific protocols

Abdominal magnetic resonance (MR) imaging has traditionally been used as a problem-solving method after a previous indeterminate imaging investigation such as computed tomography (CT) or ultrasound, frequently using organ-specific protocols to highlight the condition in question.[1] Increasingly, abdominal MR imaging is being used as a primary imaging investigation with expansion of clinical indications and increased awareness of cumulative ionizing radiation dose in medical imaging.[2] Therefore, it is important to understand the normal abdominal anatomy on MR imaging, particularly the visceral organ appearances, as well as commonly encountered variants and disease mimics. Because most abdominal MR imaging studies are targeted toward an organ or area of interest, this article discusses the protocol strategies and relevant anatomy in a segmented/organ-specific manner.

In general, abdominal MR imaging benefits substantially from the use of a high field strength magnet (1.5 Tesla or greater) and local phased-array surface coils around the anatomy of interest. Most commonly, breath-held sequences with high temporal resolution and moderate spatial resolution are frequently used in abdominal MR imaging to mitigate the effects of respiratory and bowel motion. However, when high spatial resolution and improved image signal are required, motion compensation techniques such as respiratory triggering or diaphragm-navigation can be used to facilitate longer acquisition times.[3] The diagnostic usefulness of abdominal MR imaging lies in the improved contrast resolution and ability to qualify several tissue characteristics of a specific organ or lesion. Generally, abdominal MR imaging protocols include precontrast T1-weighted images, T2-weighted images, and dynamic postcontrast T1-weighted images with sufficient imaging redundancy of the organ system in question.[4] Our institution uses organ-specific protocols to facilitate technical reproducibility and optimize scan duration. These protocols are discussed individually in this article when applicable, noting that many build on a basic protocol with slight variations (Table 1).

LIVER
Technical Considerations

General abdominal and liver imaging protocol
The general abdomen protocol at our institution serves as the base protocol for abdominal MR techniques and is frequently used for investigations of nonspecific abdominal symptoms or malignancy follow-up. First, breath-held coronal

[a] Department of Radiology, University of Michigan Health System, 1500 East Medical Center Drive, Ann Arbor, MI 48109-0030, USA
[b] Department of Radiology, Grant Medical College, Byculla, Mumbai 400018, India
[c] Department of Vascular Surgery, University of Michigan Health System, 1500 East Medical Center Drive, Ann Arbor, MI 48109-0030, USA
* Corresponding author. Departments of Radiology and Vascular Surgery, University of Michigan Health System, 1500 East Medical Center Drive, Ann Arbor, MI 48109-0030.
E-mail address: peterliu@umich.edu

Magn Reson Imaging Clin N Am 19 (2011) 521–545
doi:10.1016/j.mric.2011.05.008
1064-9689/11/$ – see front matter © 2011 Elsevier Inc. All rights reserved.

Table 1
Example protocols

Abdominal/Liver Protocol

	Coronal T2	Axial T2	Axial In/Opposed T1	Axial Fat-Suppressed T2	Axial Diffusion	Axial Pre/Post T1	Axial Dynamic Pre/Post T1
Pulse sequence	SSFSE	SSFSE	SPGR	FSE	SE EPI	SPGR	3D SPGR
Repetition time (ms)	Minimum	Minimum	150	4000	6000	150	Minimum
Echo time (ms)	180	180	2.3/4.6	90	Minimum	Minimum	Minimum
FOV (cm)	40	36	To fit	To fit	40	To fit	To fit
Slice thickness (mm)	8	6	6	6	6	6	4
Matrix	256 × 128	256 × 128	256 × 160	256–320 × 192	128 × 128	512 × 160	320 × 160
Signal averages	0.5 NEX	0.5 NEX	1 NEX	4 NEX	8 NEX	1 NEX	0.5 NEX

MRCP Sequences

	Axial MRCP	3D MRCP
Pulse sequence	SSFSE	FRFSE
Repetition true (ms)	Minimum	Minimum
Echo time (ms)	180	650
FOV (cm)	40	36
Slice thickness (mm)	5	1.4
Matrix	256 × 160	256 × 256
Signal averages	0.5 NEX	2 NEX

Kidney Sequences

	Axial Water Suppressed T1	Coronal Dynamic Pre/Post T1
Pulse sequence	SPGR	3D SPGR
Repetition time (ms)	170	Minimum
Echo time (ms)	Minimum	Minimum
FOV (cm)	To fit	To fit
Slice thickness (mm)	6	3
Matrix	256 × 160	320 × 160
Signal averages	1 NEX	0.5 NEX

Adrenal Sequences

	Coronal In/Opposed T1
Pulse sequence	SPGR
Repetition time (ms)	Minimum
Echo time (ms)	2.3/4.6
FOV (cm)	To fit
Slice thickness (mm)	5
Matrix	256 × 160
Signal averages	1 NEX

	MR Enterography Sequences		MRA Sequences	
	Axial Steady-state	Coronal Steady-state	Coronal Dynamic Pre/Post T1	3D Phase Contrast
Pulse sequence	FIESTA	FIESTA	3D SPGR	3D PC
Repetition time (ms)	Minimum	Minimum	Minimum	Minimum
Echo time (ms)	Minimum	Minimum	Minimum	Minimum
FOV (cm)	32–40	38–40	28–40 (prefer 30)	28
Slice thickness (mm)	6	3	2.4	2.5
Matrix	256 × 256	256 × 256	288 × 160	256 × 192
Signal averages	1	1	0.5–1 NEX	1 NEX

Abbreviations: EPI, echo planar imaging; FIESTA, fast imaging employing steady state acquisition; FOV, field of view; FRFSE, fast recovery fast spin echo; FSE, fast spin echo; SE, spin echo; SPGR, spoiled gradient recalled echo; SSFSE, single shot fast spin echo.

and axial T2-weighted imaging are obtained using single-shot echo-train spin-echo technique (such as single-shot fast spin-echo [SSFSE] or half-Fourier acquisition single-shot turbo spin-echo [HASTE]) with moderate T2-weighting, using an echo time (TE) of approximately 180 milliseconds (**Fig. 1**). A complementary axial fast spin-echo T2-weighted sequence is obtained using respiratory triggering, fat suppression, and a shorter TE of approximately 90 milliseconds. T1-weighted imaging is initially performed using a breath-hold spoiled gradient echo sequence in which both in-phase and opposed-phase echoes are recorded. Subsequently, breath-hold precontrast and postcontrast

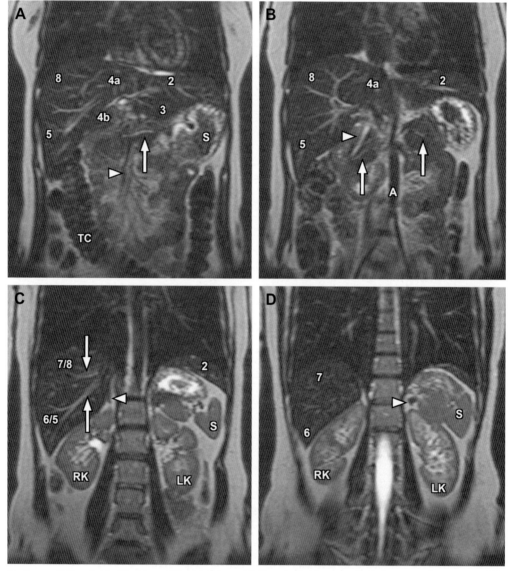

Fig. 1. Coronal T2-weighted images of the abdomen (*A–D*, anterior to posterior). Segmental anatomy of liver is labeled 2 to 8, including 4a/4b, on all images. (*A*) Anteriorly, the stomach (S) is seen with enteric contents. Transverse colon (TC) is seen crossing the midline. The pancreatic duct (*arrow*) can be well seen on coronal T2-weighted images. Superior mesenteric vessels (*arrowhead*) are seen descending in the mesentery. (*B*) The pancreatic duct is seen in piecemeal fashion on coronal T2-weighted images (*arrows*) as it courses between contiguous images. Common bile duct (*arrowhead*). Aorta, A. (*C*) Portions of the right hepatic vein are seen (*arrows*), which serves as the anatomic boundary between anterior and posterior segments of the right hepatic lobe. Note the far left lateral extent of the left hepatic lobe (2) in this patient. Right adrenal gland is seen (*arrowhead*), as is a portion of the spleen (S). LK, left kidney; RK, right kidney. (*D*) Posteriorly, the left adrenal gland can be seen (*arrowhead*). Spleen, right kidney, and left kidney as in (*C*).

T1-weighted imaging is obtained using a two-dimensional (2D) spoiled gradient echo sequence with fat suppression (**Figs. 2–6**). We also routinely obtain axial diffusion-weighted imaging using echo planar imaging because of the emerging role in various MR applications, particularly oncologic imaging.[5] However, the anatomic features of the abdomen are often less clearly seen on diffusion-weighted images than standard T1-weighted and T2-weighted sequences.

For patients undergoing specific investigations of the liver or spleen, a dynamic postcontrast technique replaces the standard precontrast and postcontrast T1-weighted imaging sequence. This dynamic sequence uses a breath-hold axial three-dimensional (3D) spoiled gradient echo technique that permits volumetric data acquisition with thinner reconstructed imaging sections.[6] The sequence usually includes a precontrast data set, followed by postcontrast data obtained in the arterial, venous, and equilibrium phases of enhancement (**Fig. 7**). There is some variability in the selected imaging matrix because of differences in patient breath-hold ability, but typical values vary between 128 × 256 and 192 × 320.

Anatomic Considerations and MR Imaging Features

The liver is the largest organ in the abdomen, occupying most of the right upper quadrant, and is the site of many metabolic processes. There are several anatomic strategies for describing the liver, which have historically bisected the liver into left and right lobes, with additional nonfunctional terminology recognizing the caudate and quadrate lobe. The more conventional segmental anatomy described by Couinaud[7] divides the liver into 8 independently functioning segments. Understanding these segments on imaging is important from surgical and transplant perspectives (see **Figs. 1–6**).

The caudate lobe (segment 1) is bordered anteriorly by the left portal vein, posteriorly by the inferior vena cava (IVC), and laterally by the ligamentum venosum. The caudate lobe is unique from other hepatic segments, given its direct venous drainage into the IVC, and it stands in the watershed area between the right and left portobiliary system. The right lobe consists of segment 5 to 8, whereas the left lobe contains segments 2 to 4. In general terms, segmental anatomy is

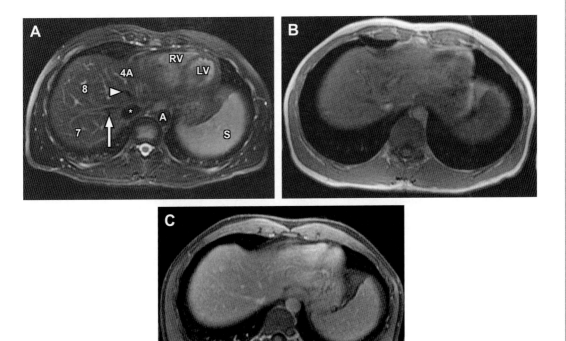

Fig. 2. Axial fat-suppressed T2-weighted (*A*), in-phase T1-weighted (*B*), and fat-suppressed postcontrast T1-weighted (*C*) imaging shows anatomy in the hepatic domes. Right hepatic lobe segments are noted (7, 8) and upper left hepatic lobe segment 4a. Right hepatic vein (*arrow*) and middle hepatic vein (*arrowhead*) are noted. A, aorta; IVC (*asterisk*); LV, left ventricle; RV, right ventricle; S, spleen.

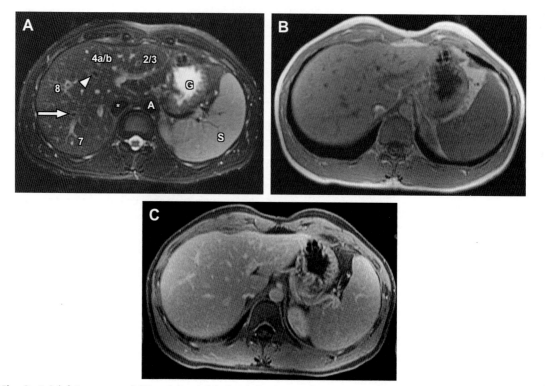

Fig. 3. Axial fat-suppressed T2-weighted (*A*), in-phase T1-weighted (*B*), and fat-suppressed postcontrast T1-weighted (*C*) imaging shows anatomy at the level of the left intrahepatic portal vein. Liver segments are numerically labeled, including boundary of left hepatic lobe segments (2/3, 4a/b). Stomach with gastric contents (G) is present. Remainder of labeled structures as in **Fig. 2**. Right hepatic vein (*arrow*); middle hepatic vein (*arrowhead*); A, aorta; IVC (*asterisk*).

bounded by vertical planes coursing through the hepatic veins, and a horizontal plane formed by the portal vein. Therefore, a vertical plane extending through the middle hepatic vein and gallbladder fossa separates the right and left hepatic lobes, at the margins of segment 8 superiorly and segment 5 inferiorly in the right lobe versus segments 4a/b in the left lobe. The left hepatic vein and falciform ligament fissure separate segments 2 and 3 in the left hepatic lobe from segments 4a/b, whereas the portal vein localizes segments 2 and 4a above the portal vein and segments 3 and 4b below the portal vein. The right hepatic vein separates the anterior segments of the right hepatic lobe, including segment 8 (superior to the portal vein) and 5 (inferior to the portal vein) from the posterior segments of the right hepatic lobe, namely segments 7 (superior) and 6 (inferior).[8,9] The porta hepatis is a deep transverse fissure situated between medial segment anteriorly and the caudate lobe posteriorly. At the porta hepatis, the portal vein and hepatic artery enter the liver, whereas the hepatic ducts emerge from the liver. The liver receives its dominant blood supply from the portal vein, with a lesser contribution

from the hepatic artery (approximately 30% of its blood supply). Hepatic drainage is through the hepatic veins into the IVC.

The normal liver shows higher signal intensity relative to normal spleen on T1-weighted images caused by increased protein synthetic activity and amount of rough endoplasmic reticulum.[4] The liver generally shows lower signal intensity versus spleen on T2-weighted images (see **Figs. 1–6**). The biliary tree courses through the liver, accompanying the portal vein and hepatic arterial segments in the portal triad, and shows linear high signal intensity on T2-weighted images; the relevant biliary anatomy and variants are discussed separately in a later section. The hepatic vessels generally show very low signal/flow voids on T2-weighted sequences, but enhance on postcontrast imaging.

Many variations are encountered with regards to shape and size of the liver, including horizontal elongated left lateral lobe wrapping around spleen, congenitally hypoplastic left lobe, or elongated tonguelike right lobe (Reidel lobe). Diaphragmatic impressions along the right lateral liver margins are also commonly encountered and present as a low signal intensity linear or

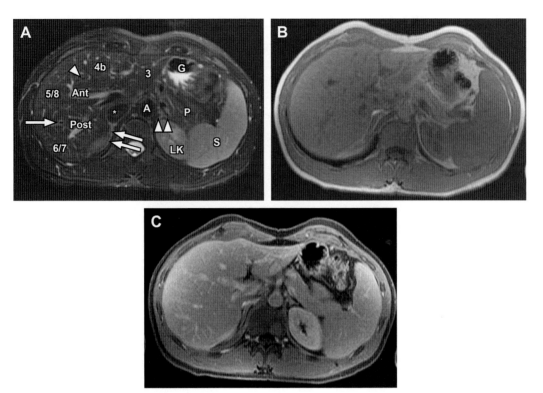

Fig. 4. Axial fat-suppressed T2-weighted (*A*), in-phase T1-weighted (*B*), and fat-suppressed postcontrast T1-weighted (*C*) imaging shows anatomy at the level of the right intrahepatic portal vein, with anterior (Ant) and posterior (Post) segments labeled. Pancreas (P) is now seen toward the splenic hilum, representing the pancreatic tail. Right adrenal gland (*double arrow*) has a slender contour, whereas the left adrenal gland (*double arrowhead*) is more triangular on axial imaging. A, aorta; LK, left kidney; right hepatic vein (*arrow*); middle hepatic vein (*arrowhead*); IVC (*asterisk*). Remainder of labeled structures as in **Fig. 3**.

wedge-shaped area on T1-weighted and T2-weighted images.[8] Hepatic steatosis is a commonly encountered abnormality in the liver with multifactorial cause. MR imaging is highly accurate in identifying focal or diffuse fatty infiltration and distinguishing focal fat from true hepatic masses.[10,11] Fat infiltration manifests as signal loss on out-of-phase gradient echo images from in-phase gradient echo T1-weighted images (**Fig. 8**), with spleen used as a reference in diffuse hepatic steatosis.[8] When multiple T2-weighted images are obtained with varying echo times, the signal intensity in the liver decreases with heavier T2 weighting. This feature can be beneficial in focal hepatic lesion detection, particularly for cystic lesions, which maintain high signal intensity even with very heavy T2 weighting, thereby increasing lesion conspicuity.

SPLEEN
Anatomic Considerations and MR Imaging Features

The spleen is a large, crescentic, encapsulated intraperitoneal organ located in the left upper quadrant posteriorly. It is composed of vascular lymphoid tissue including the reticuloendothelial cells in the white pulp and the vascular circulatory system in the red pulp. The splenic artery and vein traverse through the hilum. The splenic vein and superior mesenteric vein join to form portal vein posterior to the pancreatic neck/body region. The normal craniocaudal dimension of the spleen is 13 cm.[12]

Normal splenic parenchyma is of low signal intensity relative to liver on T1-weighted images and of high signal intensity on T2-weighted images.[13,14] In children younger than 8 months, the spleen predominantly contains vascular red pulp and less lymphoid tissue, thereby showing lower signal intensity on T2-weighted images and isointense to slightly hypointense signal relative to liver on T1-weighted images (see **Figs. 1–6**).[15] Many malignant processes are hypointense on T1-weighted images and hyperintense on T2-weighted images relative to the liver, thereby paralleling signal intensity of spleen.[16] Because of the similar precontrast characteristics between spleen and solid neoplasms, contrast-enhanced images are important in evaluation of focal lesions.[13,17,18] In postgadolinium arterial phase (45 seconds), the

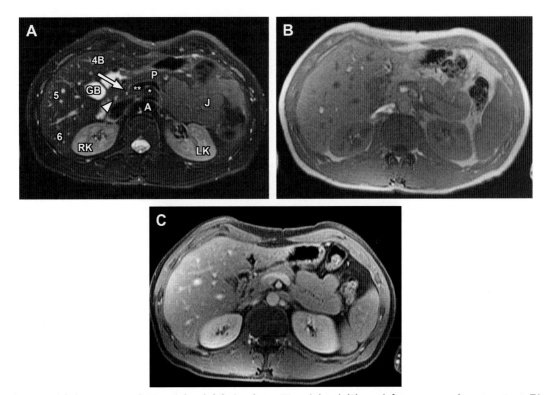

Fig. 5. Axial fat-suppressed T2-weighted (*A*), in-phase T1-weighted (*B*), and fat-suppressed postcontrast T1-weighted (*C*) imaging shows anatomy at the level of venous confluence (*double asterisk*) between splenic vein and superior mesenteric vein. Adjacent SMA (*asterisk*) is noted more medially. The pancreatic duct (*arrow*) is visible in the pancreatic head-neck region, whereas the parenchyma is seen extending across midline (P). The common bile duct is also visible (*arrowhead*). GB, gallbladder; J, jejunum; RK, right kidney. Remainder of labeled structures as in **Fig. 4.**

spleen shows a heterogeneous pattern of enhancement with the high and low serpigenous region, termed the arciform enhancement pattern, and is seen as a result of variable flow within the red pulp (see **Fig. 7**A).[19,20] However, within the portal venous phase of 60 to 70 seconds, there is homogeneous intense enhancement throughout (see **Fig. 7**B).[20]

In patients with secondary hemosiderosis, such as from repeated blood transfusions, diffuse iron deposition in the reticuloendothelial system (RES) occurs, which can be detected on MR imaging because of susceptibility effect of iron causing T2 shortening, manifesting as hypointense foci on T2-weighted and T2*-weighted images.[21] The longer echo time sequence of a dual-echo T1-weighted sequence (usually the in-phase image) shows this signal loss as enlarging low signal intensity because of the increased blooming artifact afforded by the longer echo time (**Fig. 9**). In contrast, patients with primary/genetic hemochromatosis generally show sparing of the spleen, because the RES in patients with genetic hemochromatosis is dysfunctional and does not accumulate excess iron.[22]

In portal hypertension, congestion and splenomegaly occur, resulting in development of multiple intraparenchymal hemorrhagic foci containing iron, calcium, and fibrous tissue referred to as Gamna-Gandy bodies (**Fig. 10**).[13,23]

Accessory spleen or splenules appear as spherical masses ranging from 1 to 30 mm, and are seen in up to 30% of the normal population.[13,24,25] These features are composed of splenic tissue and therefore show similar signal characteristics to the spleen itself. The most common location of an accessory spleen is in the splenic hilum. Accessory splenic tissue can simulate an adrenal mass, lymph node, or even a pancreatic mass if the accessory spleen is located within the substance of the pancreatic tail. Use of superparamagnetic iron oxide agents or nuclear scintigraphy can confirm accessory splenic tissue in uncertain cases.

GALLBLADDER AND BILE DUCTS
Technical Considerations: Pancreaticobiliary Imaging

Magnetic resonance cholangiopancreatography (MRCP) has emerged as a versatile, noninvasive

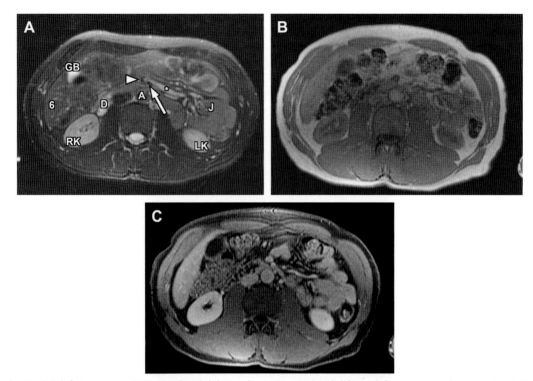

Fig. 6. Axial fat-suppressed T2-weighted (*A*), in-phase T1-weighted (*B*), and fat-suppressed postcontrast T1-weighted (*C*) imaging shows anatomy at the level of the inferior liver tip. The superior mesenteric vein (*arrowhead*) and feeding branch veins (*asterisk*) are seen. The superior mesenteric artery (*arrow*) is again adjacent to the medial aspect of the superior mesenteric vein. Duodenal C-loop (D in 6A) is seen as it approaches midline. Remainder of labeled structures as in **Fig. 5.**

method for investigation of the pancreaticobiliary tree. MRCP has assumed a primary diagnostic role over endoscopic retrograde cholangiopancreatography (ERCP) in many patient groups, particularly those with a low pretest probability of requiring biliary intervention, suspected high-grade obstruction, or complex postsurgical anatomy that would make ERCP technically challenging.[26] Several different MRCP techniques have been described with various merits, including 2D and 3D imaging.[27] At our institution, we augment our standard liver MR imaging protocol with 2 additional MRCP techniques when pancreaticobiliary disease is suspected. First, we perform a coronal 3D T2-weighted sequence using a fast-recovery fast spin-echo sequence (FRFSE) with parallel imaging to obtain a high-resolution image with an isotropic voxel (approximately 0.5–0.9 mm reconstructed voxel). Heavy T2-weighting is used (TE ≥600 milliseconds) to null signal from background tissues. Although time-consuming, this 3D dataset can then be manipulated using 3D postprocessing software to reconstruct any desired projectional view (**Fig. 11**). Studies have shown improved image

quality and diagnostic performance of 3D MRCP versus 2D imaging.[28,29] Additional breath-hold axial thin-section T2-weighted 2D imaging is performed using 4-mm to 5-mm sections with no interslice gap and moderate T2 weighting to permit some visualization of the background tissues. This 2D thin-section sequence serves both a complementary and redundant role for the primary 3D T2-weighted sequence. Optional oblique coronal T2-weighted thick-slab MRCP images can be obtained rapidly if the patient is uncooperative with breath-holding during 2D imaging or has a variable respiratory pattern that corrupts the 3D imaging.[30] Newer dual pharmacokinetic gadolinium-based contrast agents show both renal and hepatic excretion, thereby creating positive-contrast MR cholangiograms if sufficient clearance is allowed to occur in the biliary tree. The 2 available contrast agents in the United States with dual pharmacokinetic properties include gadobenate dimeglumine (Gd-BOPTA, Multihance, Bracco Diagnostics, Princeton, NJ, USA), and gadoxetic acid (Gd-EOB-DTPA, Eovist/Primovist, Bayer HealthCare Pharmaceuticals, Wayne, NJ, USA).

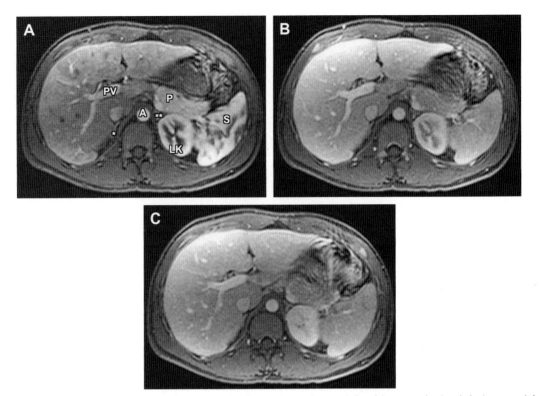

Fig. 7. Dynamic postcontrast enhancement. Axial fat-suppressed T1-weighted images obtained during arterial (*A*), venous (*B*), and equilibrium phases (*C*). Note the arciform enhancement pattern of the spleen (S) on arterial imaging. A, aorta; LK, left kidney; P, pancreas; PV, portal vein; RK, right kidney; right adrenal gland (*asterisk*); left adrenal gland (*double asterisk*).

Anatomic Considerations and MR Imaging Features

Bile is formed by hepatocytes to aid in digestion and absorption of fat and secreted into the biliary radicals that track centrally with the intrahepatic portal triad to coalesce as the paired right and left hepatic ducts. Subsequently, the paired hepatic ducts converge to form the common hepatic duct, which nominally changes to the common bile duct after the cystic duct joins along the right lateral side. The common bile duct

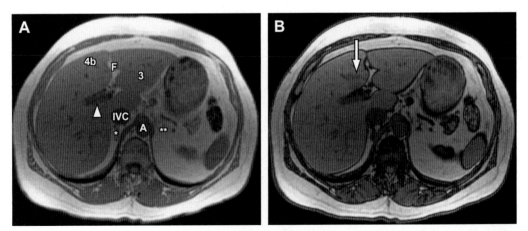

Fig. 8. Focal steatosis. Axial in-phase (*A*) and opposed-phase (*B*) images show focal loss of signal in the segment 4b on opposed-phase imaging (*arrow* in Fig. 8B) versus in-phase image. Left hepatic segmental anatomy, 3, 4b. A, aorta; F, falciform ligament fissure; portal vein (*arrowhead*); right adrenal gland (*asterisk*); left adrenal gland (*double asterisk*).

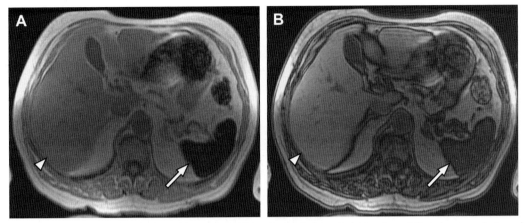

Fig. 9. Secondary hemosiderosis caused by repeated blood transfusions. Axial in-phase (*A*) and opposed-phase (*B*) images show diffuse signal loss in the spleen (*arrow*) and to a lesser degree in the liver (*arrowhead*) on in-phase image because of longer echo time, allowing greater blooming artifact/T2* effect.

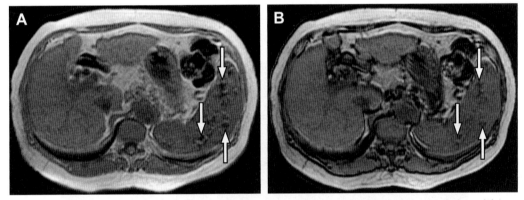

Fig. 10. Gamna-Gandy bodies caused by portal hypertension. Axial in-phase (*A*) and opposed-phase (*B*) images show multifocal signal loss in the spleen (*arrows*), which worsens on the in-phase image because of longer echo time, allowing greater blooming artifact/T2* effect.

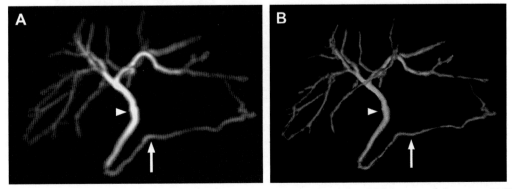

Fig. 11. Normal MRCP. Maximum intensity projection (*A*) and volume-rendered (*B*) images of the normal biliary tree show pancreatic duct (*arrow*) and common bile duct (*arrowhead*), joining in the periampullary region.

descends through the pancreatic head, communicating with the duodenum at the ampulla of Vater. The gallbladder serves as a bile reservoir, and is located in the gallbladder fossa, along the inferior surface of the liver. The cystic duct joins the gallbladder to the biliary tree, and contains characteristic folds called the spiral valves of Heister.

The signal intensity of bile within the gallbladder on noncontrast T1-weighted images depends on the concentration of bile salts, water, and cholesterol. Nonconcentrated bile is usually hypointense on T1-weighted images because of its fluid content. In a fasting state, with reabsorption of water and increased concentration of bile salts and cholesterol, bile is seen as layering high signal intensity on T1-weighted images.[30] After intravenous gadolinium contrast administration, the gallbladder wall shows thin, homogeneous enhancement. On T2-weighted images, normal bile shows high signal intensity with a thin hypointense gallbladder wall, nearly imperceptible with a thickness of approximately 3 mm. The cystic duct shows high signal as well, with a diameter of approximately 1 to 5 mm. The common bile duct usually measures less than 7 mm in diameter, although it can be larger in patients with previous cholecystectomy.[30,31]

The normal intrahepatic biliary tree shows high signal on T2-weighted images and low signal on T1-weighted images, similar to fluid (see **Fig. 11**). MRCP can be limited in patients without biliary dilation, particularly peripheral branch visualization. Evaluation of both source images and maximum intensity projection 3D reformatted images are complementary in localization of suspected disease.

Knowledge of biliary anatomic variants is important because of an increasing use of laparoscopic techniques for cholecystectomy, which can increase risk of bile duct injury.[32] The most common and important variations include aberrant right hepatic segmental duct insertions including into the left hepatic duct (**Fig. 12**A) or low in the common hepatic duct (below the bifurcation, see **Fig. 12**B) or into the cystic duct itself, variations in cystic duct length (more than 20 mm or <5 mm), aberrant cystic duct entering into the medial surface of common bile duct (see **Fig. 12**C), or low

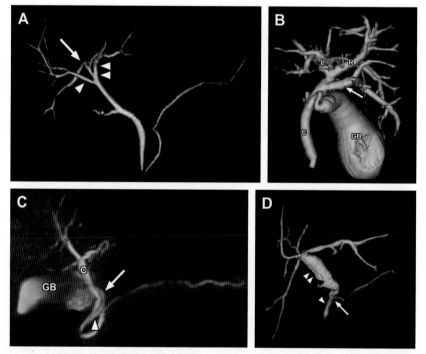

Fig. 12. Biliary variants on MRCP. (*A*) Volume-rendered image shows anomalous posterior segmental duct (*arrow*) from right hepatic lobe joining the left hepatic duct (*double arrowhead*). The normal right hepatic duct is seen (*single arrowhead*). (*B*) Volume-rendered image (viewed from posterior) shows anomalous posterior segmental duct (*arrow*) from right hepatic lobe inserting low into the common hepatic duct, just above the cystic duct. Common bile duct (C) is normal caliber. Normal left (L) and right (R) ducts are marked. GB, gallbladder. (*C*) Maximum intensity projection image shows a long parallel channel (*arrow*) and medial insertion of the cystic duct (*arrowhead*). C, common bile duct; GB, gallbladder. (*D*) Volume-rendered image shows APBJ (*arrow*) with long downstream common channel (*arrowhead*). There is a resultant choledochal cyst (*double arrowhead*).

insertion of the cystic duct into the distal third of the common duct.[31,33,34] Several described variants of the gallbladder include phrygian cap, intraluminal septations, ectopic location, or prominent mucosal fold.

Normally, the common bile duct and pancreatic duct join to form a short 4-mm to 5-mm common channel before opening at the ampulla of Vater, enveloped by a muscular sphincter called the sphincter of Oddi. Sometimes, this common channel length may be increased (>15 mm), and is called a long common channel or anomalous pancreaticobiliary junction (APBJ, see **Fig. 12D**).[35] The long common channel allows pancreaticobiliary communication before the sphincter, which can result in persistent reflux of pancreatic exocrine secretion into the common duct, predisposing to formation of choledochal cysts, stones, cholangitis, recurrent pancreatitis, and neoplasm.[36,37]

Surgical clips, metallic stents, or pneumobilia may limit evaluation of the abdomen ducts because of signal blooming artifact, particularly on gradient echo sequences.

PANCREAS
Anatomic Considerations and MR Imaging Features

Pancreas is a highly vascular mixed exocrine and endocrine gland. Grossly, it is a soft lobulated retroperitoneal organ located in the upper abdomen lying obliquely across the midline. Anatomically it is divided into head, uncinate process, neck, body, and tail. The splenic vein courses posterior to the body and tail region. The main pancreatic duct is 2 to 3 mm in diameter and is slightly more prominent in the head region relative to the tail.[38] The main pancreatic duct receives drainage from multiple side branches. Usually, the main drainage is through the duct of Wirsung, which is formed by the fusion of ducts draining from the body and tail and ducts draining from the head and uncinate process. The duct of Wirsung joins with the common bile duct at the ampulla of Vater and drains into the duodenum. In some cases, the accessory duct of Santorini, from the body and tail, drains separately into the duodenum via minor papilla.[31] Normal pancreas is high signal intensity on fat-saturated T1-weighted images because of the presence of aqueous protein in the acinar cells, intracellular paramagnetic substances (like manganese), and abundant endoplasmic reticulum in pancreatic exocrine glands.[39,40] In old age the pancreas may become more intermediate intensity on T1-weighted images, lower than the liver, because of fibrosis. Normal pancreas is only slightly hyperintense relative to muscle on T2-weighted images. Although fat-suppressed T2-weighted images may be helpful in identifying pancreatic fluid collections, there is low tissue contrast of the pancreas itself versus the adjacent nullified fat.[39,40] After intravenous gadolinium contrast administration, the pancreas shows intense homogeneous enhancement in arterial phase (30–45 seconds) of intravenous contrast, relative to the liver, and is hypointense in the equilibrium phase (150–180 seconds).[19,41,42]

Because of the fluid content, the pancreatic duct is of high signal intensity on T2-weighted images and MRCP. However, a nondilated pancreatic duct may not always be identified along its entire course.[38,43]

Congenital anomalies and normal variants of the pancreas and the pancreatic duct include pancreas divisum, annular pancreas, ectopic pancreatic tissue, variations of pancreatic contour, fatty replacement, and fat sparing of the pancreas.

Pancreas divisum is the most common congenital pancreatic ductal anatomic variant, occurring in approximately 4% to 14% of the population in 1 autopsy series.[44–46] In most cases of pancreatic divisum, no communication exists between the dorsal and ventral pancreatic ducts (**Fig. 13**); in some patients, the ventral pancreatic duct may be completely absent. Because of this configuration, pancreatic secretions drain through the minor ampulla.[47] The main features of pancreas divisum on MRCP include a dorsal pancreatic duct in direct continuity with the duct of Santorini, draining through the minor papilla. The smaller-caliber ventral duct joins the distal common bile duct to enter the major papilla, but does not communicate with the dorsal duct.[44] The clinical relevance of pancreas divisum remains controversial. Most patients with pancreas divisum are asymptomatic.[44,46,48] However, in some patients, this anomaly is associated with recurrent episodes of pancreatitis.

Annular pancreas is a rare anomaly characterized by a band of pancreatic tissue that surrounds the descending duodenum, either completely or incompletely, and is continuous with the pancreatic head (**Fig. 14**).[47,49] It results from abnormal migration and rotation of ventral anlage of the pancreas during embryogenesis.[49] Although this entity is usually identified incidentally in asymptomatic patients, it may manifest as duodenal obstruction, peptic ulcer disease, pancreatitis, or biliary obstruction.[49] Most patients present during infancy from symptoms of gastric outlet obstruction.[31,50]

Focal fatty infiltration may be seen in pancreas and may simulate a mass lesion. MR imaging is a useful tool for confirming the presence of focal

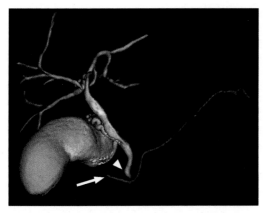

Fig. 13. Pancreas divisum. Volume-rendered image shows separate drainage (*arrow*) of the main pancreatic duct, which also had an anterior course to the common bile duct (*arrowhead*).

fatty infiltration using chemical shift. Complete pancreatic fatty replacement is commonly seen in patients with cystic fibrosis and may be diagnosed with both CT and MR imaging.[47]

Sometimes the normal pancreatic tissue may have an unusual contour, mimicking neoplasm, especially in the head and tail region. However, signal intensity of the lobular pancreas producing these contour variations follows that of normal pancreatic tissue on all unenhanced and post-contrast-enhanced images.[47]

In patients with genetic hemochromatosis (**Fig. 15**), iron deposition occurs in the pancreas late in the disease, usually after irreversible damage to the liver. Iron deposition results in loss of signal intensity on T2-weighted and T2*-weighted images, and is generally easy to recognize as blooming artifact on dual-echo T1-weighted images.[21]

KIDNEYS
Technical Considerations

Most MR studies of the kidneys at our institution involve workup of a suspected renal mass seen on either CT or ultrasound. Our renal mass protocol involves 2 additions to the general abdomen protocol. To aid in the diagnosis of fat-containing renal masses, we use an axial T1-weighted spoiled gradient echo sequence with chemical water saturation. This technique effectively highlights only fat-containing structures of the abdomen by nullifying the signal from water-based protons that comprise the normal renal parenchyma. In addition, we supplement the standard precontrast and postcontrast axial T1-weighted imaging sequence with a dynamic pre-contrast and postcontrast coronal T1-weighted spoiled gradient echo sequence to provide

additional imaging redundancy of the renal fossa. A modification of the general abdomen protocol can be used for MR urography, whereby the coronal dynamic precontrast and postcontrast T1-weighted spoiled gradient echo imaging is used with a wide field of view (FOV 40–42 cm) to cover the entire collecting system. Complementary delayed-phase T1-weighted spoiled gradient echo images are subsequently obtained in both the axial and coronal planes to ensure optimal contrast-excretion into the collecting system.

Anatomic Considerations and MR Imaging Features

The kidneys are bean-shaped paired retroperitoneal organs, situated within the fatty perirenal space, located on either side of the dorsolumbar spine. The kidneys vary in size but extend craniocaudally from approximately the T12 to L3 vertebral levels. The right kidney is slightly lower than the left kidney, because of the presence of the liver in the right upper abdomen. The kidney and the perirenal adipose tissue are enclosed by a fibrous fascia, called the Gerota fascia. The kidney is surrounded by a fibroelastic capsule, which fuses laterally to form the lateroconal fascia. The renal hilum is a dominant fissure, located along the medial aspect of each kidney that contains the vessels, nerves, and renal pelvis, and provides access to the more central fat-containing renal sinus.

The kidney is divided into 2 main areas: the outer cortex and an inner medulla. Within the medulla there are 8 or more cone-shaped sections known as renal pyramids. The apices of the pyramids converge and projects toward the renal sinus, where they form prominent papilla projecting into the calyces. The cortex arches between the pyramids and are called renal columns of Bertin. The minor renal calyces are cup-shaped, 7 to 13 in number. The calyces unite to form 2 or 3 short major calyces, which open into a funnel-shaped sac, the renal pelvis.

Renal parenchyma is of high signal intensity relative to liver on T2-weighted images and low signal intensity on T1-weighted images because of longer T1 relaxation times (see **Figs. 1–6**).[51,52] Corticomedullary differentiation is best seen on fat-suppressed noncontrast T1-weighted images and immediate postgadolinium images (see **Fig. 7**). The renal collecting system contains urine and shows fluid signal intensity, with low signal on T1-weighted images and high signal on T2-weighted images. The perinephric and renal sinus fat is also bright on T2-weighted images, whereas the

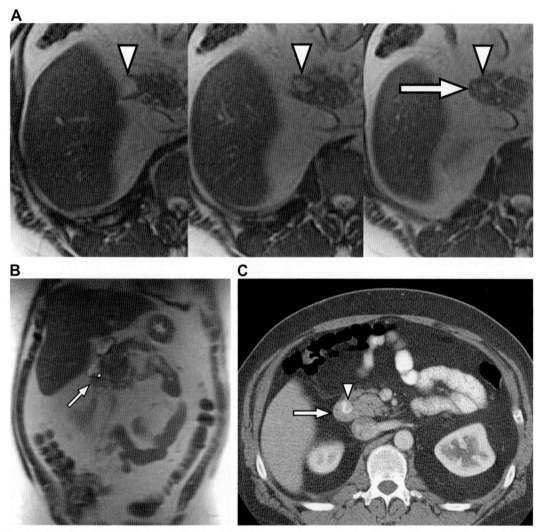

Fig. 14. Annular pancreas. (*A*) Sequential axial steady-state free precession images show the duodenal lumen (*arrowhead*) in the second portion of the duodenum. Surrounding pancreatic parenchyma is noted (*arrow*) as the duodenum courses caudally. (*B*) Coronal T2-weighted image shows abnormal pancreatic parenchyma (*arrow*) encircling the duodenal lumen (*asterisk*). (*C*) Axial CT image with oral and intravenous contrast confirms abnormal pancreatic parenchyma (*arrow*) surrounding the duodenal lumen with oral contrast (*arrowhead*).

renal fascia appears dark because of presence of fibrous tissue.[52] On opposed-phase T1-weighted images, a dark rim should be seen at the interface between kidney and perinephric fat, attributable to the chemical shift difference between the resonant frequencies of water-based and fat-based protons.[53,54]

Numerous commonly encountered anatomic variants of the kidneys include: fetal lobulations, prominent column of Bertin, and several congenital abnormalities of renal position, fusion, and number. Fetal lobulations may sometimes pose a difficulty in differentiating from renal mass on ultrasound. Because of the multiplanar nature of

MR imaging, there is clear evidence of the undulating contour showing homogeneous uniform cortical thickness on postgadolinium images. A prominent column of Bertin remains isointense to the renal cortex on all noncontrast and postcontrast images. Renal position can be ectopic with abnormal vertical ascent of the kidneys, more frequently resulting in a pelvic kidney rather than ectopic cranial location (**Fig. 16**). Abnormality of renal position is usually associated with anomalous blood supply, often associated with the adjacent local vessels. Horseshoe kidney is the most common anomaly of renal fusion. A horseshoe kidney results from an aberrant midline

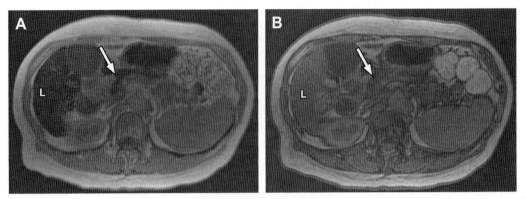

Fig. 15. Genetic hemochromatosis. Axial in-phase (*A*) and opposed-phase (*B*) images show diffuse signal loss in the pancreas (*arrow*) as well as the liver (L), which worsens on the in-phase image because of longer echo time, allowing greater blooming artifact/T2* effect.

connection/isthmus between the 2 developing kidneys, which can be comprised of normal parenchyma or fibrous tissue (**Fig. 17**). Coexistent renovascular anomalies are common and abnormal position is frequently shown with horseshoe kidney, as the isthmus fails to ascend past the inferior mesenteric artery (IMA) origin. Crossed fused renal ectopia represents a more uncommon renal fusion anomaly with joined renal parenchyma on a single side, with maintained normal/bilateral ureteral insertions into the bladder. This situation results in 1 ureter crossing the midline to insert on the contralateral aspect of the urinary bladder.[55]

ADRENAL GLANDS
Technical Considerations

MR imaging can be used to evaluate suspected adrenal disease, noting similar sensitivity and specificity as noncontrast CT for the diagnosis of adrenal adenoma.[56] The protocol for adrenal imaging at our institution builds on the general abdomen MR protocol by including a few additional sequences. First, a coronal in-phase/opposed-phase T1-weighted spoiled gradient echo imaging sequence is obtained, in addition to the axial image sequence, to provide additional chemical shift imaging redundancy of the adrenal glands. Second, instead of routine precontrast and postcontrast imaging, a coronal dynamic precontrast and postcontrast T1-weighted spoiled gradient echo sequence is obtained, including delayed-phase imaging.

Anatomic Considerations and MR Imaging Features

The adrenal glands are small paired retroperitoneal organs, each situated adjacent to the superior pole of either kidneys, hence their name adrenal or suprarenal glands. The right adrenal gland is triangular and the left adrenal gland is semilunar. The adrenal glands are composed of 2 endocrine organs, outer cortex producing steroids and inner medulla secreting catecholamines. The arterial supply to the adrenal glands is via branches from the aorta, renal artery, and inferior phrenic artery. The right suprarenal vein veins directly into the IVC, and the left suprarenal vein drains into the left renal vein.

T2-weighted images may sometimes show corticomedullary differentiation in normal adrenal gland.[57] However, T1-weighted images with fat suppression or opposed-phase gradient echo

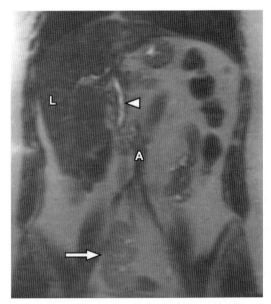

Fig. 16. Pelvic kidney. Coronal T2-weighted image show a low-lying pelvic kidney (*arrow*). Note that wide FOV images in the coronal plane may be the only chance to identify low-lying abnormalities on standard liver or renal protocol studies. A, aorta; L, liver; common bile duct (*arrowhead*).

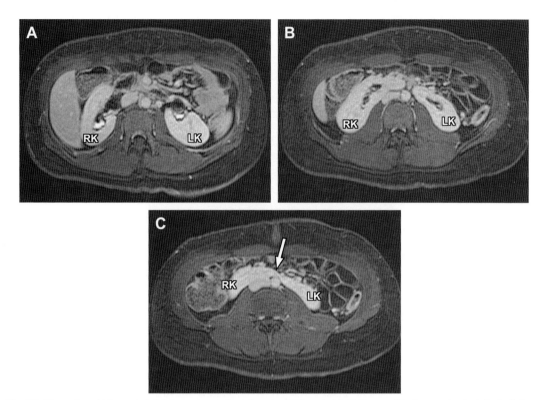

Fig. 17. Horseshoe kidney. Axial fat-suppressed postcontrast T1-weighted images (*A–C*, superior to inferior) show medial axis of the lower poles in both kidneys (LK, left kidney; RK, right kidney). There is fusion of the lower poles via a small parenchymal band (*arrow,* **Fig. 16C**).

sequence best shows the normal adrenal gland and any abnormal contour deformity or small masses.[58,59] Postgadolinium T1-weighted images in either the coronal plane or sagittal plane may be helpful in delineating renal from adrenal masses.

T2-weighted images provide information on fluid content of an adrenal lesion, with most of the metastases showing relatively higher signal intensity than adenomas.[57] The main purpose in MR imaging of adrenal glands is to further evaluate an incidentally detected mass on CT. The best approach is to compare in-phase and opposed-phase images, because adrenal adenomas lose signal on opposed-phase images because of their intracytoplasmic lipid content.[60–63] Malignant adrenal masses generally do not contain intracytoplasmic lipid. However, overlap can rarely exist with lipid-rich metastasis (such as renal cell carcinoma), whereas other benign adrenal processes like granulomatous disease may lack intracytoplasmic lipid.[64–66] Dynamic postgadolinium contrast-enhanced T1-weighted images may also be used to differentiate benign from malignant adrenal masses, with metastases enhancing more heterogeneously and retaining contrast for a longer period.[67,68]

BOWEL
Technical Considerations

There is increasing evidence that both MR imaging and CT offer advantages when compared with traditional fluoroscopic imaging studies, particularly in delineating the 3D relationship of bowel segments to one another and in evaluation of suspected extraluminal complications such as abscesses.[69] Although bowel peristalsis has traditionally limited the use of MR imaging in bowel evaluation compared with multidetector CT, newer MR imaging sequences with high temporal resolution have made bowel imaging a clinical reality. State-of-the-art MR enterography has similar diagnostic performance to that of CT enterography for the depiction of active inflammation and acute complications in Crohn disease.[70,71] The use of MR imaging for evaluation of the colon seems to be less widespread than multidetector CT, noting some discrepancy in diagnostic performance for certain-sized polyps.[72]

At our institution, the imaging protocol for bowel imaging uses sequences with very high temporal resolution to negate the effects of bowel peristalsis. Approximately 1 hour before scanning, an oral enteric contrast agent is given to promote bowel distention. A biphasic contrast agent is typically given, which is an agent that has low signal intensity on T1-weighted images and high signal intensity on T2-weighted images. At our institution, the regimen consists of 1350 mL of a sorbitol-containing barium-based oral contrast agent (VoLumen, EZ-E-M, Westbury, NY, USA) that restricts water resorption from the gut, thereby promoting bowel distention. To decrease intestinal peristalsis, 1 mg of glucagon is given intravenously. Our imaging protocol begins with axial and coronal breath-hold T2-weighted images obtained rapidly using single-shot echo-train spin-echo technique (such as SSFSE or HASTE) with full coverage of the bowel (FOV 38–42 cm). For imaging redundancy, the T2-weighted images are supplemented with axial and coronal balanced gradient echo steady-state free precession imaging such as fast imaging employing steady-state acquisition (FIESTA) or true fast imaging with steady-state procession (**Fig. 18**A). Precontrast and postcontrast imaging is performed using a coronal dynamic fat-suppressed T1-weighted spoiled gradient echo sequence (see **Fig. 18**B), followed by a delayed-phase axial fat-suppressed T1-weighted spoiled gradient echo sequence. Standardization of delayed-phase imaging within an institution has been highlighted as a means to producing consistent bowel wall

enhancement within the same patient on serial examinations.[73]

Anatomic Considerations and MR Imaging Features

The normal anatomy of the intra-abdominal gastrointestinal tract begins with the stomach, which is classically J-shaped and located in the epigastrium or left upper quadrant.[74] The stomach functions as a reservoir for ingested food and is the chief site of enzymatic digestion. Different named parts of the stomach include the gastric cardia, fundus, body, antrum, and pylorus. The cardia surrounds the cardial orifice near the gastroesophageal junction. The fundus corresponds to the raised portion of stomach above the horizontal plane of the cardial orifice. The body constitutes the dominant component of the stomach, with 2 curvatures formed from the J shape (the lesser curve comprising the shorter concave border and the greater curve comprising the longer convex border). The antrum is the wide portion of the funnel-shaped distal stomach, leading to the narrow pyloric canal with distal sphincter. The gastric mucosa forms longitudinal ridges during contraction, called gastric rugae. When filled with fluid, T2-weighted images show normal impressions of the gastric rugae and can be used to localize abnormal outpouchings such as diverticula. Postcontrast

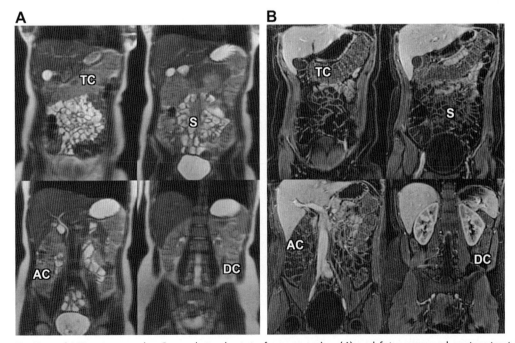

Fig. 18. Normal MR enterography. Coronal steady-state free precession (A) and fat-suppressed postcontrast (B) imaging. Note small bowel distention on using a biphasic contrast agent, resulting in high signal in (A) and low signal in (B). AC, ascending colon; DC, descending colon; S, small bowel; TC, transverse colon.

T1-weighted images show intense mucosal enhancement in the stomach, more so than other segments of bowel.[19,73]

The duodenum is located immediately downstream from the pylorus, and forms a characteristic C-shaped loop with 4 named components. The first portion, also called the duodenal bulb, has a mesentery and is the only intraperitoneal portion of the duodenum; the other segments are located in the retroperitoneum.[73] Several important anatomic relationships with neighboring structures are important to consider when looking at the retroperitoneal segments of the duodenum, including the pancreatic head, common bile duct, pancreatic duct, superior mesenteric artery (SMA), and left renal vein. The duodenojejunal junction is formed as the duodenum courses anteriorly, supported by the ligament of Treitz.[74] The jejunum and ileum comprise the largest portion of the small bowel, approximately 6 to 7 m in length. These midgut-derived structures normally fixate after 270° rotation during embryogenesis such that the jejunum lies in the left upper quadrant and the ileum occupies much of the right lower quadrant.[74] Normal bowel wall thickness is approximately 3 to 4 mm.[73] The small bowel folds or plicae circulares increase the surface area of the small bowel, with increased fold density in the jejunum and decreased fold density in the ileum.[75] With adequate bowel distention using a biphasic contrast agent, the bowel lumen is high signal intensity on T2-weighted images and balanced gradient echo steady-state free precession images with low signal intensity in the wall and folds.[69] On postcontrast imaging, the bowel wall normally shows some enhancement, but should always enhance to a lesser degree than renal cortex; this internal imaging control can be used in cases of suspected bowel inflammation.[76]

The colon is located along the periphery of the abdomen and plays an important role in fluid resorption. Several segments are generally recognized, including the cecum, ascending, transverse, descending, and sigmoid colon. Three longitudinal muscular bands called teniae coli are seen from the base of the appendix through the rectosigmoid junction. The teniae result in the characteristic bowel sacculation or haustration that occurs between the longitudinal muscle bands. The ascending and descending colon are retroperitoneal structures, whereas the transverse and sigmoid colon are intraperitoneal structures.[74] The normal bowel wall thickness of the colon is less than 4 mm, frequently imperceptible on T2-weighted images.[73] Postcontrast imaging shows some degree of enhancement, similar to small bowel.

ABDOMINAL VASCULATURE
Technical Considerations

At our institution, the abdominal vascular system is well seen on most of the standard protocols performed for other indications, particularly those with dynamic postcontrast imaging. For patients presenting for primary vascular evaluation using MR angiography, our protocol typically is based on a breath-hold precontrast and dynamic postcontrast 3D spoiled gradient echo imaging obtained in the coronal plane (**Fig. 19**). Precontrast imaging provides important information about hemorrhagic complications of aortic disease, such as intramural hematoma, which can be visually less impressive after intravenous contrast administration.[77] Because of the rapid acquisition of multiple phases of enhancement, this sequence provides both arterial and venous imaging sequences. Additional breath-hold axial balanced steady-state free precession gradient echo imaging is obtained for imaging redundancy, which provides high signal in both arteries and veins. When selectivity of flow is required, an axial 2D time-of-flight MR angiography sequence is used with a selective saturation band that can be placed superiorly for venography purposes and inferiorly for arteriography purposes. Patients with impaired renal function who cannot receive intravenous gadolinium contrast caused by a potential risk of nephrogenic systemic fibrosis can still have time-of-flight and balanced steady-state free precession MR angiography images obtained, using supplemental planes to account for the lack of 3D postcontrast imaging.

Anatomic Considerations and MR Imaging Features

The abdominal arterial circulation is generally focused on the abdominal aorta and branch vessels. The aorta is generally constant in position, averaging 2.0 cm in the suprarenal portion and 1.5 cm in the infrarenal portion.[78] Near the L4 to L5 vertebral levels, the aorta bifurcates into the bilateral common iliac arteries, which then give rise to the external and internal iliac arteries further into the pelvis. The mesenteric circulation arises along the anterior aspect of the aorta, including the celiac axis, SMA, and IMA. The celiac usually arises around the T12 level, and classically gives rise to 3 branches: the left gastric artery, common hepatic artery, and splenic artery (see **Fig. 19**).[79] An important downstream branch of the common hepatic artery is the gastroduodenal artery which courses inferiorly and gives rise to the superior pancreaticoduodenal arcade. Substantial anatomic variability is present about the celiac branches,

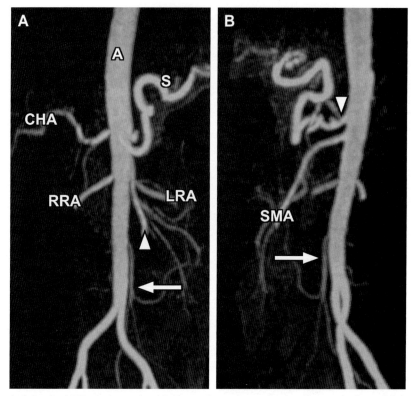

Fig. 19. Normal abdominal MR angiography. Maximum intensity projection images in frontal (*A*) and lateral (*B*) views. A, aorta; CHA, common hepatic artery; LRA, left renal artery; RRA, right renal artery; S, splenic artery. (*A*) Frontal projection easily shows the laterally oriented renal arteries, but masks evaluation of the mesenteric circulation because it is seen en face. IMA (*arrow*); SMA (*arrowhead*). (*B*) Lateral projection now shows mesenteric circulation in profile, allowing better evaluation of vessel origins. Celiac axis (*arrowhead*); IMA (*arrow*).

which may arise from the aorta discretely or from the SMA, which has been attributed to a common peritoneal embryology.[80] The SMA arises 1 to 2 cm downstream in the aorta from the celiac takeoff, coursing above the left renal vein and third portion of the duodenum. The degree of anterior angulation between the SMA and aorta has been variably reported between 38° and 90° in normal healthy individuals, with a more acute angulation noted in patients suffering from symptomatic compression of the duodenum or left renal vein.[81,82] The SMA supplies a large distribution of bowel, extending from the distal duodenum through to the splenic flexure. The inferior pancreaticoduodenal arcade is 1 of the first branches of the SMA, representing an important collateral anastomosis with the celiac axis. The IMA arises approximately 2 to 3 cm above the iliac bifurcation with a marked caudal course along its proximal segment. The IMA supplies branches to the left colon and sigmoid colon via named branches, and to the rectum through the superior hemorrhoidal artery.[80] Important collateral circulation is made with the SMA in the left

abdomen through the laterally located marginal artery of Drummond and the medially located arcade of Riolan (**Fig. 20**). Another important collateral route to consider is the arterial arcade around the rectum, which provides communication between the IMA and internal iliac artery flow via the hemorrhoidal arteries. The renal arteries are frequently located just below the takeoff of SMA, and are classically single to each kidney. The renal artery is approximately 5 to 6 mm in diameter and bifurcates into an anterior and posterior division. However, there is substantial reported variability in the number, location, and bifurcation pattern of renal arteries, including accessory renal arteries or early bifurcation patterns.[83] Several other smaller arterial branches also arise from the abdominal aorta, including paired phrenic, gonadal, and middle adrenal arteries, which are variably seen depending on scan technique and patient cooperation.

The normal venous configuration of the abdomen, seen in approximately 97% of the population, has a single IVC that forms from at the confluence of bilateral common iliac veins.[18] The IVC courses vertically along a plane situated slightly right of midline, and can nominally be divided into intrahepatic, infrahepatic-suprarenal, and infrarenal segments. The IVC contains no valves and varies in size/shape based on volume status and venous pressure. Standard venous anatomy of the abdomen evolves from a complex embryology that involves selected persistence and regression of the fetal venous circulation. Absence of the intrahepatic IVC can be attributed to inappropriate regression of the right subcardinal vein, whereas a double infrarenal IVC is associated with failed regression of the left supracardinal vein (**Figs. 21** and **22**).[84] The renal and hepatic veins constitute major venous circulations draining into the IVC; other smaller veins are variably seen on

MR venography such as gonadal, phrenic, and lumbar veins. The left renal vein is necessarily longer than the right renal vein because of anatomic location, and normally crosses anterior to the aorta. There is substantial variability of renal vein location, including a split circumaortic course of the left renal vein, reportedly seen in approximately 17% of cadaveric specimens in 1 study, as well as a solely retroaortic course, which has been reported in 2% to 3% of the population.[85,86] Duplicated renal veins are also frequently encountered because of the embryology of renovascular development, reported in up to 28% of patients.[84] The portal system is formed through venous inflow from the gastrointestinal tract, pancreas, and spleen. The extrahepatic portal vein originates at the confluence of the superior mesenteric vein and splenic vein. The inferior mesenteric vein has a variable drainage pattern, most commonly directly into the splenic vein, as is seen in 68% of the population, and less commonly into the superior mesenteric vein or directly into the splenoportal confluence.[87] The main portal vein approaches the porta hepatis and divides to provide right and left intrahepatic portal branches that subsequently arborize in the hepatic parenchyma. Several variants have been described, including a trifurcation caused by absence of the right portal trunk (seen in 10%–16% of the population) and aberrant right portal supply to segment intravenously.[88,89] The hepatic veins are traditionally comprised of the right, middle, and left hepatic veins. Anatomic variants of the hepatic venous circulation have been described, most commonly with accessory veins. In 1 series, 40% of patients had a surgically relevant accessory hepatic vein when evaluating potential preoperative liver donors, with most

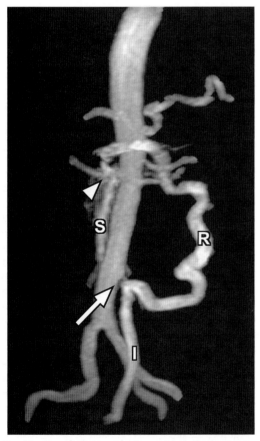

Fig. 20. Arc of Riolan. Maximum intensity projection image in frontal projection shows an enlarged collateral between the SMA (S) and engorged IMA (I), called the arc of Riolan (R), which runs in the medal aspect of the mesentery. The patient had multiple severe stenoses of the mesenteric branch origins, including the IMA (*arrow*). Reconstituted flow in the SMA (*arrowhead*).

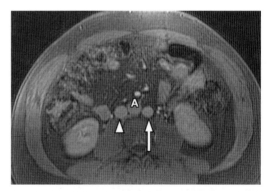

Fig. 21. Duplicated infrarenal IVC. Axial postcontrast fat-suppressed T1-weighted image shows an additional venous channel along the left para-aortic station (*arrow*), compatible with a duplicated/left-sided IVC. A, aorta; standard right-sided IVC (*arrowhead*).

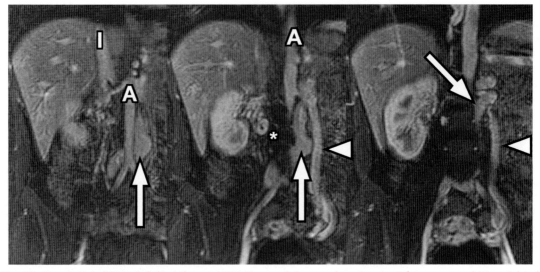

Fig. 22. Congenital absence of the infrarenal IVC. Sequential coronal postcontrast fat-suppressed T1-weighted images show absence of the expected infrarenal IVC (*asterisk*). The intrahepatic IVC is present (I). Tortuous retroperitoneal collaterals (*arrows*) and enlargement of the left gonadal vein (*arrowheads*) provide a route for venous return from the lower extremities. A, aorta.

arising in the posterior segments of the right hepatic lobe (segments VI and VII).[89]

OTHER NONVISCERAL ANATOMY OF THE ABDOMEN

There are several muscles of the abdomen that are generally included in imaging for abdominal MR imaging studies. Although high-resolution imaging of the muscles and their tendinous insertions can be performed using MR imaging, this level of detail is not frequently obtained in most abdominal MR imaging protocols. These muscles can be divided into those primarily associated with the anterior abdominal wall and posterior abdominal wall. The external oblique, internal oblique, and transversus abdominis muscles are 3 anterior abdominal wall muscles with oblique horizontal orientations, each terminating in a medially located aponeurosis.[90] The aponeuroses of the different muscles become intertwined to form an anterior and incomplete posterior rectus sheath around the vertically oriented rectus abdominis muscles.[91] The posterior abdominal wall muscles include the psoas, iliacus, and quadratus lumborum muscles. The psoas and iliacus muscles become contiguous along their inferior portion, forming the iliopsoas muscle, which acts as the primary flexor for the thigh.[74]

Because of the superior contrast resolution of MR imaging, normal lymph nodes can be easily visualized as low to intermediate signal intensity on T1-weighted imaging and intermediate to high

signal intensity on T2-weighted imaging.[92] Numerous lymph node stations are present throughout the abdomen, many of which correspond anatomically to adjacent vascular structures such as the left para-aortic or aortocaval stations. Differentiating benign from malignant lymph nodes is difficult by imaging grounds alone, and short axis size is usually applied as a discriminating feature. Most lymph nodes in the abdomen can measure up to 10 mm in short axis.[92] Nodes in the retrocrural space and porta hepatis are allowed to measure only up to 6 mm in the short axis, whereas those in the gastrohepatic ligament may measure up to 8 mm. Conversely, lymph nodes in the inguinal stations are permitted short axis dimensions of up to 15 mm. Frank internal necrosis, manifest as increased T2-weighted signal with lack of central enhancement, is highly suggestive of pathologic involvement, often by malignancy.

Most lymphatic channels are below the spatial resolution of MR imaging at conventional resolutions prescribed for abdominal indications. However, the cisterna chyli is a normal dilation of the lymphatic channels coursing through the retrocrural space, which can be seen in up to 20% of autopsy studies.[93] It can be seen in up to 15% of patients undergoing abdominal MR imaging studies, noting a higher reported frequency than with CT, which is likely because of the improved contrast resolution of MR imaging.[94] The cisterna chyli appears as a linear or saccular focus of high signal intensity on T2-weighted imaging located near the L1 to L2 vertebral levels, with no internal enhancement on postcontrast T1-weighted imaging obtained within 5 minutes from injection.[93,95]

SUMMARY

Knowledge of the normal and variant abdominal anatomy is critical for appropriate interpretation of abdominal MR imaging. Because of the large anatomic coverage required for imaging the entire abdomen, most MR imaging protocols are organ specific or targeted. Therefore, a detailed knowledge of the visceral organ anatomy complements an understanding of focused MR imaging protocols to optimize anatomic visibility and tissue contrast for each organ system in the abdomen.

REFERENCES

1. Fisher A, Siegelman ES. Body MR techniques and MR of the liver. In: Siegelman ES, editor. Body MRI. 1st edition. Philadelphia: Elsevier; 2005. p. 1–62.
2. Amis ES Jr, Butler PF, Applegate KE, et al. American College of Radiology white paper on radiation dose in medicine. J Am Coll Radiol 2007;4(5):272–84.
3. Ivancevic MK, Kwee TC, Takahara T, et al. Diffusion-weighted MR imaging of the liver at 3.0 Tesla using TRacking Only Navigator echo (TRON): a feasibility study. J Magn Reson Imaging 2009;30(5):1027–33.
4. Semelka RC, Hussain SM, Firat Z. Diagnostic approach to protocoling and interpreting MR studies of the abdomen and pelvis. In: Semelka RC, editor. Abdominal-pelvic MRI. 2nd edition. Hoboken (NJ): Wiley; 2006. p. 1–46.
5. Koh DM, Collins DJ. Diffusion-weighted MRI in the body: applications and challenges in oncology. AJR Am J Roentgenol 2007;188(6):1622–35.
6. Bitar R, Leung G, Perng R, et al. MR pulse sequences: what every radiologist wants to know but is afraid to ask. Radiographics 2006;26(2):513–37.
7. Couinaud C. Le foie: études anatomiques et chirurgicales. Paris (France): Masson; 1957. p. 74–5.
8. Braga L, Semelka RC, Armao D. Liver. In: Semelka RC, editor. Abdominal pelvic MRI. 2nd edition. Hoboken (NJ): John Wiley; 2006. p. 47–445.
9. Heiken J. Liver. In: Lee JKT, Stanley RJ, Heiken JP, editors. Computed body tomography with MR correlation. 3rd edition. Philadelphia: Lippincott-Raven; 1998. p. 701–77.
10. Mitchell DG. Focal manifestations of diffuse liver disease at MR imaging. Radiology 1992;185(1):1–11.
11. Mitchell DG, Kim I, Chang TS, et al. Fatty liver. Chemical shift phase-difference and suppression magnetic resonance imaging techniques in animals, phantoms, and humans. Invest Radiol 1991;26(12): 1041–52.

12. Taylor AJ, Dodds WJ, Erickson SJ, et al. CT of acquired abnormalities of the spleen. AJR Am J Roentgenol 1991;157(6):1213–9.
13. Carucci L, Siegelman ES. MRI of spleen. In: Siegelman ES, editor. Body MRI. 1st edition. Philadelphia: Elsevier; 2005. p. 185–205.
14. Torres GM, Terry NL, Mergo PJ, et al. MR imaging of the spleen. Magn Reson Imaging Clin N Am 1995; 3(1):39–50.
15. Donnelly LF, Emery KH, Bove KE, et al. Normal changes in the MR appearance of the spleen during early childhood. AJR Am J Roentgenol 1996;166(3): 635–9.
16. Hahn PF, Weissleder R, Stark DD, et al. MR imaging of focal splenic tumors. AJR Am J Roentgenol 1988; 150(4):823–7.
17. Runge VM, Williams NM. Dynamic contrast-enhanced magnetic resonance imaging in a model of splenic metastasis. Invest Radiol 1998;33(1):45–50.
18. Nyman R, Rhen S, Ericsson A, et al. An attempt to characterize malignant lymphoma in spleen, liver and lymph nodes with magnetic resonance imaging. Acta Radiol 1987;28(5):527–33.
19. Hamed MM, Hamm B, Ibrahim ME, et al. Dynamic MR imaging of the abdomen with gadopentetate dimeglumine: normal enhancement patterns of the liver, spleen, stomach, and pancreas. AJR Am J Roentgenol 1992;158(2):303–7.
20. Ito K, Mitchell DG, Honjo K, et al. Gadolinium-enhanced MR imaging of the spleen: artifacts and potential pitfalls. AJR Am J Roentgenol 1996; 167(5):1147–51.
21. Siegelman ES, Mitchell DG, Semelka RC. Abdominal iron deposition: metabolism, MR findings, and clinical importance. Radiology 1996;199(1):13–22.
22. Siegelman ES, Mitchell DG, Outwater E, et al. Idiopathic hemochromatosis: MR imaging findings in cirrhotic and precirrhotic patients. Radiology 1993; 188(3):637–41.
23. Sagoh T, Itoh K, Togashi K, et al. Gamna-Gandy bodies of the spleen: evaluation with MR imaging. Radiology 1989;172(3):685–7.
24. Robertson F, Leander P, Ekberg O. Radiology of the spleen. Eur Radiol 2001;11(1):80–95.
25. Sica GT, Reed MF. Case 27: intrapancreatic accessory spleen. Radiology 2000;217(1):134–7.
26. Barish MA, Yucel EK, Ferrucci JT. Magnetic resonance cholangiopancreatography. N Engl J Med 1999;341(4):258–64.
27. Yeh BM, Liu PS, Soto JA, et al. MR imaging and CT of the biliary tract. Radiographics 2009;29(6):1669–88.
28. Sodickson A, Mortele KJ, Barish MA, et al. Three-dimensional fast-recovery fast spin-echo MRCP: comparison with two-dimensional single-shot fast spin-echo techniques. Radiology 2006;238(2):549–59.
29. Zhang J, Israel GM, Hecht EM, et al. Isotropic 3D T2-weighted MR cholangiopancreatography with

parallel imaging: feasibility study. AJR Am J Roentgenol 2006;187(6):1564–70.

30. Adusumilli S, Siegelman ES. MR imaging of the gallbladder. Magn Reson Imaging Clin N Am 2002; 10(1):165–84.

31. Adusumilli S, Siegelman ES. MRI of the bile ducts, gallbladder, and pancreas. In: Siegelman ES, editor. Body MRI. 1st edition. Philadelphia: Elsevier Saunders; 2005. p. 63–128.

32. Davidoff AM, Pappas TN, Murray EA, et al. Mechanisms of major biliary injury during laparoscopic cholecystectomy. Ann Surg 1992;215(3):196–202.

33. Taourel P, Bret PM, Reinhold C, et al. Anatomic variants of the biliary tree: diagnosis with MR cholangiopancreatography. Radiology 1996;199(2):521–7.

34. Mortele KJ, Ros PR. Anatomic variants of the biliary tree: MR cholangiographic findings and clinical applications. AJR Am J Roentgenol 2001;177(2): 389–94.

35. Rizzo RJ, Szucs RA, Turner MA. Congenital abnormalities of the pancreas and biliary tree in adults. Radiographics 1995;15(1):49–68 [quiz: 147–8].

36. Sugiyama M, Baba M, Atomi Y, et al. Diagnosis of anomalous pancreaticobiliary junction: value of magnetic resonance cholangiopancreatography. Surgery 1998;123(4):391–7.

37. Sugiyama M, Atomi Y. Anomalous pancreaticobiliary junction without congenital choledochal cyst. Br J Surg 1998;85(7):911–6.

38. Fulcher AS, Turner MA. MR pancreatography: a useful tool for evaluating pancreatic disorders. Radiographics 1999;19(1):5–24 [discussion: 41–4]; [quiz: 148–9].

39. Semelka RC, Ascher SM. MR imaging of the pancreas. Radiology 1993;188(3):593–602.

40. Winston CB, Mitchell DG, Outwater EK, et al. Pancreatic signal intensity on T1-weighted fat saturation MR images: clinical correlation. J Magn Reson Imaging 1995;5(3):267–71.

41. Brailsford J, Ward J, Chalmers AG, et al. Dynamic MRI of the pancreas–gadolinium enhancement in normal tissue. Clin Radiol 1994;49(2):104–8.

42. Kanematsu M, Shiratori Y, Hoshi H, et al. Pancreas and peripancreatic vessels: effect of imaging delay on gadolinium enhancement at dynamic gradient-recalled-echo MR imaging. Radiology 2000;215(1): 95–102.

43. Soto JA, Barish MA, Yucel EK, et al. Pancreatic duct: MR cholangiopancreatography with a three-dimensional fast spin-echo technique. Radiology 1995;196(2):459–64.

44. Bret PM, Reinhold C, Taourel P, et al. Pancreas divisum: evaluation with MR cholangiopancreatography. Radiology 1996;199(1):99–103.

45. Kozu T, Suda K, Toki F. Pancreatic development and anatomical variation. Gastrointest Endosc Clin N Am 1995;5(1):1–30.

46. Morgan DE, Logan K, Baron TH, et al. Pancreas divisum: implications for diagnostic and therapeutic pancreatography. AJR Am J Roentgenol 1999; 173(1):193–8.

47. Yu J, Turner MA, Fulcher AS, et al. Congenital anomalies and normal variants of the pancreaticobiliary tract and the pancreas in adults: part 2, Pancreatic duct and pancreas. AJR Am J Roentgenol 2006; 187(6):1544–53.

48. Lehman GA, Sherman S. Diagnosis and therapy of pancreas divisum. Gastrointest Endosc Clin N Am 1998;8(1):55–77.

49. Lecesne R, Stein L, Reinhold C, et al. MR cholangiopancreatography of annular pancreas. J Comput Assist Tomogr 1998;22(1):85–6.

50. Urayama S, Kozarek R, Ball T, et al. Presentation and treatment of annular pancreas in an adult population. Am J Gastroenterol 1995;90(6):995–9.

51. Hricak H, Crooks L, Sheldon P, et al. Nuclear magnetic resonance imaging of the kidney. Radiology 1983;146(2):425–32.

52. Newhouse JH, Markisz JA, Kazam E. Magnetic resonance imaging of the kidneys. Cardiovasc Intervent Radiol 1986;8(5–6):351–66.

53. Runge VM, Clanton JA, Partain CL, et al. Respiratory gating in magnetic resonance imaging at 0.5 Tesla. Radiology 1984;151(2):521–3.

54. Soila KP, Viamonte M Jr, Starewicz PM. Chemical shift misregistration effect in magnetic resonance imaging. Radiology 1984;153(3):819–20.

55. Zagoria R. Genitourinary radiology–the requisites. 2nd edition. St Louis (MO): Mosby; 2004. p. 53–61.

56. Blake MA, Cronin CG, Boland GW. Adrenal imaging. AJR Am J Roentgenol 2010;194(6):1450–60.

57. Mitchell DG, Nascimento AB, Alam F, et al. Normal adrenal gland: in vivo observations, and high-resolution in vitro chemical shift MR imaging-histologic correlation. Acad Radiol 2002;9(4):430–6.

58. Semelka RC, Shoenut JP, Lawrence PH, et al. Evaluation of adrenal masses with gadolinium enhancement and fat-suppressed MR imaging. J Magn Reson Imaging 1993;3(2):337–43.

59. Lee MJ, Mayo-Smith WW, Hahn PF, et al. State-of-the-art MR imaging of the adrenal gland. Radiographics 1994;14(5):1015–29 [discussion: 1029–32].

60. Fujiyoshi F, Nakajo M, Fukukura Y, et al. Characterization of adrenal tumors by chemical shift fast low-angle shot MR imaging: comparison of four methods of quantitative evaluation. AJR Am J Roentgenol 2003;180(6):1649–57.

61. Korobkin M, Giordano TJ, Brodeur FJ, et al. Adrenal adenomas: relationship between histologic lipid and CT and MR findings. Radiology 1996; 200(3):743–7.

62. Mitchell DG, Crovello M, Matteucci T, et al. Benign adrenocortical masses: diagnosis with chemical shift MR imaging. Radiology 1992;185(2):345–51.

63. Tsushima Y, Ishizaka H, Matsumoto M. Adrenal masses: differentiation with chemical shift, fast low-angle shot MR imaging. Radiology 1993;186(3):705–9.

64. Ferrozzi F, Bova D. CT and MR demonstration of fat within an adrenal cortical carcinoma. Abdom Imaging 1995;20(3):272–4.

65. Shinozaki K, Yoshimitsu K, Honda H, et al. Meta-static adrenal tumor from clear-cell renal cell carcinoma: a pitfall of chemical shift MR imaging. Abdom Imaging 2001;26(4):439–42.

66. Yamada T, Saito H, Moriya T, et al. Adrenal carcinoma with a signal loss on chemical shift magnetic resonance imaging. J Comput Assist Tomogr 2003; 27(4):606–8.

67. Krestin GP, Freidmann G, Fishbach R, et al. Evaluation of adrenal masses in oncologic patients: dynamic contrast-enhanced MR vs CT. J Comput Assist Tomogr 1991;15(1):104–10.

68. Korobkin M, Dunnick NR. Characterization of adrenal masses. AJR Am J Roentgenol 1995; 164(3):643–4.

69. Fidler J. MR imaging of the small bowel. Radiol Clin North Am 2007;45(2):317–31.

70. Siddiki HA, Fidler JL, Fletcher JG, et al. Prospective comparison of state-of-the-art MR enterography and CT enterography in small-bowel Crohn's disease. AJR Am J Roentgenol 2009;193(1):113–21.

71. Schmidt S, Guibal A, Meuwly JY, et al. Acute complications of Crohn's disease: comparison of multidetector-row computed tomographic enterography with magnetic resonance enterography. Digestion 2010;82(4):229–38.

72. Thornton E, Morrin MM, Yee J. Current status of MR colonography. Radiographics 2010;30(1):201–18.

73. Martin DR, Lauenstein TC, Ascher SM, et al. Gastrointestinal tract. In: Semelka RC, editor. Abdominal-pelvic MRI. 2nd edition. Hoboken (NJ): Wiley; 2006. p. 677–812.

74. Moore KL, Dalley AF. Abdomen. Clinically oriented anatomy. 4th edition. Baltimore (MD): Lippincott Williams & Wilkins; 1999. p.174–330.

75. Levine MS, Rubesin SE, Laufer I. Pattern approach for diseases of mesenteric small bowel on barium studies. Radiology 2008;249(2):445–60.

76. Messaris E, Chandolias N, Grand D, et al. Role of magnetic resonance enterography in the management of Crohn disease. Arch Surg 2010;145(5):471–5.

77. Sakamoto I, Sueyoshi E, Uetani M. MR imaging of the aorta. Radiol Clin North Am 2007;45(3):485–97, viii.

78. Kaufman J. Abdominal aorta and iliac arteries. In: Vascular and interventional radiology. The requisites. 1st edition. Philadelphia: Mosby; 2004. p. 246–85.

79. Rao AS, Rhee RY. Coverage of the celiac artery during TEVAR: is it ever appropriate? Semin Vasc Surg 2009;22(3):152–8.

80. Kaufman J. Visceral arteries. In: Vascular and interventional radiology. The requisites. 1st edition. Philadelphia: Mosby; 2004. p. 286–322.

81. Kurklinsky AK, Rooke TW. Nutcracker phenomenon and nutcracker syndrome. Mayo Clin Proc 2010; 85(6):552–9.

82. Cuellar I, Calabria H, Quiroga Gomez S, et al. Nutcracker or left renal vein compression phenomenon: multidetector computed tomography findings and clinical significance. Eur Radiol 2005;15(8): 1745–51.

83. Liu PS, Platt JF. CT angiography of the renal circulation. Radiol Clin North Am 2010;48(2):347–65, viii–ix.

84. Kaufman J. Inferior vena cava and tributaries. In: Vascular and interventional radiology. The requisites. 1st edition. Philadelphia: Mosby; 2004. p. 350–76.

85. Kawamoto S, Fishman EK. MDCT angiography of living laparoscopic renal donors. Abdom Imaging 2006;31(3):361–73.

86. Kawamoto S, Montgomery RA, Lawler LP, et al. Multi-detector row CT evaluation of living renal donors prior to laparoscopic nephrectomy. Radiographics 2004;24(2):453–66.

87. Sakaguchi T, Suzuki S, Morita Y, et al. Analysis of anatomic variants of mesenteric veins by 3-dimensional portography using multidetector-row computed tomography. Am J Surg 2010;200(1):15–22.

88. Atri M, Bret PM, Fraser-Hill MA. Intrahepatic portal venous variations: prevalence with US. Radiology 1992;184(1):157–8.

89. Guiney MJ, Kruskal JB, Sosna J, et al. Multi-detector row CT of relevant vascular anatomy of the surgical plane in split-liver transplantation. Radiology 2003; 229(2):401–7.

90. Bendavid R, Howarth D. Transversalis fascia rediscovered. Surg Clin North Am 2000;80(1):25–33.

91. Fukuda T, Sakamoto I, Kohzaki S, et al. Spontaneous rectus sheath hematomas: clinical and radiological features. Abdom Imaging 1996;21(1):58–61.

92. Torigian DA, Siegelman ES. MRI of the retroperitoneum and peritoneum. In: Siegelman ES, editor. Body MRI. 1st edition. Philadelphia: Elsevier; 2005. p. 63–127.

93. Pinto PS, Sirlin CB, Andrade-Barreto OA, et al. Cisterna chyli at routine abdominal MR imaging: a normal anatomic structure in the retrocrural space. Radiographics 2004;24(3):809–17.

94. Smith TR, Grigoropoulos J. The cisterna chyli: incidence and characteristics on CT. Clin Imaging 2002;26(1):18–22.

95. Restrepo CS, Eraso A, Ocazionez D, et al. The diaphragmatic crura and retrocrural space: normal imaging appearance, variants, and pathologic conditions. Radiographics 2008;28(5):1289–305.

Normal and Variant Pelvic Anatomy on MRI

Ashish P. Wasnik, MBBS, MD[a], Michael B. Mazza, MD[a],
Peter S. Liu, MD[a,b],*

KEYWORDS
- Pelvic anatomy • MRI • Variant anatomy • Pelvic viscera

Because of its superior tissue contrast, native multiplanar capabilities, and nonionizing technique, magnetic resonance imaging (MRI) is well suited for evaluation of the pelvis. Although ultrasound is frequently indicated for the primary evaluation of suspected genitourinary pathology in both men and women, it can be limited by body habitus, depth of acoustic penetration, and ability to discriminate between specific tissue types.[1,2] Knowledge of normal pelvic anatomy on MRI is critical for proper interpretation, in particular the standard visceral organ appearances, commonly encountered variants, and pathology mimics. Because most pelvic MRI studies are targeted toward an organ or area of interest, this article discusses the protocol strategies and relevant anatomy in a segmented/organ-specific manner, using gender as a broad split given the substantial variance in relevant organs.

FEMALE PELVIS
Technical Considerations

At the authors' institution, the female pelvis protocol is performed for suspected ovarian, uterine, vaginal, or bladder pathology; a separate protocol is used for high-resolution imaging of the female urethra. Studies are performed using a phased-array surface coil and intramuscular injection of an antiperistaltic agent to suppress bowel motion, which improves visualization of the adnexal and peritoneal surfaces.[2,3]

The basic female pelvis protocol begins with a coronal T2-weighted single-shot echo-train spin-echo technique (such as single-shot fast spin-echo [SSFSE] or half-Fourier acquisition single-shot turbo spin-echo [HASTE]), with wide field of view (FOV) to include portions of the kidneys, due to the coexistent risk of renal anomalies in the setting of suspected genitourinary developmental disorders.[4] Subsequently, a sagittal T2-weighted fast spin-echo sequence is used to delineate the uterine lie, demonstrate the zonal anatomy of the uterus, and provide improved anatomic landmarks for subsequent uterine image planning (**Fig. 1**). Both short-axis and long-axis T2-weighted fast spin-echo images are then obtained to provide redundant detail of the uterine zonal anatomy and optimize evaluation of the external uterine contour (**Figs. 2 and 3**). T1-weighted imaging is initially accomplished using a breath-hold spoiled gradient-echo sequence in which both in-phase and opposed-phase echoes are recorded (**Figs. 4–6**). Subsequently, T1-weighted imaging using chemical fat suppression is performed, which aids in the differentiation of lipid and hemorrhagic/proteinaceous pathologies on T1-weighted imaging. Additional postcontrast images are obtained using the same sequence (see **Figs. 4–6**). If a patient is evaluated for fibroid disease and potential uterine artery embolization, a dynamic oblique coronal magnetic resonance angiography sequence augments the normal precontrast and postcontrast axial imaging, which

[a] Department of Radiology, University of Michigan Health System, 1500 East Medical Center Drive, Ann Arbor, MI 48109-0030, USA
[b] Department of Vascular Surgery, University of Michigan Health System, 1500 East Medical Center Drive, Ann Arbor, MI 48109-0030, USA
* Corresponding author. Department of Radiology, University of Michigan Health System, 1500 East Medical Center Drive, Ann Arbor, MI 48109-0030.
E-mail address: peterliu@umich.edu

Magn Reson Imaging Clin N Am 19 (2011) 547–566
doi:10.1016/j.mric.2011.05.001

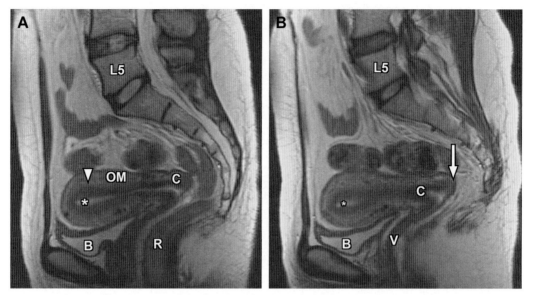

Fig. 1. Sagittal T2-weighted images of the female pelvis in midline (*A*) and paramidline (*B*) locations. The zonal anatomy of the uterus is well demonstrated on T2-weighted images, with high signal intensity in the endometrium (*asterisk*) and characteristic low signal intensity of the junctional zone (*arrowhead*). Outer myometrium demonstrates intermediate signal intensity between the two other uterine layers. The cervix is well seen in longitudinal dimension, noting contiguity of the dark fibromuscular stroma with the uterine junctional zone. The posterior fornix (*arrow*) is formed from the posterior reflection/interface of the exocervix and the vagina. B, bladder; C, cervix; L5, L5 vertebral level; OM, outer myometrium; R, rectum; V, vagina.

aids in prediction of anomalous ovarian arterial supply to uterine fibroids.[5]

For specific evaluation of the female urethra, a high-resolution protocol is employed. Most patients are examined using an endoluminal coil placed in the vagina to improve signal-to-noise ratio at higher spatial resolutions.[6] The protocol begins with axial, sagittal, and coronal T2-weighted fast spin-echo imaging sequences using a focused small FOV (**Fig. 7**A, C). Subsequently, precontrast axial T1-weighted spin-echo imaging is performed with a similar small FOV. Chemical fat suppression is then added to this T1-weighted sequence, which is repeated for both precontrast and postcontrast imaging (see **Fig. 7**B). In patients who are unable to tolerate local coil placement in the vagina, the female pelvis protocol with phased-array surface coil can be substituted, focusing mostly on the perineum rather than the uterus; in this setting, long-axis and short-axis T2-weighted imaging is converted to traditional axial and coronal planes.

Anatomic Considerations and MRI Features

Magnetic resonance has a significant role in evaluation of the pelvic abnormalities, including uterine, ovarian, cervical, adnexal, and congenital abnormalities. A better understanding of anatomy remains crucial in the evaluation of congenital abnormalities as well as in characterization of a lesion and its extent.

Uterus and cervix

The uterus can be divided into 3 segments: fundus, body, and cervix. The uterine body or corpus consists of 3 layers; from central to peripheral, these include the endometrium, junctional zone, and myometrium.

The endometrium is the central most portion of the uterus, with a varying thickness that changes during the menstrual cycle—it is wider during the secretory phase than during follicular phase or menstruation.[7–9] The normal endometrial thickness varies depending on age, with thickness of less than 10 mm considered normal in reproductive age women, whereas a thickness of less than 5 mm is considered normal in postmenopausal women.[7] Women on hormonal replacement therapy can have endometrial thickness ranging from 5 to 8 mm. The endometrium is typically high signal on T2-weighted images (see **Figs. 1–3**), although not as high signal as simple fluid in the adjacent urinary bladder and homogeneous low signal intensity on precontrast T1-weighted images (see **Figs. 4–7**).

The junctional zone represents the innermost layer of the myometrium and demonstrates a characteristic low signal intensity relative to myometrium

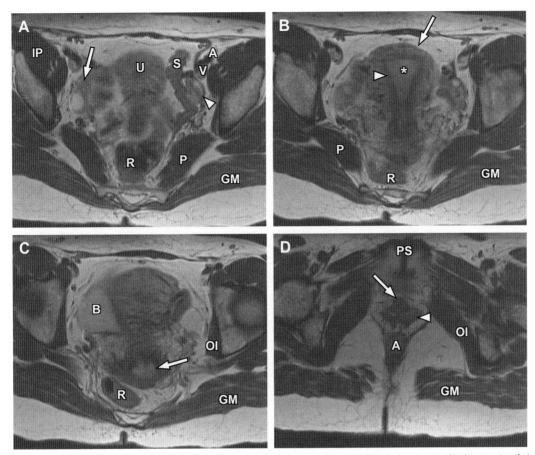

Fig. 2. (*A*) Oblique T2-weighted long-axis image of the pelvis, superior cut through uterus. The long-axis of the uterus is partially visualized on this image. Several pelvic structures are well delineated, including right ovary (*arrow*) and left ovary (*arrowhead*). (*B*) Oblique T2-weighted long-axis image of the pelvis, middle cut through uterus. This long-axis view of the uterus shows the external uterine contour (*arrow*) in a single image, in this case slightly convex outward. The zonal anatomy is well seen on this central uterine image, including endometrium (*asterisk*) and junctional zone (*arrowhead*). (*C*) Oblique T2-weighted long-axis image of the pelvis, inferior cut through uterus. The uterus is only partially visualized at this level. The cervix and upper vagina, however, are now in plane (exocervix [*arrow*]). (*D*) Oblique T2-weighted long-axis image of the pelvis toward the perineum. At this level, the urethra (*arrow*) and vagina (*arrowhead*) are well seen. The anal canal is also visible. A (*A*), external iliac artery; A (*C*), anal canal; B, bladder; GM, gluteus maximus muscle; IP, iliopsoas muscle; OI, obturator internus muscle; PS, pubic symphysis; P, piriformis muscle; R, rectum; S, sigmoid colon; V, external iliac vein.

on T2-weighted images (see **Figs. 1–3**), likely from a multifactorial basis.[10] These described factors include the presence of compact smooth muscles, decreased water content of the cells versus the outer myometrium, and increased number and size of nuclei compared with outer myometrium.[10–12] The normal junctional zone can vary in size, but a thickness greater than 12 mm is considered abnormal.[10,13,14] The junctional zone can be poorly demarcated in postmenopausal women.

The outer myometrium is structurally different than the junctional zone, with increased cellular free water and decreased cell packing/density. This results in intermediate increased signal intensity on T2-weighted images (see **Figs. 1–3**),

substantially higher than the junctional zone but generally lower than the hyperintense endometrium. The entire uterus is of intermediate signal intensity on T1-weighted images relative to muscle with no clear demarcation of different zones (see **Figs. 4–7**).[15]

The cervix is separated from the uterine body by the internal os. Three discrete cervical zones can be identified on high-resolution T2-weighted images. The central hyperintense zone is formed by the endocervical canal with its mucosa, secretions, and plica palmatae/longitudinal folds. Peripheral to this, there is a middle layer, which represents the inner fibromuscular stroma, characterized by hypointense features on T2-weighted imaging due to

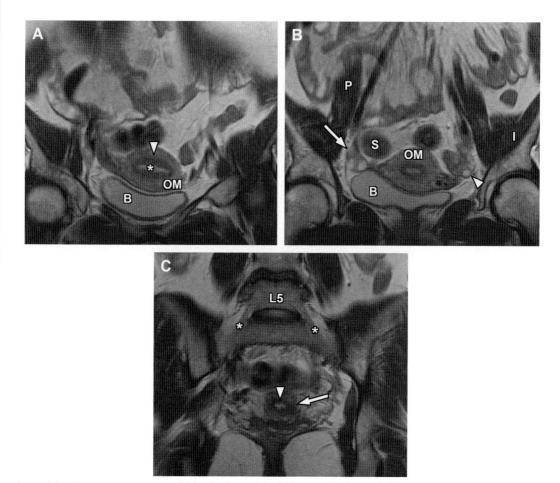

Fig. 3. (*A*) Oblique T2-weighted short-axis image of the pelvis, anterior cut through the uterus. Zonal anatomy is well demonstrated on short-axis imaging, including endometrium (*asterisk*), junctional zone (*arrowhead*), and outer myometrium. (*B*) Oblique T2-weighted short-axis image of the pelvis, central cut through the uterus. Zonal anatomy is gain well seen though uterine size is decreasing toward the lower uterine segment; only the outer myometrium is marked. Both ovaries are demonstrated (right ovary [*arrow*]; left ovary [*arrowhead*]). (*C*) Oblique T2-weighted short-axis image of the pelvis, posterior cut through the uterus. Cervix is now seen (*arrow*). Longitudinal fold of the cervical folds/plicae palmatae is well seen in cross section (*arrowhead*). Exiting nerve L5 roots (*asterisk*) are well seen given slight obliquity of image. B, bladder; I, iliacus muscle; L5, L5 vertebral body; OM, outer myometrium; P, psoas muscle; S, sigmoid colon.

fibrous stroma and dense smooth muscle. The peripheral outer layer demonstrates a more modest signal intensity, often low-intermediate signal on T2-weighted images, corresponding to the outer fibromuscular stroma. The inner fibromuscular stroma/middle layer is frequently contiguous with the junctional zone in many women, whereas the outermost layer may be contiguous with the outer uterine myometrium.[16–18] On T1-weighted images, there is no apparent distinction between different layers of the cervix; however, after the administration of intravenous gadolinium contrast, the endocervical mucosa enhances more rapidly than the fibromuscular stroma.[17,19]

Congenital uterine anomalies comprise a wide spectrum of variant anatomy. The true prevalence of uterine anomalies has been difficult to assess, with varying reported rates between 0.16% and 10%, often confounded by selection bias or variance in classification schemes.[4] Abnormal uterine configurations are typically related to developmental problems of the paramesonephric or müllerian ducts in the first trimester fetus. The paired müllerian ducts join together to form the uterus and upper vagina. After fusion, a midline septum is resorbed as the uterus assumes its normal configuration. Conceptually, müllerian fusion abnormalities can be broadly characterized into 3 categories: agenesis/hypoplasia, defects in vertical fusion, and defects in lateral fusion.[18] The modern and widely used classification scheme developed by the American Fertility Society

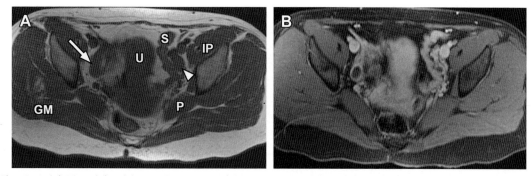

Fig. 4. Axial T1-weighted image in upper pelvis, precontrast (*A*) and fat-suppressed postcontrast (*B*). Zonal anatomy of the uterus (U) is not well seen on T1-weighted images. The follicular architecture of the ovaries (right ovary [*arrow*], left ovary [*arrowhead*]) is also not as well seen as T2-weighted images, although some follicles are more easily seen on postcontrast imaging due to lack of internal enhancement. Muscular architecture is well depicted, including iliopsoas muscle (IP), gluteus maximus muscle (GM), and piriformis muscle (P). S, sigmoid colon.

divides congenital anomalies into 7 discrete classes; associated vaginal or cervical abnormalities are reported as subsets of the major classes.[20] Although many cases can be placed into a single category, it is possible for individual cases to overlap classes or fall along a spectrum of classical disease.

Disorders of agenesis and hypoplasia form the basis for class I anomalies, usually resulting from failure of müllerian duct development before potential fusion. Class I anomalies account for approximately 5% to 10% of all müllerian fusion anomalies.[4] Classically, complete bilateral agenesis of the entire uterus and upper vagina is termed, *Mayer-Rokitansky-Küster-Hauser syndrome* (**Fig. 8**). In 10% of such cases, isolated vaginal agenesis may be present with a rudimentary or obstructed uterine remnant in place.[4,18] Clinically, these patients present with normal female phenotype but demonstrate primary amenorrhea. MRI demonstrates normal female gonads/ovaries but agenesis of the uterus and upper vagina (see **Fig. 8**).

Class II anomalies result from failure of a single müllerian duct to develop normally, causing an asymmetry of the mature uterus called a unicornuate uterus (**Fig. 9**). This accounts for approximately 20% of all müllerian fusion anomalies.[4] There are 3 general subtypes, occurring in approximately similar frequencies, including an isolated single horn, a rudimentary second horn without functional endometrium, and a rudimentary second horn containing an endometrial segment.[18] In the latter situation, the endometrial tissue/cavity may or may not communicate with the endometrial space in the normal horn on the contralateral side—noncommunication is more common than communication by approximately a 2:1 ratio. Unicornuate uterus can be clinically occult, but the presence of a noncommunicating rudimentary

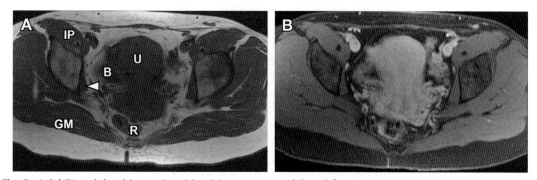

Fig. 5. Axial T1-weighted image in mid pelvis, precontrast (*A*) and fat-suppressed postcontrast (*B*). The uterus remains relatively homogeneous is signal intensity, with only subtle differential signal on postcontrast imaging to suggest zonal anatomy. Bladder is partially visualized, with low signal intensity expected for normal urine. Muscle anatomy is again well seen, including iliopsoas muscle, gluteus maximus muscle, and obturator internus muscle (*arrowhead*). B, bladder; GM, gluteus maximum; IP, iliopsoas muscle; R, rectum; U, uterus.

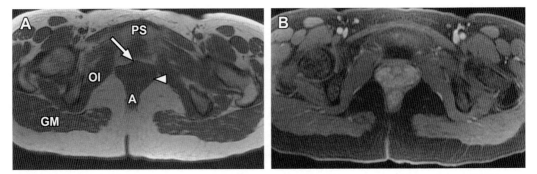

Fig. 6. Axial T1-weighted image in lower pelvis, precontrast (*A*) and fat-suppressed postcontrast (*B*). The structural anatomy seen at this level on T2-weighed images is more difficult to appreciate, particularly on precontrast T1-weighted images. Urethra (*arrow*) and vagina (*arrowhead*) are present anteriorly, whereas anal canal is present posteriorly. A, anal canal; GM, gluteus maximus muscle; OI, obturator Internus muscle; PS, pubic symphysis.

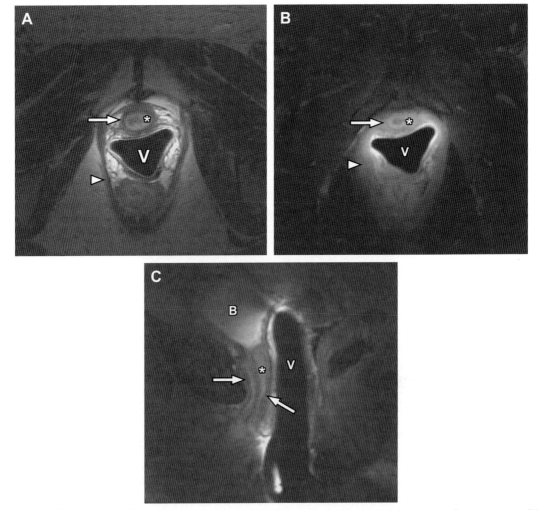

Fig. 7. Small FOV urethral imaging, including axial T2 weighted (*A*), axial fat-suppressed postcontrast T1 weighted (*B*), and sagittal T2 weighted (*C*). The concentric layers of the female urethra are well depicted, including high signal intensity submucosa (*asterisk*) and low signal intensity outer muscular layer (*arrows*). Vagina is distended with air due to indwelling receiver coil. Levator ani muscle group (*arrowhead*). B, bladder; V, vagina.

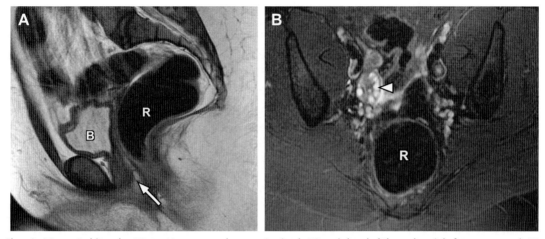

Fig. 8. Mayer-Rokitansky-Küster-Hauser syndrome. Sagittal T2-weighted (*A*) and axial fat-suppressed T2-weighted (*B*) images demonstrate urinary bladder (B) and rectum (R). There is no uterus, however, seen in the midline. Diminutive outer vagina/introitus (*arrow*) was seen on physical examination. Higher in the pelvis, normal ovaries were demonstrated (right ovary [*arrowhead*]), confirming female gonads.

horn is often associated with dysmenorrhea and hematometra. Surgery is often indicated for rudimentary horns that have associated endometrial tissue, regardless of whether or not they communicate, due to potential pregnancy issues and symptomatic relief, respectively. On MRI, unicornuate uterus has a curvilinear shape resembling a banana with normal zonal differentiation in the mature horn. The presence of a rudimentary horn should be noted, though the zonal anatomy may be absent if there is no functional endometrial tissue.[4]

Class III and IV anomalies represent fusion defects between the paired müllerian ducts, including incomplete midline fusion (class III,

bicornuate uterus) and near total failure of midline fusion (class IV, uterus didelphys). Together, these account for approximately 15% of all müllerian fusion anomalies, with bicornuate uterus more common than uterus didelphys by approximately a 2:1 ratio.[4] A bicornuate uterus has cephalad separation of the uterine horns, with some midline fusion seen along the caudal margin of the uterine body or lower uterine segment (**Fig. 10**). Duplication of the cervix is variable in bicornuate uterus, offering both single (unicollis) and double (bicollis) cervix subtypes. Uterus didelphys has 2 widely splayed uterine horns with almost no observed midline fusion (**Fig. 11**) extending through the

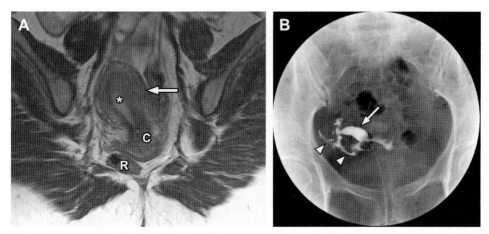

Fig. 9. Unicornuate uterus. Oblique T2-weighted long-axis image (*A*) and fluoroscopic spot image from hysterosalpingography (*B*). Rather than assuming a normal triangular shape, the uterus (*arrow*) has a curvilinear shape, similar to a banana. Normal zonal anatomy is seen, including hyperintense endometrium (*asterisk*). Cervix (C) and rectum (R) are both demonstrated on MRI image. Unicornuate uterine configuration is confirmed on hysterosalpingogram with free spill of contrast through the single horn and tube (*arrowheads*).

lower uterine segment; duplicated cervices are present.[18] On MRI, both entities are characterized by a split uterine horns that demonstrate zonal uterine anatomy. The key feature is a deep concavity of the expected uterine fundus, with a cleft of at least 1 cm diagnostic. Because of the multiplanar nature of MRI, this determination is straightforward on oblique imaging obtained along the uterine long axis. Once the fundal cleft is established, attention is turned to degree of midline fusion, either partial or near absent, to differentiate between bicornuate uterus and uterus didelphys. Presence of 2 cervices cannot be relied on for differentiation because it is present in both bicornuate uterus bicollis subtype and uterus didelphys.

Accounting for approximately 55% of all müllerian fusion anomalies, the septate uterus (class V) is the most common uterine anomaly (Fig. 12).[4] The developmental defect associated with septate uterus occurs after midline fusion, during the septal resorption phase, including both partial and total failure of septal resorption. The resultant longitudinal septum extends caudally from the uterine fundus and is termed complete if it extends to the external cervical os; approximately 25% of patients have septal extension into the upper vagina.[4] Because of differences in treatment for patients with septate uterus versus those with bicornuate or didelphys configurations, differentiating these entities is critical. On MRI, a septate uterus shows a normal configuration, either convex outward, flat, or minimally concave with a fundal cleft/depth of less than 1 cm on long-axis imaging. The signal intensity of the septum is important, because muscular septa demonstrate similar characteristics to background myometrium, whereas fibrous septa are generally thinner with dark signal on T2-weighted images.

The final 2 classes of müllerian fusion anomalies are unique. Class VI refers to an arcuate configuration, which some authors consider a normal variant rather than a müllerian fusion anomaly. On MRI, an arcuate configuration has a broad-based shallow bulge of the inner fundal myometrial contour, with a normal outer fundal contour. Class VII is a specific uterine configuration related to in utero exposure to diethylstilbestrol (DES), a synthetic estrogen that was thought to decrease the rate of pregnancy loss in patients with prior spontaneous abortions or premature deliveries. In utero DES exposure was shown to interfere with embryologic genital tract development, causing resultant structural abnormalities in the term fetus, and was discontinued in 1971. Classically, the anomaly linked to prior DES exposure was a hypoplastic uterus with a T-shaped configuration of the endometrial cavity. Several other anomalies of the cervix and fallopian tubes have also been reported.

Both physiologic events and acquired defects can alter the apparent uterine anatomy. Functional myometrial contractions occur in the junctional zone and can distort the endometrium, but generally do not affect the myometrium (Fig. 13).[21–23] Although commonly seen in gravid uterus, they can be present in the nongravid uterus as well.

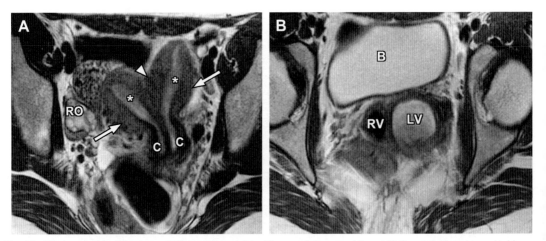

Fig. 10. Bicornuate bicollis uterus. Oblique T2-weighted long-axis images (A and B) through the uterus and lower pelvis, demonstrating 2 uterine horns (arrows) with deep fundal cleft (arrowhead) but some maintained midline fusion. Normal zonal anatomy is present in both horns (endometrium [asterisk]). Duplicated cervices are present, and lower images demonstrate duplication of the upper vagina with tampon in right hemivagina and obstructed left hemivagina. B, bladder; C, cervices; LV, left hemivagina; RO, right ovary; RV, right hemivagina.

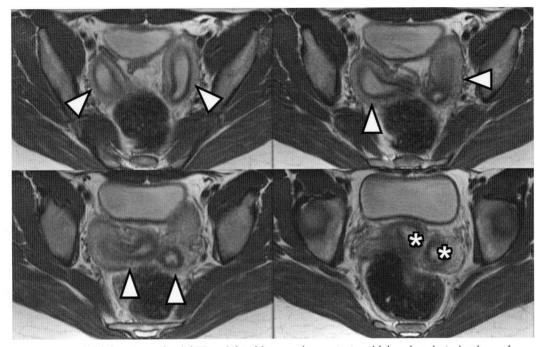

Fig. 11. Uterus didelphys. Several axial T2-weighted images demonstrate widely splayed uterine horns (*arrowheads*) with no midline fusion. Duplicated cervices are also present (*asterisk*).

The rounded nature of a contraction can mimic a fibroid or adenomyosis.[22] Contractions should resolve or change, however, during the course of the MRI study. After cesarean section, a small scar/defect is present along the lower uterine segment (**Fig. 14**). During the early postpartum period, this scar may demonstrate high signal on both T1-weighted and T2-weighted images due to subacute hematoma in the uterine incision.[24]

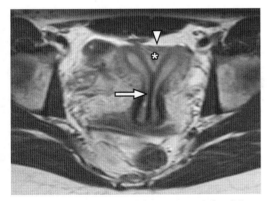

Fig. 12. Septate uterus. Oblique T2-weighted long-axis image demonstrates flat outer uterine contour (*arrowhead*) with mixed muscular (*asterisk*) and fibrous (*arrow*) septum coursing through the midline, including extension into the cervix.

Vagina

The vagina is a fibromuscular tube measuring approximately 7 to 9 cm in length, extending from the vulva inferiorly to the cervix superiorly and lying between the bladder and rectum. It is attached to the levator ani at the level of the urogenital diaphragm. It is lined by estrogen-sensitive stratified squamous epithelium. The layers of the vagina are the inner mucosal layer, middle submucosal/muscular layer, and outer adventitial layer consisting of a vaginal venous plexus. For descriptive purposes the vagina is divided into thirds, with the lower third defined as below the level of the bladder base with the urethra seen immediately anterior to it. The middle third corresponds to the level of the bladder base, whereas the upper third corresponds to the lateral vaginal fornices. The arterial supply is from a network of vessels formed by anastomosis between the vaginal and uterine branches of the internal iliac artery, with the mid and lower thirds of the vagina supplied by the middle rectal artery and internal pudendal arteries. Venous drainage is via the uterine and vaginal venous plexuses into the internal iliac veins.

The vulva is comprised of the mons pubis, the labia majora and minora, the clitoris, the vestibular bulb, vestibular glands, and the vestibule of the vagina. Blood supply is from branches of the external and internal pudendal arteries.

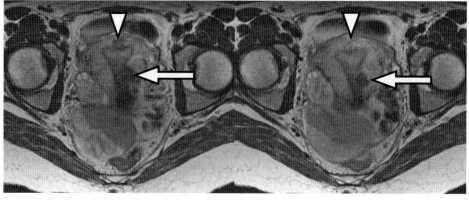

Fig. 13. Functional myometrial contraction. Oblique T2-weighted long-axis images taken several minutes apart demonstrate a focal low signal intensity near the uterine fundus (*arrowhead*), which is present on the first image (*left*) but not seen on the repeat image several minutes later (*right*), compatible with a myometrial contraction. Note slight indentation on the endometrial surface associated with this contraction. Fibroid (*arrow*).

The vaginal layers are best seen on T2-weighted images.[25] The vaginal mucosa with intraluminal fluid demonstrates high signal intensity on T2-weighted images and low signal intensity on T1-weighted images. The submucosal and the muscularis layer are low signal intensity on both

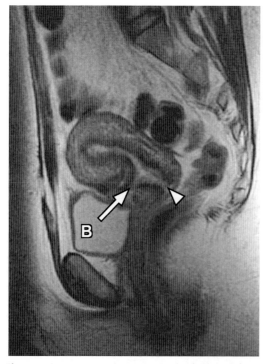

Fig. 14. Cesarean section scar. Sagittal T2-weighted image demonstrates anterior linear defect in the lower uterine segment (*arrow*) compatible with cesarean section scar. Normal cervix is noted more posteriorly (*arrowhead*), in line with the longitudinal axis of the uterus. B, bladder.

T1-weighted and T2-weighted imaging. The adventitial layer demonstrates high signal intensity on T2-weighted images due to presence of well-developed venous plexus that has slow flow.[18,25–27] After intravenous gadolinium administration, the vaginal mucosa enhances. Signal characteristics of the vaginal wall and thickness of the mucosal layer vary depending on the phase of the menstrual cycle, paralleling estrogen levels.[25,28] The vulva shows low to intermediate signal intensity on T1-weighted imaging and slightly higher signal intensity on T2-weighted imaging.[28]

Female urethra

Female urethra is thin-walled tubular muscular channel, measuring approximately 40 mm in length, coursing anteroinferiorly from internal urethral meatus located at bladder trigone and terminating in an external urethral meatus anterior to the vagina. Tiny glands in the periurethral tissues (Skene glands) secrete mucus during sexual intercourse. The lower two-thirds of the urethra is lined by stratified squamous epithelium and the proximal one-third is lined by transitional epithelium. The urethra has 3 layers, including an inner mucosal layer, a vascular submucosal layer, and an outer muscular layer. Urethropelvic ligaments provide structural support to the urethra.

T2-weighted sequence using endoluminal coils is best suited for demonstration the urethral zonal anatomy.[26,29,30] The zonal anatomy is almost similar to the vaginal layers on T2-weighted images, with low signal intensity inner mucosal layer, a high signal intensity vascular submucosal layer and low signal intensity outer muscular layer, giving a target appearance on transverse images (see **Fig. 7**A).[31,32] The intraluminal fluid or urine is high signal intensity on T2-weighted images.[18]

The zonal anatomy is indistinct on noncontrast T1-weighted images with increased enhancement of the submucosal layer on postgadolinium T1-weighted images (see **Fig. 7**B). In postmenopausal women, the zonal anatomy may be poorly defined. In patients with stress incontinence, atrophy of the outer muscular layer can be noted.[33]

Ovaries

The ovaries are located within a depression in pelvic sidewall, called the ovarian fossa. The location of the ovaries may vary based on multiparity, size of uterus, and bladder distension. The ovaries are held in position by several ovarian suspensory ligaments.[34] Arterial vascular supply to the ovaries is provided by an ovarian artery, directly branching from the abdominal aorta below the origin of renal arteries. Small anastomoses exist with channels originating from the uterine arteries. The venous drainage occurs through the gonadal vein, with the right gonadal vein draining directly into the inferior vena cava just below the right renal vein insertion and the left gonadal vein draining into the left renal vein.

In premenopausal women, T2-weighted images reveal zonal anatomy of the ovary, demonstrating hypointense cortex and intermediate to high signal intensity medulla.[18,35,36] The high intensity of the medulla is secondary vascularloose connective tissue. In postmenopausal women, there is decreased signal on T2-weighted images in the medulla due to paucity of follicles and decreased vascular connective tissue.[37,38] Several high signal intensity cysts are identified within the cortex on T2-weighted images. In the premenopausal age group, the normal ovary demonstrates multiple peripherally located follicles, generally measuring less than 3 cm—these are low signal intensity on T1-weighted images and high signal intensity on T2-weighted images with thin enhancing walls.[38] The corpus luteum cyst is an involuting dominant functional cyst and tend to have a more irregular wall. When hemorrhage is present within the corpus luteum cyst, it demonstrates intermediate to high signal intensity on T1-weighted and T2-weighted images depending on the phase of hemorrhage. These cysts demonstrate heterogeneous postgadolinium enhancement in the wall.[36,37]

MALE PELVIS
Technical Considerations

The use of MRI in evaluation of the male genitourinary tract/pelvis is less common due to the inherent differences in internal anatomy. With much of the male genitourinary tract located superficially, ultrasound is the preferred method for cross-sectional imaging of the scrotum and penis; MRI can be a useful problem solving modality for sonographically equivocal or discordant clinical findings.[39,40] A circular/ring-shaped surface coil is preferred, although a short phased-array surface coil can also be used (such as a cardiac coil). The penis is frequently dorsiflexed against the lower midabdomen and taped to reduce motion.[41] Axial, coronal, and sagittal T2-weighted fast spin-echo imaging is performed, using a small FOV, high-resolution matrix, and thin section imaging (**Figs. 15**A and **16**); coronal imaging is often performed using chemical fat-suppression as well. Axial precontrast T1-weighted spin-echo is obtained similar parameters to the T2-weighted imaging sequences. Finally, precontrast and postcontrast sagittal T1-weighted spoiled gradient echo imaging is performed with chemical fat suppression to increase visual detection of subtle enhancement (see **Fig. 15**B).

Few studies at the authors' institution are specifically ordered for primary evaluation of the male bladder—more frequently, such investigations are performed as part of a magnetic resonance urography study. Additionally, the urinary bladder can typically be well seen on the general female pelvis protocol, which can be modified for the male gender by converting long-axis and short-axis T2-weighted imaging into traditional axial and coronal planes.

There is mounting evidence that imaging patients with a suspected perianal fistula can have substantial benefit, including better initial depiction of fistula geometry, improved triage for surgical management, and superior monitoring for treatment failures.[13,14] At the authors' institution, a high field strength magnet (3.0 Tesla [T]) is used in combination with a surface phased-array coil for perianal imaging; the improved signal at 3.0 T and lack of substantial bowel motion facilitates high spatial resolution imaging of this area. A high-resolution axial T2-weighted fast spin-echo sequence is obtained, using a wide FOV (36 cm) with high 600 × 800 matrix. Similarly, a high-resolution fat-suppressed sagittal T2-weighted sequence is centered on the perianal region with smaller FOV (20 cm) with a 400 × 400 matrix providing high spatial detail. Parallel imaging with acceleration factors of 1.5 to 3.0 are used to decrease imaging times. Other lower-resolution, water-sensitive sequences with fat suppression complement these 2 sequences, including short TI inversion recovery (STIR) imaging. High-resolution precontrast and post-contrast axial T1-weighted 3-D spoiled gradient-echo imaging is performed, using small FOV (25 cm), thin 1-mm reconstructed slice thickness,

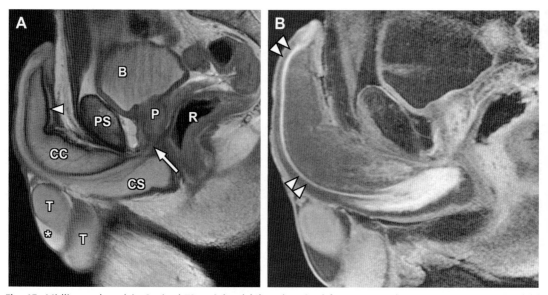

Fig. 15. Midline male pelvis. Sagittal T2-weighted (*A*) and sagittal fat-suppressed postcontrast T1-weighted (*B*) images demonstrate normal penis and scrotal structures. The paired dorsal corpora cavernosa and single ventral corpus spongiosum. Dark surrounding tunica albuginea/fascial layer (*arrowhead*). Testes show homogeneous signal on both T2-weighted images and postcontrast images; note small hydrocele (*asterisk*). Prostate and portion of the posterior urethra (*arrow*) are seen. There is intense mucosal enhancement associated with the urethra on postcontrast imaging (*arrowheads*). B, bladder; CC, corpora cavernosa; CS, corpus spongiosum; P, prostate; PS, pubic symphysis; R, rectum; T, testes.

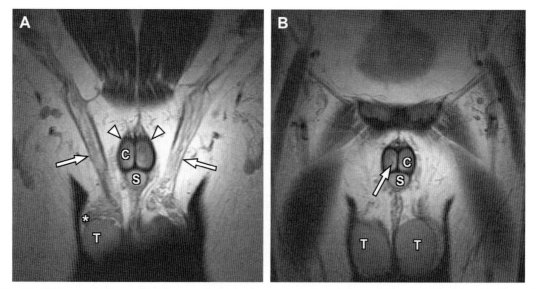

Fig. 16. (*A*) Coronal T2-weighted images through the penis and scrotum, anterior cut. The coronal plane of imaging displays the cross-sectional anatomy of the penis as it approaches the perineum, with right corpus cavernosa and corpus spongiousm marked. Tunica albuginea fascia (*arrowheads*) shows stark hypointensity on T2-weighted images. Spermatic cords (*arrows*) are seen coursing through the inguinal canals. Right testis and epididymis (*asterisk*) are partially visualized. (*B*) Coronal T2-weighted images through the penis and scrotum, middle cut. The testes are now well seen bilaterally, with uniform homogeneous internal signal on T2-weighted images. The right cavernosal artery can be seen as a small flow void (*arrow*) in the right corpus cavernosa. C (*A*), right corpus cavernosa; C (*B*), left corpus cavernosa; S, corpus spongiosum; T, testes.

and a 256 × 512 matrix. Similar high-resolution postcontrast sagittal and coronal planes are also routinely obtained.

Anatomic Considerations and MRI Features

Testes

The testes lie within the scrotal sac, encased by fibrous tunica albuginea that invaginates the testis posteriorly to form mediastinum testis. The processes vaginalis is an extension of the peritoneum into the scrotal sac. The efferent ductules are formed from 400 to 600 seminiferous tubules, which converge in the epididymal head and course through the epididymal body and tail to the vas deferens. The spermatic cord contains vas deferens, testicular artery, venous plexus, and lymphatics as it crosses the inguinal canal. The vas deferens merges with the ejaculatory ducts carrying seminal fluid from the seminal vesicles and opens to the prostatic urethra near the verumontanum.

Even though sonography remains primary modality of choice for evaluation of scrotum and penis, MRI may be used as problem-solving modality in cases where ultrasound is suboptimal or equivocal.[42,43] The testicles are distinctly identified on both T1-weighted and T2-weighted images, enveloped by the tunica albuginea which is low signal intensity on both T1-weighted and T2-weighted images. Normal testes are ovoid structures with homogeneous intermediate signal intensity on T1-weighted images and high signal intensity relative to skeletal muscle on T2-weighted images (see **Figs. 15** and **16**).[44] The mediastinum testis is seen as a low T2 signal intensity band.[41,45] T2-weighted images are best used in evaluation of focal lesion or mass due to better tissue contrast. T1-weighted images are useful in evaluation of hematoma or fat containing tumors. Normally, a small amount of simple fluid is present between the tunica vaginalis, demonstrating high signal on T2-weighted images. The epididymis is isointense to the testis on T1-weighted images and lower in signal intensity on T2-weighted images.[41] The pampiniform plexus lies superior to the epididymal head and may be demonstrated by multiple flow voids depending on flow speeds. When varicoceles are present, dilation and sluggish flow in the pampiniform plexus are expected, resulting in increased high signal on T2-weighted images.

Penis

The penis is comprised of 3 tubular compartments, namely a single ventral corpus spongiosum and paired dorsal corpora cavernosa, enveloped by a thin layer of connective tissue called the tunica albuginea. Peripheral to the tunica albuginea is an additional connective tissue layer, called the Buck fascia, which also serves to separate the dorsal and ventral compartments of the penis.[45,46] The posterior segments of the corpora cavernosa are referred to as the crura and attach to the ischiopubic ramus, becoming contiguous with ischiocavernosus muscle inferiorly. The corpus spongiosum forms the glans penis anteriorly and the penile bulb posteriorly, which is attached to the urogenital diaphragm.[39,41,46] The urethra originates from the bladder base and is generally divided into posterior and anterior segments. The posterior urethra is anatomically divided into 2 subcomponents, namely the prostatic and membranous segments, where the urethra traverses the prostate and urogenital diaphragm, respectively. As the urethra courses from the urogenital diaphragm into the penis itself, it is referred to as the anterior urethra, surrounded by the corpus spongiosum along its entire length and nominally divided into bulbous and pendulous segments. Several of the small vessels supplying the penis can be identified on dedicated small FOV imaging, including the centrally located cavernosal arteries within the substance of the corpora cavernosa, the deep dorsal vein which lies between the tunica albuginea and the Buck fascial layers, and sometimes the paired deep dorsal arteries that run adjacent to the lateral aspects of the deep dorsal vein.

The corpora cavernosa and spongiosa are of intermediate signal intensity on T1-weighted images. On T2-weighted images, the corpus spongiosum demonstrates homogeneous high signal intensity relative to the skeletal muscle (see **Figs. 15** and **16**). The corpora cavernosa may have a heterogeneous signal intensity versus that of the corpus spongiosum, depending on the perfusion distribution. The bulb of the penis demonstrates high signal intensity on T2-weighted images. The tunica albuginea, which surrounds the corpus spongiosum and corpora cavernosa, is of low signal intensity on T1 and T2-weighted images; it can be difficult to separate the tunica lbuginea fascia from the Buck fascia, particularly around the corpora cavernosa, such that the 2 fascia actually form a single thick hypointense rim on T1-weighted and T2-weighted sequences.[39,45,46] The cavernosal arteries are located medially within the corpora cavernosa and are seen as a flow void on T2-weighted images. Postgadolinium images show increased signal intensity of corpora cavernosa, proceeding both from central to peripheral and from proximal to distal, as expected given the location of the cavernosal arteries (see **Fig. 15**B).

Urinary bladder

The bladder is a muscular sac located in the lower pelvis posterior and superior to the pubis. The superior surface of the bladder is covered with peritoneum, which dips down posteriorly and forms the vesicouterine pouch in females and rectovesical pouch in males. From the bladder apex to the umbilicus is a fold of peritoneum, which is remnant of the urachus.

The thickness of bladder wall depends on its distension, varying between 2 and 8 mm.[47] From central to peripheral, the layers of the bladder include the mucosa, submucosa, muscularis containing circular, and longitudinal muscle fibers, and the outer serosa, consisting of adventitious layer. The trigone is the smooth triangular region between the openings of the 2 ureters and urethra and does not feature mucosal folds, even when the bladder is empty.

The bladder receives arterial supply from the internal iliac arteries via superior and inferior vesical arteries. The bladder is also in part supplied by the branches from obturator, uterine, and vaginal arteries. Venous drainage is via a complex plexus draining into the internal iliac vein. Lymphatic drainage is to the common and internal iliac chain.[48,49]

The urine within the bladder appears as low signal on T1-weighted images whereas the bladder wall is also low signal intensity but slightly higher than intraluminal fluid. On T2-weighted images the urine is of high signal intensity and the bladder wall remains of low signal intensity. Bladder mucosa and submucosa may enhance early during dynamic postcontrast T1-weighted images, whereas the muscularis can enhance on delayed imaging.[44] Excreted gadolinium in the bladder has variable signal intensity depending on the concentration of the contrast.[47]

Several normal variants and congenital anomalies of the bladder have been described, including bladder diverticulum, duplication, patent urachus, bladder exstrophy, or agenesis. A bladder diverticulum can be congenital or acquired from chronic outlet obstruction and is usually well depicted on MRI as a focal outpouching from the bladder wall containing urine. Diverticula lead to localized urine stasis, which may result in inflammation, chronic infection, and dysplasia/metaplasia. Incomplete obliteration of the urachus may persist as urachal cyst, sinus, or diverticulum. A ureterocele is a congenital dilation of the submucosal component of distal ureter as it crosses through the urinary bladder wall. Generally, ureteroceles are classified into orthotopic or ectopic in location (**Fig. 17**). Orthotopic ureteroceles can be clinically occult and noted only incidentally on imaging

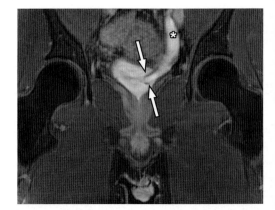

Fig. 17. Incidental left orthotopic ureterocele. Coronal fat suppressed postcontrast T1-weighted image demonstrates bulging intramural segment of the distal left ureter (*arrows*) with some mild upstream collecting system dilation (*asterisk*).

studies. Alternatively, ectopic ureteroceles are often associated with a duplicated collection system, frequently representing the aberrant insertion of an upper pole moiety. In such cases, patients often present clinically with a urinary tract infection, often due to obstruction of the upper tract system.[44]

Prostate and seminal vesicles

Technical considerations The role of imaging in the setting of suspected prostatic malignancy has historically been of relatively minor value to treating physicians, most frequently using transrectal ultrasound for guidance during biopsy. Unfortunately, even biopsy can be a misleading standard, with reported false-negative rates of up to 40%.[50] As MRI technology and techniques have advanced, the use of MRI for evaluation of prostate cancer has become more clinically relevant. Local imaging of the prostate by MRI yields images with high spatial and contrast resolution, permitting excellent morphologic depiction of the prostate. Emerging functional techniques, such as diffusion-weighted imaging, MR spectroscopy, and dynamic contrast-enhanced MRI, are areas of active investigation, because these may be useful adjuncts to morphologic imaging.[50,51] At the authors' institution, prostate MRI is performed for local tumor morphologic depiction in the setting of known prostate carcinoma. The standard protocol uses a 1.5-T scanner with an endorectal coil for local imaging and a phased-array surface coil for whole pelvis imaging. The protocol consists of axial, coronal, and sagittal T2-weighted fast spin-echo imaging with small FOV (14 cm) and high resolution (**Figs. 18** and **19**).

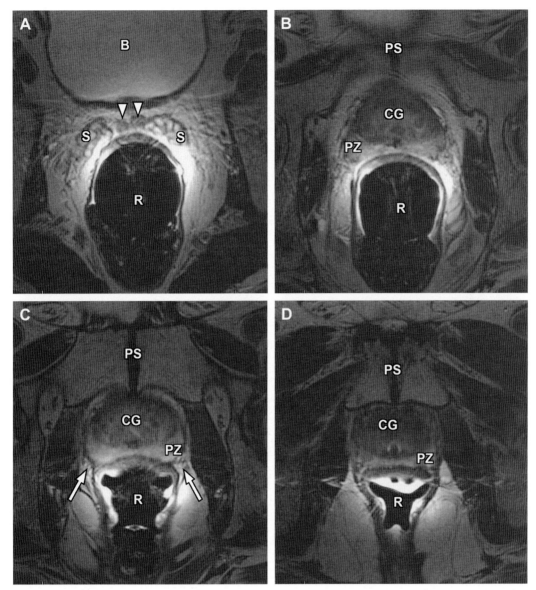

Fig. 18. Small FOV prostate examination with endorectal coil. Axial T2-weighted images from superior to inferior, including above the prostate (*A*), at the prostatic base (*B*), at the midgland (*C*), and at the apex (*D*). Note the zonal anatomy of the prostate, which can include the central gland and peripheral zone following the practical integrated approach. The peripheral zone demonstrates uniform high signal intensity, while the central gland is more heterogeneously low signal. The seminal vesicles and vas deferens (*arrowheads*) are seen toward the superior aspect of the gland. Neurovascular bundles (*arrows*) run in the periprostatic fat at the 5:00 and 7:00 positions relative to the prostate. B, bladder; CG, central gland; PS, pubic symphysis; PZ, peripheral zone; R, rectum with receiver coil; S, seminal vesicles.

Matched axial spin-echo T1-weighted imaging with small FOV, similar to the T2-weighted imaging, is critical for delineating postbiopsy change or hemorrhage. Finally, whole-pelvis imaging is performed using a wide FOV in conjunction with the surface coil. Although prostatic imaging can be performed using a high field strength magnet (3.0 T) with a surface phased-array coil in patients who cannot tolerate endorectal coil placement, published data regarding image quality are conflicting.[52,53] As such, this is considered a secondary option at the authors' institution, with preference given to 1.5-T imaging using an endorectal coil.

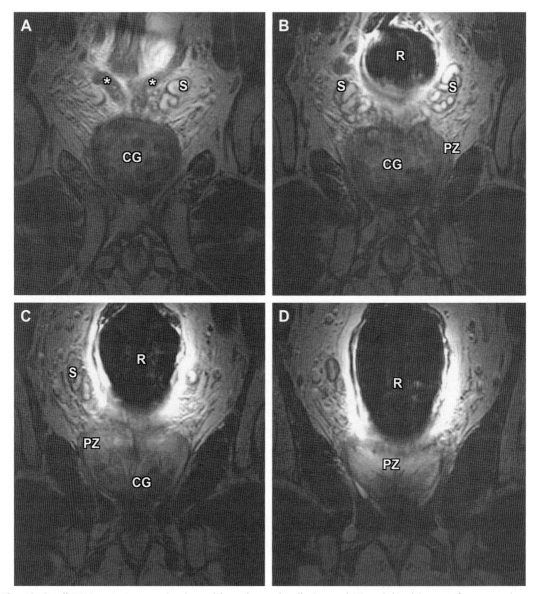

Fig. 19. Small FOV prostate examination with endorectal coil. Coronal T2-weighted images from anterior to posterior (*A–D*). Zonal anatomy of prostate is more difficult to appreciate in the coronal plane, as the transition from central gland to peripheral zone is somewhat subtle given the geometry of the imaging plane. The high signal intensity of the peripheral zone, however, is again conspicuous versus the heterogeneous low signal central gland. Seminal vesicles and vas deferens (*astrisk*) are demonstrated. CG, central gland; PZ, peripheral zone; R, rectum with receiver coil; S, seminal vesicles.

Anatomic considerations and MRI features The prostate is an exocrine gland found only in males and consists of a glandular part (70%) and fibromuscular stroma (30%).[41] It is located just below the urinary bladder and almost equals the size of a walnut. The prostate gland surrounds the proximal urethra (also called prostatic urethra). The ejaculatory ducts coming from the seminal vesicles opens into the prostatic urethra at a site called verumontanum. The seminal vesicle receives sperm

from the testicles via vas deferens. The main function of prostate gland is to secrete alkaline fluid that aids in liquefying semen. There are several anatomic classifications of prostatic anatomy, including traditional lobar divisions and a more contemporary zonal classification.[54] The zonal description divides the prostate into glandular and nonglandular elements, the latter of which includes the anterior fibromuscular stroma and the prostatic urethra. The glandular elements can be further

Table 1
Example protocols

Female Pelvis

	Coronal T2 Wide FOV	Sagittal T2	Long-Axis T2	Short-Axis T2	Axial In/ Opposed T1	Axial Pre-/ Post-T1 FS
Pulse Sequence	SSFSE	FSE	FSE	FSE	SPGR	SPGR, FS
Repetition Time (ms)	Minimum	3000–4000	3000–4500	3000–4500	205	190
Echo Time (ms)	180	96	96	96	2.3/4.6	Minimum
FOV (cm)	40	24–32	20–24	20–24	28–34	24–32
Slice Thickness (mm)	8	5	5	5	6	6
Matrix	256 × 128	512 × 224	512 × 224	512 × 224	256 × 160	320 × 160
Signal Averages	0.5	4	4	4	1	1

Female Urethra

	Axial Small FOV	Sagittal Small FOV	Axial Pre-/Post-T1 FS
Pulse Sequence	FSE	FSE	SE, FS
Repetition Time (ms)	4200	3000	450
Echo Time (ms)	85	85	Minimum
FOV (cm)	18	20	18
Slice Thickness (mm)	4	5	4
Matrix	512 × 224	256 × 224	256 × 224
Signal Averages	4	4	2

Male Penis/Scrotum

	Coronal T2 Wide FOV	Axial T1	Axial T2	Sagittal T2	Sagittal Pre-/Post-T1 FS
Pulse Sequence	SSFSE	SE	FSE	FSE	SPGR, FS
Repetition Time (ms)	Minimum	650	4200	3000	220
Echo Time (ms)	90	Minimum	85	85	Minimum
FOV (cm)	30	18	18	20	20
Slice Thickness (mm)	6	4	4	5	6
Matrix	256 × 128	256 × 224	256 × 224	256 × 224	512 × 160
Signal Averages	0.5	2	4	4	2

Fistula

	Axial T2 HR	Sagittal T2 FS	Axial Pre-/Post-T1 HR FS
Pulse Sequence	TSE	SE	3-D FFE
Repetition Time (ms)	Minimum	Minimum	Minimum
Echo Time (ms)	80	80	Minimum
FOV (cm)	36	20	25
Slice Thickness (mm)	6	6	1
Matrix	800 × 600	400 × 400	512 × 256
Signal Averages	4	4	8

Prostate

	Axial T2	Coronal T2	Sagittal T2	Axial T1	Axial T1 Whole Pelvis
Pulse Sequence	FSE	FSE	FSE	SE	SE
Repetition Time (ms)	5100	5000	5000	675	700
Echo Time (ms)	120	120	120	Minimum	Minimum
FOV (cm)	14	14	14	14	38
Slice Thickness (mm)	3	3	3	3	6
Matrix	256 × 192	256 × 192	256 × 192	256 × 160	256 × 192
Signal Averages	4	4	4	2	2

Abbreviations: FFE, fast field echo; FOV, field of view; FS, fat saturation; FSE, fast spin echo; HR, high resolution; SE, spin echo; SPGR, spoiled gradient recalled echo; SSFSE, single shot fast spin echo; TSE, turbo spin echo.

divided into inner and outer components. Subdivisions of the inner component include the periurethral tissue and the transition zone, whereas the outer components can be divided into the smaller central zone and the larger peripheral zone. The transitional zone comprises 5% of the prostate volume in young adults and surrounds the anterior-lateral aspect of the proximal urethra in a curvilinear fashion. The central zone constitutes 25% of the prostate volume in young adults and abuts the posterior-superior aspect of the proximal urethra.[45] The volumetric contribution of the transitional zone and central zone change with age, because the transitional zone is primarily involved by benign prostatic hyperplasia, leading to growth and compression of the central zone in older.[54] The peripheral zone accounts for 70% of the volume of the prostate and contains most of the glandular tissue; 70% of the prostate cancer originates in the peripheral zone, 20% in transitional zone, and 10% in central zone.[41,45,55,56] The zonal classification is often modified for radiologic use, where the term, *central gland*, collectively refers to the periurethral tissues, transitional zone, and the central zone. The peripheral zone is, therefore, referenced independently of the central gland, often in the practical integrated approach to prostatic anatomy.[45,54] Some investigators group the central zone and peripheral zone together as the peripheral gland, although this subtle nomenclature difference can confuse readers versus the practical integrated approach and is not used in this article.

On T1-weighted image, the normal prostate has relatively homogeneous low to intermediate signal intensity with poor differentiation of zonal anatomy.[45] The zonal anatomy is better defined on T2-weighted sequence. On T2-weighted images, the prostatic signal intensity depends on the proportion of glandular tissue versus stromal or muscular components, with glandular tissue normally demonstrating high signal intensity whereas fibromuscular stromal elements have low signal intensity. Thus, the normal peripheral zone is relatively high signal intensity due to presence of rich glandular tissue whereas the central and transitional zones are more hypointense due to increased stromal components. The central gland is separate from the peripheral zone by a low T2 signal intensity band of tissue known as the surgical capsule. The true prostate capsule is comprised of fibromuscular tissue that is of low signal intensity on T2-weighted image and separates the high signal intensity peripheral zone of the prostate from the periprostatic soft tissues.[41,45]

The neurovascular bundles are located posterolaterally within the rectoprostatic region at the 5:00 and 7:00 positions and include the nerves innervating the corpora cavernosa and venous plexuses. These bundles are of low signal intensity relative to the surrounding periprostatic fat (see **Fig. 18C**).

The seminal vesicles are paired structure located above the prostate. Each seminal vesicle is composed of multiple lobules containing high T2 signal intensity simple fluid with hypointense wall, giving a cluster of grapes appearance.[41,45] After 60 years of age, the fluid content in the seminal vesicles may decrease symmetrically, thereby causing lower signal intensity on T2WI.[45]

SUMMARY

The superior tissue contrast and flexible imaging planes afforded by MRI versus competing technologies permits optimal depiction of the pelvic viscera. Targeted protocols developed for specific pelvic visceral organs highlight important anatomic features that may not be imaged by other modalities (**Table 1**). Therefore, a solid understanding of normal and variant pelvic anatomy is crucial for appropriate interpretation of pelvic MRI studies.

REFERENCES

1. Rezvani M, Shaaban A. Imaging of cervical pathology. Clin Obstet Gynecol 2009;52(1):94–111.
2. Jeong YY, Outwater EK, Kang HK. Imaging evaluation of ovarian masses. Radiographics 2000;20(5):1445–70.
3. Imaoka I, Wada A, Kaji Y, et al. Developing an MR imaging strategy for diagnosis of ovarian masses. Radiographics 2006;26(5):1431–48.
4. Troiano RN, McCarthy SM. Mullerian duct anomalies: imaging and clinical issues. Radiology 2004;233(1):19–34.
5. Kroencke TJ, Scheurig C, Kluner C, et al. Uterine fibroids: contrast-enhanced MR angiography to predict ovarian artery supply—initial experience. Radiology 2006;241(1):181–9.
6. Chou CP, Levenson RB, Elsayes KM, et al. Imaging of female urethral diverticulum: an update. Radiographics 2008;28(7):1917–30.
7. Chaudhry S, Reinhold C, Guermazi A, et al. Benign and malignant diseases of the endometrium. Top Magn Reson Imaging 2003;14(4):339–57.
8. Nalaboff KM, Pellerito JS, Ben-Levi E. Imaging the endometrium: disease and normal variants. Radiographics 2001;21(6):1409–24.
9. McCarthy S, Tauber C, Gore J. Female pelvic anatomy: MR assessment of variations during the menstrual cycle and with use of oral contraceptives. Radiology 1986;160(1):119–23.

10. Brown HK, Stoll BS, Nicosia SV, et al. Uterine junctional zone: correlation between histologic findings and MR imaging. Radiology 1991;179(2):409–13.

11. McCarthy S, Scott G, Majumdar S, et al. Uterine junctional zone: MR study of water content and relaxation properties. Radiology 1989;171(1):241–3.

12. Scoutt LM, Flynn SD, Luthringer DJ, et al. Junctional zone of the uterus: correlation of MR imaging and histologic examination of hysterectomy specimens. Radiology 1991;179(2):403–7.

13. Reinhold C, McCarthy S, Bret PM, et al. Diffuse adenomyosis: comparison of endovaginal US and MR imaging with histopathologic correlation. Radiology 1996;199(1):151–8.

14. Lee JK, Gersell DJ, Balfe DM, et al. The uterus: in vitro MR-anatomic correlation of normal and abnormal specimens. Radiology 1985;157(1):175–9.

15. Hricak H, Alpers C, Crooks LE, et al. Magnetic resonance imaging of the female pelvis: initial experience. AJR Am J Roentgenol 1983;141(6):1119–28.

16. Brown MA, Kubik-huch RA, Reinhold C, et al. Uterus and cervix. In: Semelka RC, editor. 2nd edition, Abdominal pelvic MRI, vol. 1. New Jersey: John Wiley & Sons, Inc; 2006. p. 1251–332.

17. Scoutt LM, McCauley TR, Flynn SD, et al. Zonal anatomy of the cervix: correlation of MR imaging and histologic examination of hysterectomy specimens. Radiology 1993;186(1):159–62.

18. Siegelman ES. MRI of the female pelvis. In: Siegelman ES, editor. Body MRI. 1st edition. Philadelphia: Elsevier Saunders; 2005. p. 269–342.

19. deSouza NM, Hawley IC, Schwieso JE, et al. The uterine cervix on in vitro and in vivo MR images: a study of zonal anatomy and vascularity using an enveloping cervical coil. AJR Am J Roentgenol 1994;163(3):607–12.

20. The American Fertility Society classifications of adnexal adhesions, distal tubal occlusion, tubal occlusion secondary to tubal ligation, tubal pregnancies, mullerian anomalies and intrauterine adhesions. Fertil Steril 1988;49(6):944–55.

21. Ascher SM, Scoutt LM, McCarthy SM, et al. Uterine changes after dilation and curettage: MR imaging findings. Radiology 1991;180(2):433–5.

22. Togashi K, Kawakami S, Kimura I, et al. Uterine contractions: possible diagnostic pitfall at MR imaging. J Magn Reson Imaging 1993;3(6):889–93.

23. Togashi K, Kawakami S, Kimura I, et al. Sustained uterine contractions: a cause of hypointense myometrial bulging. Radiology 1993;187(3):707–10.

24. Woo GM, Twickler DM, Stettler RW, et al. The pelvis after cesarean section and vaginal delivery: normal MR findings. AJR Am J Roentgenol 1993;161(6):1249–52.

25. Hricak H, Chang YC, Thurnher S. Vagina: evaluation with MR imaging. Part I. Normal anatomy and congenital anomalies. Radiology 1988;169(1):169–74.

26. Eisenberg LB, Semelka RC, Firat Z. Female urethra and vagina. In: Semelka RC, editor. Abdominal pelvic MRI. 2nd edition. New Jersey: John Wiley & Sons. Inc; 2006. p. 1219–49.

27. Siegelman ES, Outwater EK, Banner MP, et al. High-resolution MR imaging of the vagina. Radiographics 1997;17(5):1183–203.

28. Griffin N, Grant LA, Sala E. Magnetic resonance imaging of vaginal and vulval pathology. Eur Radiol 2008;18(6):1269–80.

29. Preidler KW, Tamussino K, Szolar DM, et al. Staging of cervical carcinomas. Comparison of body-coil magnetic resonance imaging and endorectal surface coil magnetic resonance imaging with histopathologic correlation. Invest Radiol 1996;31(7):458–62.

30. Nurenberg P, Zimmern PE. Role of MR imaging with transrectal coil in the evaluation of complex urethral abnormalities. AJR Am J Roentgenol 1997;169(5):1335–8.

31. Siegelman ES, Banner MP, Ramchandani P, et al. Multicoil MR imaging of symptomatic female urethral and periurethral disease. Radiographics 1997;17(2):349–65.

32. Hricak H, Secaf E, Buckley DW, et al. Female urethra: MR imaging. Radiology 1991;178(2):527–35.

33. Kim JK, Kim YJ, Choo MS, et al. The urethra and its supporting structures in women with stress urinary incontinence: MR imaging using an endovaginal coil. AJR Am J Roentgenol 2003;180(4):1037–44.

34. Brown MA, Ascher SM, Semelka RC. Adnexa. In: Semelka RC, editor. Abdominal pelvic MRI. 2nd edition. New Jersey: John Wiley & Sons, Inc; 2006. p. 1333–82.

35. Togashi K. MR imaging of the ovaries: normal appearance and benign disease. Radiol Clin North Am 2003;41(4):799–811.

36. Outwater EK, Mitchell DG. Normal ovaries and functional cysts: MR appearance. Radiology 1996;198(2):397–402.

37. Outwater EK, Talerman A, Dunton C. Normal adnexa uteri specimens: anatomic basis of MR imaging features. Radiology 1996;201(3):751–5.

38. Sala EJ, Atri M. Magnetic resonance imaging of benign adnexal disease. Top Magn Reson Imaging 2003;14(4):305–27.

39. Pretorius ES, Siegelman ES, Ramchandani P, et al. MR imaging of the penis. Radiographics 2001;21(Spec No):S283–98 [discussion: S298–9].

40. Muglia V, Tucci S Jr, Elias J Jr, et al. Magnetic resonance imaging of scrotal diseases: when it makes the difference. Urology 2002;59(3):419–23.

41. Pretorius ES, Siegelman ES. MRI of the male pelvis and the bladder. Body MRI. 1st edition. Philadelphia: Elsevier Saunders; 2005. p. 371–424.

42. Woodward PJ, Schwab CM, Sesterhenn IA. From the archives of the AFIP: extratesticular scrotal

masses: radiologic-pathologic correlation. Radiographics 2003;23(1):215–40.

43. Patel MD, Silva AC. MRI of an adenomatoid tumor of the tunica albuginea. AJR Am J Roentgenol 2004; 182(2):415–7.

44. Sica GT, Teeger S. MR imaging of scrotal, testicular, and penile diseases. Magn Reson Imaging Clin N Am 1996;4(3):545–63.

45. Noone TC, Semelka RC, Firat Z, et al. Male pelvis. In: Semelka RC, editor. Abdominal pelvic MRI. 2nd edition. New Jersey: John Wiley & Sons, Inc; 2006. p. 1179–217.

46. Hricak H, Marotti M, Gilbert TJ, et al. Normal penile anatomy and abnormal penile conditions: evaluation with MR imaging. Radiology 1988;169(3): 683–90.

47. Duerdulian C, Firat Z, Brown ED, et al. Bladder. In: Semelka RC, editor. Abdominal-pelvic MRI. 2nd edition. New Jersey: John Wiley & Sons, Inc; 2006. p. 1141–78.

48. Banson ML. Normal MR anatomy and techniques for imaging of the male pelvis. Magn Reson Imaging Clin N Am 1996;4(3):481–96.

49. Teeger S, Sica GT. MR imaging of bladder diseases. Magn Reson Imaging Clin N Am 1996;4(3):565–81.

50. Turkbey B, Albert PS, Kurdziel K, et al. Imaging localized prostate cancer: current approaches and new developments. AJR Am J Roentgenol 2009; 192(6):1471–80.

51. Coakley FV, Qayyum A, Kurhanewicz J. Magnetic resonance imaging and spectroscopic imaging of prostate cancer. J Urol 2003;170(6 Pt 2):S69–75 [discussion: S75–6].

52. Beyersdorff D, Taymoorian K, Knosel T, et al. MRI of prostate cancer at 1.5 and 3.0 T: comparison of image quality in tumor detection and staging. AJR Am J Roentgenol 2005;185(5):1214–20.

53. Sosna J, Pedrosa I, Dewolf WC, et al. MR imaging of the prostate at 3 Tesla: comparison of an external phased-array coil to imaging with an endorectal coil at 1.5 Tesla. Acad Radiol 2004;11(8):857–62.

54. Coakley FV, Hricak H. Radiologic anatomy of the prostate gland: a clinical approach. Radiol Clin North Am 2000;38(1):15–30.

55. Choi YJ, Kim JK, Kim N, et al. Functional MR imaging of prostate cancer. Radiographics 2007; 27(1):63–75 [discussion: 75–7].

56. Hricak H, Dooms GC, McNeal JE, et al. MR imaging of the prostate gland: normal anatomy. AJR Am J Roentgenol 1987;148(1):51–8.

Magnetic Resonance Imaging of the Long Bones of the Upper Extremity

Esben S. Vogelius, MD*, Waad Hanna, MD,
Mark Robbin, MD

KEYWORDS

- Magnetic resonance imaging • Upper extremity • Humerus
- Radius • Ulna • Normal anatomy

The long bones of the upper extremity are often overlooked in favor of addressing their intervening joints. However, there are a wide variety of pathologic processes that can involve these anatomic segments. To better understand the complex anatomy of the upper extremity, the following discussion is divided into sections describing the osseous, muscular, and neurovascular anatomy of the arm and forearm using a compartmental approach. The discussion touches on a few common normal variants and their potential functional consequences. The upper extremity joints of the shoulder, elbow, and wrist are addressed separately.

IMAGING

Applications of MR imaging of the musculoskeletal system have expanded enormously from the initial narrow indications of infection and tumor evaluation.[1] Examinations are now routinely performed for the assessment of sports-related or other injury. Most musculoskeletal examinations at our institution are performed on a standard 1.5-Tesla scanner; however, higher-field (3.0T) imaging offers many potential advantages. The potential advantages include increased signal-to-noise ratio (SNR) and decreased imaging time. Higher field imaging shortens the time required for chemical fat saturation sequences but this advantage is offset by the higher field inhomogeneity that degrades chemically selected fat-saturation sequences. Various parameters need to be adjusted to optimize 3T imaging. Because T1 relaxation time is increased, TR needs to be increased to maintain contrast. Additionally, the decreased T2 relaxation time needs to be compensated by decreasing the TE. The TI for short tau inversion recovery (STIR) imaging also needs to be increased for 3T imaging.[2]

The images presented in this article were obtained of a 30-year-old asymptomatic healthy male volunteer on a 3T Verio Scanner (Siemens Medical, Erlangen, Germany). The pulse sequences obtained on the 3T are similar to those obtained with lower field strength. The examinations are obtained using a 6-channel standard body surface coil with the patient in anatomic position. T2 HASTE sequences are obtained in 3 orthogonal planes to act as a localizer. T1 fast spin-echo (FSE) images are obtained in all 3 orthogonal planes. Fluid-sensitive STIR images are obtained in the coronal and sagittal planes and intermediate TE T2 FSE fat-saturated images were obtained for the smaller field of view axial images. When indicated, contrast (Magnevist, gadopentetate dimeglumine, Bayer Schering Pharma AG, Berlin, Germany) is administered intravenously at a dose of 0.1 mmol/kg and saturated T1 FSE images are also obtained in the 3 orthogonal planes. Patients

The authors have nothing to disclose.
Department of Radiology, Case Western Reserve Medical School, 11100 Euclid Avenue, Cleveland, OH 44106, USA
* Corresponding author.
E-mail address: Esben.Vogelius@uhhospitals.org

Magn Reson Imaging Clin N Am 19 (2011) 567–579
doi:10.1016/j.mric.2011.05.004

with compromised renal function (stage 4 or 5 renal failure) are informed of the risk of nephrogenic systemic fibrosis and consented before contrast administration if the examination is deemed clinically necessary and of favorable risk-benefit ratio.[3] A complete examination of the arm or the forearm takes approximately 28 minutes to complete with contrasted sequences requiring another 12 minutes.

ADVANTAGES OF SEQUENCES

MR can detect marrow abnormalities earlier than competing modalities including computed tomography (CT) and bone scan.[4] STIR images are particularly useful for depiction of marrow pathology. Intermediate TE T2 FSE fat-saturated images offer better anatomic detail and similar sensitivity for fluid signal abnormalities when compared with STIR. However, T2 FSE images suffer from inhomogeneous fat suppression with larger fields of view, a problem that is compounded at higher field strength.[5] T1 FSE images are useful in delineating muscles and other structures by their separating fat planes and are therefore the predominate sequence used in this pictorial essay. Post contrast images are useful in differentiating solid and cystic lesions and increase the sensitivity for abscess detection.[6]

NORMAL MR SIGNAL

Bone marrow signal is variable among patients depending on age and hematopoietic stressors. Bone marrow is referred to as red or yellow according to its relative hematopoietic content. Red marrow is composed of 60% hematopoietic cells, whereas yellow marrow is almost entirely adiopocytic.[7,8] Bone marrow converts to its mature distribution in an orderly and predictable manner. The epiphyses followed by the diaphyses and then the metaphyses convert from red to yellow marrow. The conversion of the appendicular skeleton to yellow marrow should be complete within the third decade of life.[7,9] Marrow can reconvert at times of stress with re-conversion proceeding in the reverse order of the initial conversion. On MR imaging, the signal characteristics of yellow marrow are similar to those of fat. Red marrow demonstrates intermediate signal on both T1-weighted and T2-weighted sequences secondary to its lesser fat content and T1 shortening.[7,10]

Tendons and ligaments are normally of homogeneously low signal on all pulse sequences. Some of the larger tendons, including the triceps, can normally demonstrate internal high signal striations.[11,12]

Nerves in the arm and forearm demonstrate similar signal characteristics to other peripheral nerves. Nerves are normally intermediate in signal on both T1-weighted and T2-weighted images, similar to that of adjacent muscle. Nerves are made more conspicuous by peri-neural fat. Routine axial images with the elbow in full extension should allow consistent visualization of the major nerves. Specialized axial views with the elbow in flexion for ulnar nerve or pronation for the median and radial nerves may be helpful for further characterization or to assess for impingement.[13]

Vessels have a variable appearance depending on their internal flow. High-flow vessels normally demonstrate signal voids, whereas smaller low-flow vessels demonstrate increased signal on T2-weighted images.[14]

NORMAL ANATOMY

The upper limb consists of 4 segments, which are from proximal to distal: the pectoral girdle, the arm, the forearm, and the hand. These segments are separated by the joints of the shoulder, elbow, and wrist, respectively. In this article, we address the normal MR appearance of the arm and the forearm with the intervening joints being addressed separately.

OSSEOUS ANATOMY

The humerus (**Fig. 1**) is the largest bone of the upper limb. The proximal spherical humeral head articulates with the glenoid to form the scapulo-humeral (shoulder joint). The anatomic neck of the humerus circumscribes the head and separates it from the tuberosities. The lesser and greater tuberosities project off the anterior and lateral aspects of the proximal humerus respectively and form the intervening intertubercular (bicipital) groove. The narrowing of the humerus just distal to the tubercles is referred to as the surgical neck, a common site of humeral fracture.[15] The body of the humerus has 2 prominent features: the deltoid tuberosity and the radial groove. The deltoid tuberosity, located laterally, is the insertion site of the deltoid muscle. The radial groove, located posteriorly, accommodates the radial nerve and the deep brachial artery as they course between the medial and lateral heads of the triceps muscle. The distal humerus flares out forming the supracondylar ridges, which end distally as the epicondyles, the medial of which is more prominent. The distal end of the humerus, including the epicondyles and articular surfaces of the trochlea and the capitellum, is referred to as the condyle of the humerus. The lateral

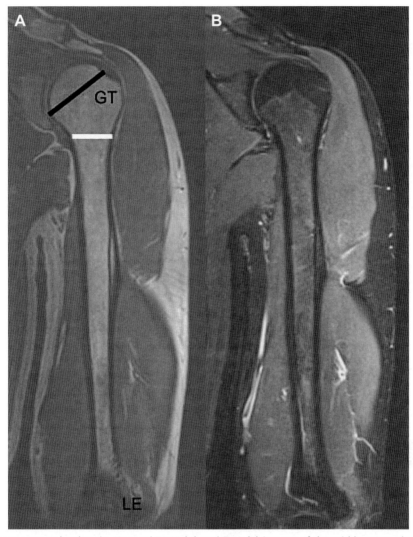

Fig. 1. Humerus osseous landmarks. Coronal T1WI (*A*) and STIR (*B*) images of the mid humerus demonstrate the anatomic neck of the humerus (*black solid line*), surgical neck (*white line*), greater tuberosity (GT) and the lateral epicondyle (LE).

capitellum articulates with the radial head. The capitellum resembles a sphere with a distinct contour change where the anterior capitellum intersects the posterior lateral epicondyle. This normal appearance has been termed the "pseudo-defect of the capitellum," which may be confused for an osteochondral lesion (**Fig. 2**).[16] Superior to the capitellum anteriorly is the radial fossa, which accommodates the radial head in full flexion. The medial trochlea articulates with the trochlear notch of the proximal ulna. Superior to the trochlea anteriorly is the coronoid fossa, which accommodates the coronoid process of the ulna in full flexion. Posteriorly, the more prominent olecranon fossa accommodates the olecranon in full extension.

There is an osseous excrescence off the anterior humerus that can be seen as a normal variant. This is referred to as the "supracondylar process," found approximately 7 cm proximal to the medial epicondyle in 0.3% to 2.7% of asymptomatic human subjects. The ligament of Struthers, a fibrous band passing from the supracondylar process to the medial epicondyle creates a fibro-osseous tunnel through which the brachial artery and median nerve pass. Compression of the median nerve at this location can cause numbness of the hand and weakness of the muscles of the anterior compartment of the forearm.[17]

The ulna is the medial and longer of the 2 fore-arm bones. The proximal ulna has 2 prominent projections, the olecranon and the coronoid process coming off the posterior and anterior aspects of the proximal ulna, respectively, and forming the trochlear groove. Lateral to the

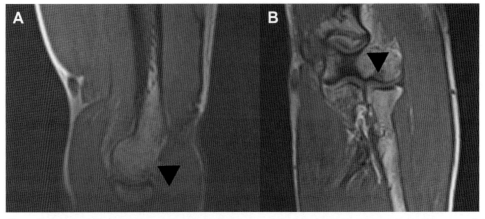

Fig. 2. "Pseudodefect of the capitellum." Sagittal T1WI image (*A*) of the distal humerus shows the normal abrupt contour change of the capitellum (*black arrowhead*). Coronal T1-weighted image (*B*) of the proximal radius re-demonstrates the cortical irregularity (*black arrowhead*) at this location that could be misinterpreted as an osteochondral lesion.

coronoid process is the radial groove, which forms the articulation with the radial head. Inferior to the radial groove is the supinator groove and crest, the attachment site of the supinator muscle. The body of the ulna is thick and cylindrical and tapers distally. At its end it abruptly enlarges forming the discoid head with the styloid process medially. Ulnar variance denotes the length of the ulna relative to the adjacent radius. Negative ulnar variance indicates that the ulna is shorter than the radius and, conversely, positive ulnar variance indicates that it is longer. Typically, a 3-mm difference is required to denote significant ulnar variance.[18]

The radius is the lateral and shorter of the 2 forearm bones. The proximal discoid radial head articulates with the capitellum and the radial notch of the ulna. The radial tuberosity serves as the insertion of the biceps muscle and separates the proximal head and neck from the distal body. The body

of the radius has a lateral convexity and enlarges in width distally. The distal end of the radius is rectangular when viewed in axial sections. At its distal medial aspect, it forms the concave ulnar notch, which accommodates the head of the ulna. At its distal lateral aspect, it forms the radial styloid process, which is larger and distal to its ulnar counterpart. The dorsal tubercle (Lister tubercle) projects posteriorly forming grooves for the posterior compartment muscles (**Fig. 3**).

MUSCLE ANATOMY, ARM

The arm can be divided into anterior and posterior compartments. The anterior compartment contains the flexors (biceps brachii, brachialis, and coracobrachialis) and is supplied by the musculocutaneous nerve (**Figs. 4–6**). The posterior compartment contains the extensor triceps brachii

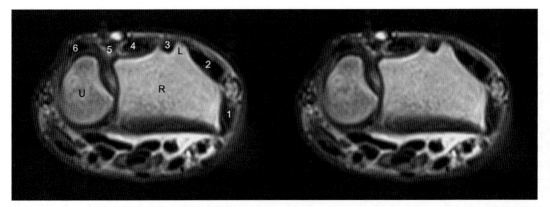

Fig. 3. Dorsal extensor compartments. Axial T1-weighted image just proximal to the wrist illustrates the 6 extensor compartments of the posterior forearm. 1, extensor pollicis brevis and abductor pollicis longus; 2, extensor carpi radialis brevis and longus; 3, extensor pollicis longus; 4, extensor digitorum and indicis; 5, extensor digiti minimi; 6, extensor carpi ulnaris; U, ulna; R, radius; L, Lister tubercle.

Color Key for arm diagrams:

Color	Compartment	Innervation
Red	Anterior	Musculocutaneous nerve
Green	Posterior	Radial nerve
Yellow	Mobile Wad	Radial/deep radial nerve

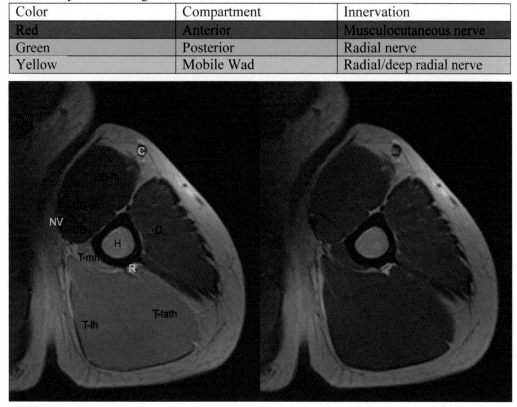

Fig. 4. Axial T1-weighted image anatomy of the upper arm just distal to the pectoralis insertion. Black text: H, humerus; D, deltoid muscle; T-lath, triceps lateral head; T-lh, triceps long head; T-mh, triceps medial head; CB, coracobrachialis; BB-sh, biceps brachii short head; BB-lh, biceps brachii long head. White text: R, radial nerve and deep brachial artery; NV, neurovascular bundle (median and ulnar nerves, brachial artery, and vein); C, cephalic vein. Red area: anterior compartment, innervation by musculocutaneous nerve; Green area: posterior compartment, innervation by radial nerve.

and the lateral anconeus and is supplied by the radial nerve.

Anterior Compartment

The short and long heads of the biceps originate on the coracoid and supraglenoid tubercle respectively. The long head passes though the bicipital groove under the transverse humeral ligament. The biceps muscle bellies unite approximately 7 cm proximal to the elbow and insert on the radial tuberosity. The distal biceps tendon has no tendon sheath, like that of the Achilles tendon. There is a relatively hypovascular zone of the distal biceps tendon, which may subject to degeneration and tearing secondary to mechanical impingement between the radial tuberosity and the ulna.[19–21] The biceps muscle serves as both a flexor and supinator of the forearm. Approximately 10% of the population has a third head of the biceps

originating from the superomedial portion of the brachialis. This normal variant is of uncertain functional or clinical significance.[22]

The brachialis is the main flexor of the forearm. It lies deep to the biceps originating from the distal half of the anterior humerus and inserting on the tuberosity of the ulna.

The coracobrachialis helps to flex and abduct the arm and stabilize the glenoid joint. The elongated muscle is located at the superomedial aspect of the arm originating from the coracoid tip and inserting on the mid medial humerus.

Posterior Compartment

The triceps is the main extensor of the elbow joint and has 3 heads. The long, lateral, and medial heads originate from the infraglenoid tubercle, superior posterior surface of the humerus, and inferior posterior surface of the humerus respectively.

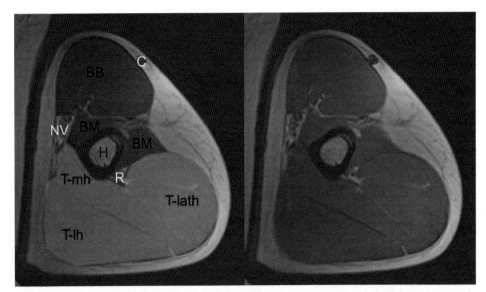

Fig. 5. Axial T1-weighted image of anatomy of the mid arm just distal to the deltoid insertion. Black text: H, humerus; T-lath, triceps lateral head; T-lh, triceps long head; T-mh, triceps medial head; BB, biceps brachii; BM, brachialis muscle. White text: R, radial nerve and deep brachial artery; NV, neurovascular bundle (median and ulnar nerves, brachial artery, and vein); C, cephalic vein. Red area: anterior compartment, innervation by musculocutaneous nerve; Green area: posterior compartment, innervation by radial nerve.

They insert as a common tendon on the proximal olecranon. This common tendon may normally have a striated appearance.[11] Rarely, the medial triceps may insert on the medial epicondyle, potentially causing ulnar nerve compression.[23]

The anconeus is a diminutive relatively unimportant muscle at the posterolateral aspect of the distal humerus. It originates from the posterior aspect of the lateral epicondyle and courses medially, inserting on the lateral olecranon. The anconeus is thought to help with extension and resist elbow abduction.[16] The anconeus also serves as a landmark for the lateral aspect of the elbow.

The anconeus epitrochearis (accessory anconeus) is an anomalous accessory muscle, which arises from the medial humeral condyle, passes superficial to the ulnar nerve and inserts on the olecranon. This variant may occur in up to 11%

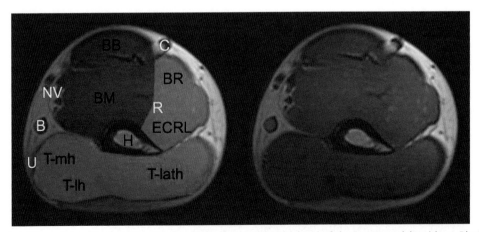

Fig. 6. Axial T1-weighted image of anatomy of the distal arm at the level of the supracondylar ridges. Black text: H, humerus; T-lath, triceps lateral head; T-lh, triceps long head; T-mh, triceps medial head; BB, biceps brachii; BM, brachialis muscle; BR, brachioradialis muscle; ECRL, extensor carpii radialis longus. White text: R, radial nerve and deep brachial artery; U, ulnar nerve; B, basilic vein, NV, neurovascular bundle (median nerve, brachial artery, and vein); C, cephalic vein. Red area: anterior compartment, innervation by musculocutaneous nerve; Green area: posterior compartment, innervation by radial nerve; Yellow area: mobile wad compartment, innervation by radial/deep radial nerve.

of the population and is one of the potential causes of cubital tunnel syndrome owing to ulnar nerve compression.[24] The small muscle is not palpable and requires imaging for its depiction. During elbow flexion, it can impinge on the underlying nerve and cause compression. Excision without anterior transposition of the ulnar nerve is the treatment in symptomatic patients.[25]

MUSCLE ANATOMY, FOREARM

The forearm is separated into 2 compartments by the interosseous membrane (**Figs. 7–9, Tables 1 and 2**). The anteromedial ("anterior") compartment contains the flexor-pronators and is supplied predominately by the median nerve (with the ulnar nerve supplying the remaining one and a half muscles as detailed later in this article). The deep muscles of the anterior compartment are supplied by a median nerve branch, the anterior interosseous nerve. The posterolateral ("posterior") compartment contains the extensor-supinators and is supplied by the radial nerve and its branches.

Anterior Compartment

The muscles of the anterior compartment can be divided into superficial and deep groups. The 5 superficial muscles originate from the medial epicondyle (the common flexor tendon), cross the elbow joint, and include the pronator teres, flexor carpi radialis, palmaris longus, flexor carpi ulnaris, and flexor digitorum superficialis. The deep muscles do not cross the joint and include the flexor digitorum profundus, flexor pollicis longus, and pronator quadratus.

Superficial

The pronator teres is a forearm pronator and allows flexion at the elbow. It has 2 proximal attachments at coronoid process of the ulna in addition to the medial epicondyle. It attaches distally at the mid

Color Key for arm diagrams:

Color	Compartment	Innervation
Red	Anterior, deep	Anterior interosseous nerve (branch of median)
Pink	Anterior, superficial	Predominately median nerve, minor supply from ulnar nerve
Green	Posterior, deep	Deep radial and posterior interosseous nerves (branches of radial)
Blue	Posterior, superficial	Posterior interosseous nerve (branch of radial)
Yellow	Mobile Wad	Radial/deep radial Nerves

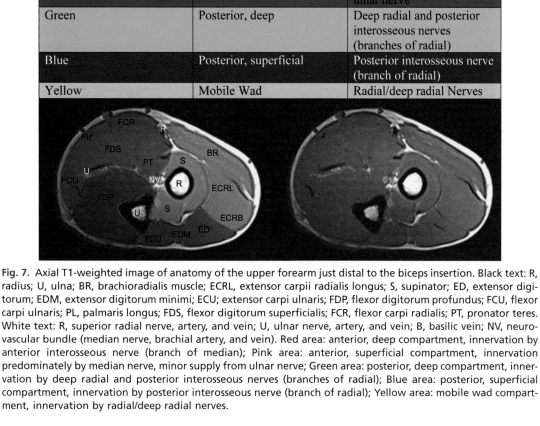

Fig. 7. Axial T1-weighted image of anatomy of the upper forearm just distal to the biceps insertion. Black text: R, radius; U, ulna; BR, brachioradialis muscle; ECRL, extensor carpii radialis longus; S, supinator; ED, extensor digitorum; EDM, extensor digitorum minimi; ECU; extensor carpi ulnaris; FDP, flexor digitorum profundus; FCU, flexor carpi ulnaris; PL, palmaris longus; FDS, flexor digitorum superficialis; FCR, flexor carpi radialis; PT, pronator teres. White text: R, superior radial nerve, artery, and vein; U, ulnar nerve, artery, and vein; B, basilic vein; NV, neurovascular bundle (median nerve, brachial artery, and vein). Red area: anterior, deep compartment, innervation by anterior interosseous nerve (branch of median); Pink area: anterior, superficial compartment, innervation predominately by median nerve, minor supply from ulnar nerve; Green area: posterior, deep compartment, innervation by deep radial and posterior interosseous nerves (branches of radial); Blue area: posterior, superficial compartment, innervation by posterior interosseous nerve (branch of radial); Yellow area: mobile wad compartment, innervation by radial/deep radial nerves.

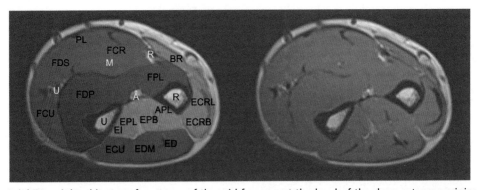

Fig. 8. Axial T1-weighted image of anatomy of the mid forearm at the level of the deep extensor origins. Black text: R, radius; U, ulna; BR, brachioradialis muscle; ECRL, extensor carpii radialis longus; ED, extensor digitorum; EDM, extensor digitorum minimi; ECU, extensor carpi ulnaris; EI, extensor indicis; EPL, extensor pollicis longus; EPB, extensor pollicis brevis; APL, abductor pollicis longus; FDP, flexor digitorum profundus; FPL, flexor pollicis longus; FCU, flexor carpi ulnaris; PL, palmaris longus; FDS, flexor digitorum superficialis; FCR, flexor carpi radialis. White text: R, superior radial nerve, artery, and vein; A, anterior interosseous nerve; M, median nerve; U, ulnar nerve, artery, and vein. Red area: anterior, deep compartment, innervation by anterior interosseous nerve (branch of median); Pink area: anterior, superficial compartment, innervation predominately by median nerve, minor supply from ulnar nerve; Green area: posterior, deep compartment, innervation by deep radial and posterior interosseous nerves (branches of radial); Blue area: posterior, superficial compartment, innervation by posterior interosseous nerve (branch of radial); Yellow area: mobile wad compartment, innervation by radial/deep radial nerves.

lateral aspect of the radius. Its lateral border forms the medial margin of the cubital fossa.

The flexor carpi radialis (FCR) is a long cylindrical muscle located medial to the pronator teres, which flexes and abducts the wrist. To reach its distal attachment at the base of the second metatarsal, the FCR passes through a canal in the lateral flexor retinaculum and lies just medial to the radial artery.

The palmaris longus is a small fusiform muscle that flexes the wrist and is often congenitally absent (in up to 13% of the population, more often on the left side), generally without substantial functional loss.[26] Normally, it has a short proximal belly and long distal tendon that passes superficial to the flexor retinaculum to insert at the apex of the palmar aponeurosis. However, the palmaris longus is one of the most variable muscles in the

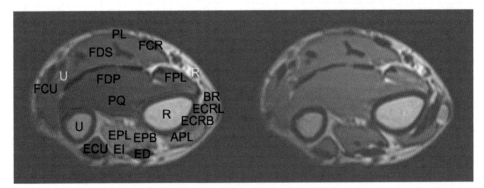

Fig. 9. Axial T1-weighted image of anatomy of the distal forearm at the level of the proximal radial metaphysis. Black text: R, radius; U, ulna; BR, brachioradialis muscle; ECRL, extensor carpii radialis longus; ED, extensor digitorum; EDM, extensor digitorum minimi; ECU, extensor carpi ulnaris; EI, extensor indicis; EPL, extensor pollicis longus; EPB, extensor pollicis brevis; APL, abductor pollicis longus; FDP, flexor digitorum profundus; FPL, flexor pollicis longus; FCU, flexor carpi ulnaris; PL, palmaris longus; FDS, flexor digitorum superficialis; FCR, flexor carpi radialis. White text: R, radial artery; U, ulnar nerve, artery, and vein. Red area: anterior, deep compartment, innervation by anterior interosseous nerve (branch of median); Pink area: anterior, superficial compartment, innervation predominately by median nerve, minor supply from ulnar nerve; Green area: posterior, deep compartment, innervation by deep radial and posterior interosseous nerves (branches of radial); Blue area: posterior, superficial compartment, innervation by posterior interosseous nerve (branch of radial); Yellow area: mobile wad compartment, innervation by radial/deep radial nerves.

Table 1
Standard protocol for imaging the forearm on a 3T scanner

Pulse Sequence	Plane	Matrix	ST, mm	TE	TR	TI	ETL	NEX
T1 FSE	Axial	192 × 256	4.0	10–15	700–750	—	4	4
	Coronal	290 × 384	2.5	10–15	700–750	—	4	1
	Sagittal	237 × 384	2.5	10–15	700–750	—	4	3
STIR	Coronal	290 × 384	2.5	10–15	3000	220	8	1
	Sagittal	237 × 384	2.5	10–15	3000	220	8	2
T2 FSE with fat saturation	Axial	192 × 256	4.0	60–65	5000	—	28	3

Abbreviations: ETL, echo train length; FSE, fast spin echo; NEX, number of excitations (number of signal averages); ST, slice thickness; STIR, short tau inversion recovery.

forearm. Occasionally, its muscle belly lies centrally between proximal and distal tendons (digastric variant) or even distally having a long proximal tendon ("reversed" palmaris). This can present as a contractile mass at the level of the wrist superficial to the flexor retinaculum and the flexor digitorum superficialis (FDS). The muscle can cause compression of the underlying flexor tendons or median nerve. Treatment is by muscle excision.[25]

The flexor carpi ulnaris (FCU) is the most medial of the superficial flexor muscles. It flexes and adducts the wrist and is unique among the anterior compartment muscles in that it is supplied entirely by the ulnar nerve. The FCU has 2 proximal attachments attaching at the medial olecranon in addition to the medial epicondyle. A fibrous arch between the 2 heads forms the roof of the cubital tunnel which has variously been referred to as the arcuate ligament, Osborne band, and the cubital tunnel retinaculum.[16] This structure may be absent in up to 23% of subjects.[24] The FCU is a guide to the ulnar artery, which is situated immediately lateral to it and it inserts distally on the pisiform, hook of the hamate, and fifth metacarpal.

The FDS is the largest superficial muscle of the forearm. Typically considered with the superficial muscles because it crosses the elbow joint, it actually forms an intermediate layer between the superficial and deep muscles of the anterior compartment. The FDS has 2 heads, humeroulnar and radial, between which pass the median nerve and ulnar artery. Near the wrist the FDS gives rise to 4 tendons that pass deep to the flexor retinaculum within the carpal tunnel. The tendons are enclosed in the common flexor synovial sheath and insert on the bodies of the middle phalanges of the medial 4 digits. The FDS flexes both the middle phalanges and proximal phalanges in addition to the wrist.

Deep

The flexor digitorum profundus (FDP) has an extensive attachment to the proximal anterior and medial ulna and anterior interosseous membrane. It separates into 4 separate tendons that course deep to the flexor retinaculum and is located posterior to the FDS tendons within the shared common flexor synovial sheath. The tendons distally insert at the bases of the distal phalanges and allow for the flexion of the distal interphalangeal joint in addition to flexion of the wrist. The FDP has a dual nerve supply with the ulnar nerve supplying its medial aspect (innervating digits 4 and 5) and the median nerve supplying the remainder.

Table 2
Standard protocol for imaging the arm on a 3T scanner

Pulse Sequence	Plane	Matrix	ST, mm	TE	TR	TI	ETL	NEX
T1 FSE	Axial	240 × 256	5	10–15	700–750	—	4	3
	Coronal	401 × 448	3	10–15	700–750	—	4	1
	Sagittal	231 × 448	3	10–15	700–750	—	4	3
STIR	Coronal	401 × 448	3	10–15	3000	220	8	1
	Sagittal	231 × 448	3	10–15	3000	220	8	2
T2 FSE with fat saturation	Axial	240 × 256	5	60–65	5000	—	28	2

Abbreviations: ETL, echo train length; FSE, fast spin echo; NEX, number of excitations (number of signal averages); ST, slice thickness; STIR, short tau inversion recovery.

The flexor pollicis longus (FPL) lies lateral to the FDP, originating from the anterior radius distal to the supinator. Its flat tendon passes deep to the flexor retinaculum and has its own synovial sheath just lateral to the common flexor synovial sheath. Its tendon inserts at the base of the distal phalanx of the thumb and is therefore the only muscle capable of flexing the interphalangeal joint of the thumb. In addition, it may assist in flexion of the first metacarpophalangeal, first carpometacarpal, and wrist joints. An accessory slip ("head") of the FPL muscle (also referred to as the Gantzer muscle) can be seen in up to 45% of healthy subjects and may impinge on the anterior interosseous branch of the median nerve.[27,28] MR can demonstrate the resultant atrophy of the supplied deep muscles of the anterior compartment of the forearm.[25]

The pronator quadratus is a quadrilateral muscle that originates from the anterior distal fourth of the ulna and inserts on the anterior distal fourth of the radius. The pronator quadratus initiates pronation at the radioulnar joint and is assisted by the pronator teres when more power is needed. The pronator quadratus also helps the interosseous membrane keep the distal radius and ulna together, particularly when upward thrusts are transmitted through the wrist (eg, fall on the hand).

Posterior Compartment

The muscles of the posterior compartment can be divided into the mobile wad, superficial, and deep groups. The lateral mobile wad is composed of 2 wrist extensors (extensor carpi radialis brevis and longus) and a forearm flexor (brachioradialis). The proximal attachment of the brachioradialis and extensor carpi radialis longus is the lateral supracondylar ridge. The third muscle of the mobile wad, the extensor carpi radialis brevis and the 3 muscles of the superficial group (extensor digitorum, extensor digiti minimi, and the extensor carpi ulnaris) originate from the common extensor tendon of the lateral epicondyle. The deep extensors of the forearm originate distal to the elbow in an outcropping dividing the extensors. They include the APL, EPB, EPL, and the extensor indicis. The extensors are divided into 6 compartments, which can be seen on the most distal axial images of the forearm (see **Fig. 3**).

The mobile wad
The brachioradialis is a fusiform muscle that lies superficial on the anterolateral aspect of the forearm. As mentioned previously, it originates from the lateral supracondylar ridge of the humerus and attaches distally to the distal lateral radius. The brachioradialis flexes the forearm at the elbow. It is exceptional in that it is the only elbow

flexor located in the posterior compartment and supplied by the radial nerve.

The extensor carpi radialis longus (ECRL) is a fusiform muscle sharing its origin at the lateral supracondylar ridge with the brachioradialis. Its tendon passes distal and posterior to the brachioradialis to insert on the base of the second metacarpal. The ECRL extends and abducts the wrist, indispensable when clenching the fist.

The extensor carpi radialis brevis (ECRB) is a short muscle that shares the common extensor origin of the lateral epicondyle. It passes deep to the ECRL, inserting on the base of the third metacarpal and assisting in the flexion and abduction of the wrist. The ECRB is the initial site of signal abnormality in lateral epicondylitis (tennis elbow) and should therefore be carefully scrutinized.[29]

Superficial
The extensor digitorum is the main extensor of the medial 4 digits. From the common extensor origin, its 4 tendons pass through a common synovial sheath deep to the extensor retinaculum to insert on the extensor expansion of the medial 4 digits. The extensor digitorum is the main extensor of the medial 4 digits at the metacarpophalangeal joints and also assists with extension at the wrist.

The extensor digiti minimi (EDM) is a slip of muscle partially detached from the medial aspect of extensor digitorum. It has a separate tendon sheath and inserts at the extensor expansion of the fifth digit and similarly extends the fifth digit at the metacarpophalangeal joint. It also likewise assists in extension of the wrist.

The extensor carpi ulnaris (ECU) is a long fusiform muscle located at the medial border of the forearm. The ECU originates from the posterior ulna, as well as the lateral epicondyle. It courses down the medial forearm with its distal insertion on the base of the fifth metacarpal. It functions to extend and adduct the wrist.

Deep
The supinator lies deep in the cubital fossa and along with the brachioradialis forms its floor. The supinator originates from the lateral epicondyle with extensive attachments to the proximal third of the radius. It serves as the main muscle of supination of the forearm by rotating the radius and in this capacity is assisted by the biceps brachii.

The other deep extensor muscles of the forearm originate distally and deep to the superficial muscles from an outcropping that divides the extensors. They are therefore also referred to as outcropping (thumb) muscles.

The abductor pollicis longus (APL) is a long fusiform muscle that typically inserts on the base of the first metacarpal, although it can also insert on the trapezium. It serves to abduct and extend the thumb at the carpometacarpal joint.

The extensor pollicis brevis (EPB) originates distal to the APL but attaches distally at the base of the first proximal phalanx. It shares a common synovial sheath with the APL, and together they form the lateral margin of the anatomic snuff box. It serves mainly to extend the first digit at the meta-carpophalangeal joint.

The extensor pollicis longus (EPL) originates distal to the APL. It inserts on the base of the distal phalanx of the thumb and therefore allows extension of the interphalangeal joint of the thumb. The EPL also passes medial to the Lister tubercle to form the medial border of the anatomic snuff box, an important clinical landmark.

The extensor indicis has the most distal origin of the deep muscles of the posterior compartment. It inserts on the extensor expansion of the digit allowing for independent extension of the index finger and assisting extension of the wrist.

Neurovascular Anatomy

The brachial artery provides the main arterial supply to the arm. The brachial artery is the continuation of the axillary artery distal to the inferior margin of the teres minor. It lies anterior to the triceps and brachialis, and medial to the humerus for most of its course. The brachial artery gives off the deep brachial artery and several smaller side branches. It turns in the antecubital fossa to lie anterior to the humerus and shortly thereafter divides into the radial and ulnar arteries. Shortly after the brachial bifurcation, the ulnar artery gives off the common interosseous artery. The short common interosseous artery quickly branches into the anterior and posterior interosseous arteries that supply the anterior and posterior compartments of the forearm respectively. The radial and ulnar arteries continue to the hand, terminating in the superficial and deep palmar arches respectively.

The 4 main nerves of the arm and forearm are the musculocutaneous, median, ulnar and radial nerves.

The musculocutaneous nerve is the terminal branch of the lateral cord of the brachial plexus and courses between the brachialis and the biceps without accompanying artery. The musculocutaneous nerve innervates all muscles of the anterior compartment of the arm.

The median nerve follows the course of the brachial artery in its course through the arm. At the level of the cubital fossa it passes between the heads of the pronator teres to supply most of the muscles of the anterior compartment of the forearm. Nerve impingement can occur as the nerve passes between the heads of the heads of the pronator teres (referred to as pronator syndrome). Less commonly the median nerve may be entrapped by a thickened lacertus fibrosis (bicipital aponeurosis), fibrous arch of the FDS, or the fibro-osseous tunnel created by the ligament of Struthers. The anterior interosseous is the major branch of the median nerve in the forearm arising approximately 5 cm distal to the elbow, coursing distally along the interosseous membrane to supply the deep muscles of the anterior compartment. Impingement of the anterior interosseous nerve is referred to as Kiloh-Nevin syndrome and may clinically mimic pronator syndrome.[30]

The ulnar nerve accompanies the proximal brachial artery but then pierces the intramuscular septum to enter the posterior compartment of the arm, passing posterior to the medial epicondyle through the cubital tunnel. The nerve then passes between the FCU and FDP, innervating the FCU and the medial aspect of the FDP. The cubital tunnel at the medial aspect of the elbow is a potential location for ulnar nerve impingement. In healthy individuals, elbow flexion causes narrowing of the cubital tunnel with resultant increased intraneural pressure. This phenomenon likely accounts for the frequent occurrence of cubital tunnel syndrome in occupations where patients are subject to repeated elbow flexion.[31] The ulnar nerve may also sublux or dislocate from the cubital tunnel. However, subluxation may be seen in 10% to 16% of healthy subjects and therefore correlation with symptoms is required.[32] The ulnar nerve at the level of the cubital tunnel is best evaluated on axial images.

The radial nerve accompanies the deep brachial artery through the radial groove of the humerus. It supplies all of the muscles of the posterior compartment of the arm. It crosses into the anterior compartment at the level of the cubital fossa between the brachialis and brachioradialis. Soon after entering the forearm it branches into a cutaneous superficial branch and a deep muscular branch. The radial nerve and its deep muscular branch (also referred to distal to the supinator as the posterior interosseous nerve) innervate all muscles of the posterior compartment of the forearm, including the brachioradialis. The deep muscular branch of the radial nerves course through a fibromuscular tunnel referred to as the radial tunnel innervating the ECRB and supinator. The tunnel begins near the proximal border of the supinator and extends to its distal margin. The supinator tunnel refers to the distal portion of the radial tunnel corresponding to the fatty space between the superficial and deep portions of the supinator muscle. The roof of the radial tunnel is formed by fibrous bands from adjacent muscles, the leash of Henry (recurrent radial artery vessels) and the arcade of Frohse (fibrous arch of the superficial portion of the proximal supinator). In most (70%) individuals, the deep radial nerve passes through the body of the supinator; in the remainder of individuals, it passes via the arcade of Frohse.[28] The radial tunnel is prone to compression at these sites and potentially by the ECRB muscle.[33] Many different terms have been used to describe the impingement of the deep branch of the radial nerve within the radial tunnel, including posterior interosseous nerve syndrome, supinator syndrome, and radial tunnel syndrome.[34]

The veins of the arm can be divided into superficial and deep. The main superficial veins are the basilar and the cephalic and median antebrachial veins. The median antebrachial vein, which drains the superficial palmar arch, usually drains into the basilic vein. The basilic and cephalic veins join the deep axillary vein at the level of the upper arm to form the axillary vein. The deep veins follow their analogous arteries and are relatively small, usually paired and connected by intervening transverse branches. Although this is the most common pattern, there is considerable variability of the veins of the upper extremity.[35]

SUMMARY

Knowledge of normal anatomy is imperative for the diagnosis of musculoskeletal pathology of the upper extremity. This knowledge allows for the recognition of normal variants to prevent misdiagnosis.

REFERENCES

1. Sofka CM, Pavlov H. The history of clinical musculoskeletal radiology. Radiol Clin North Am 2009;47(3):349–56.
2. Meyer JS, Jaramillo D. Musculoskeletal MR imaging at 3 T. Magn Reson Imaging Clin N Am 2008;16(3):533–45, vi.
3. Kuo PH, Kanal E, Abu-Alfa AK, et al. Gadolinium-based MR contrast agents and nephrogenic systemic fibrosis 1. Radiology 2007;242(3):647–9.
4. Schmidt GP, Reiser MF, Baur-Melnyk A. Whole-body imaging of the musculoskeletal system: the value of MR imaging. Skeletal Radiol 2007;36(12):1109–19.
5. Pui MH, Chang SK. Comparison of inversion recovery fast spin-echo (FSE) with T2-weighted fat-saturated FSE and T1-weighted MR imaging in bone marrow lesion detection. Skeletal Radiol 1996;25(2):149–52.
6. Harkens KL, Moore TE, Yuh WT, et al. Gadolinium-enhanced MRI of soft tissue masses. Australas Radiol 1993;37(1):30–4.
7. Vogler J III, Murphy W. Bone marrow imaging. Radiology 1988;168(3):679–93.
8. Steiner RM, Mitchell DG, Rao VM, et al. Magnetic resonance imaging of diffuse bone marrow disease. Radiol Clin North Am 1993;31(2):383–409.
9. Vande Berg BC, Malghem J, Lecouvet FE, et al. Magnetic resonance imaging of the normal bone marrow. Skeletal Radiol 1998;27(9):471–83.
10. Moulopoulos LA, Dimopoulos MA. Magnetic resonance imaging of the bone marrow in hematologic malignancies. Blood 1997;90(6):2127.
11. Rosenberg ZS, Bencardino J, Beltran J. MR imaging of normal variants and interpretation pitfalls of the elbow. Magn Reson Imaging Clin N Am 1997;5(3):481–99.
12. Stevens KJ. Magnetic resonance imaging of the elbow. J Magn Reson Imag 2010;31(5):1036–53.
13. Kim YS, Yeh LR, Trudell D, et al. MR imaging of the major nerves about the elbow: cadaveric study examining the effect of flexion and extension of the elbow and pronation and supination of the forearm. Skeletal Radiol 1998;27(8):419–26.
14. Wedeen VJ, Weisskoff RM, Poncelet BP. MRI signal void due to in-plane motion is all-or-none. Magn Reson Med 1994;32(1):116–20.
15. Lind T, Krøner K, Jensen J. The epidemiology of fractures of the proximal humerus. Arch Orthop Trauma Surg 1989;108(5):285–7.
16. Fowler KA, Chung CB. Normal MR imaging anatomy of the elbow. Magn Reson Imaging Clin N Am 2004;12(2):191–206, v.
17. Pećina M, Borić I, Antičević D. Intraoperatively proven anomalous Struthers' ligament diagnosed by MRI. Skeletal Radiol 2002;31(9):532–5.
18. Yu JS, Habib PA. Normal MR imaging anatomy of the wrist and hand. Magn Reson Imaging Clin N Am 2004;12(2):207–19, v.
19. Seiler JG III, Parker LM, Chamberland PD, et al. The distal biceps tendon. Two potential mechanisms involved in its rupture: arterial supply and mechanical impingement. J Shoulder Elbow Surg 1995;4(3):149–56.
20. Williams BD, Schweitzer ME, Weishaupt D, et al. Partial tears of the distal biceps tendon: MR appearance and associated clinical findings. Skeletal Radiol 2001;30(10):560–4.
21. Fitzgerald SW, Curry DR, Erickson SJ, et al. Distal biceps tendon injury: MR imaging diagnosis. Radiology 1994;191(1):203.
22. Nayak SR, Krishnamurthy A. An unusual supernumerary head of biceps brachii muscle. Clin Anat 2008;21(8):788–9.
23. Matsuura S, Kojima T, Kinoshita Y. Cubital tunnel syndrome caused by abnormal insertion of triceps brachii muscle. J Hand Surg Br 1994;19(1):38–9.
24. Dellon L. Musculotendinous variations about the medial humeral epicondyle. J Hand Surg Br 1986;11(2):175–81.

25. Martinoli C, Perez MM, Padua L, et-al. Muscle variants of the upper and lower limb (with anatomical correlation). Semin Musculoskelet Radiol 2010;14(2):106–21.

26. Mallisee TA, Boynton MD, Erickson SJ, et al. Normal MR imaging anatomy of the elbow. Magn Reson Imaging Clin N Am 1997;5(3):451–79.

27. Rosenberg ZS, Bencardino J, Beltran J. MR features of nerve disorders at the elbow. Magn Reson Imaging Clin N Am 1997;5(3):545–65.

28. Boles CA, Kannam S, Cardwell AB. The forearm: anatomy of muscle compartments and nerves. Am J Roentgenol 2000;174(1):151.

29. Potter HG, Hannafin JA, Morwessel RM, et al. Lateral epicondylitis: correlation of MR imaging, surgical, and histopathologic findings. Radiology 1995;196(1):43.

30. Wertsch JJ, Melvin J. Median nerve anatomy and entrapment syndromes: a review. Arch Phys Med Rehabil 1982;63(12):623–7.

31. Gelberman RH, Yamaguchi K, Hollstien SB, et al. Changes in interstitial pressure and cross-sectional area of the cubital tunnel and of the ulnar nerve with flexion of the elbow. An experimental study in human cadavera. J Bone Joint Surg Am 1998; 80(4):492.

32. Bozentka DJ. Cubital tunnel syndrome pathophysiology. Clin Orthop 1998;351:90.

33. Mazurek MT, Shin AY. Upper extremity peripheral nerve anatomy: current concepts and applications. Clin Orthop 2001;383:7.

34. Resnick D, Kang H, Pretterklieber M. Shoulder. In: Resnick D, Kang H, Pretterklieber M, editors. Internal derangements of joints: emphasis on MR imaging. Philadelphia: Saunders; 1997. p. 163–333.

35. Weber TM, Lockhart ME, Robbin ML. Upper extremity venous Doppler ultrasound. Ultrasound Clin 2009;4(2):181–92.

Normal and Variant Anatomy of the Shoulder on MRI

Tessa S. Cook, MD, PhD*, Joel M. Stein, MD, PhD,
Stephanie Simonson, MD, Woojin Kim, MD

KEYWORDS

- Normal shoulder anatomy
- Shoulder magnetic resonance imaging • Normal variants

New developments in musculoskeletal magnetic resonance (MR) imaging, including improved spatial resolution and MR arthrography, have led to an increasing frequency in the performance of shoulder MR imaging. As a result, radiologists' understanding of the normal and variant anatomy of the shoulder visible on MR imaging has also become more important. In this article, the authors review the normal arrangement and appearance of osseous and soft-tissue structures in the shoulder, as well as nonpathologic osseous and nonosseous variants that should be recognized.

PROTOCOLS

When imaging the shoulder with MR imaging, patients are placed in a supine position with their arm on the side of the body in partial external rotation. Initially, the localizer images are obtained, followed by coronal-oblique, sagittal-oblique, and axial images. The coronal-oblique plane is selected parallel to the course of the supraspinatus tendon. Because the supraspinatus tendon may have a degree of obliquity that is different than the supraspinatus muscle, it is important to select the course of the tendon itself when prescribing the coronal-oblique plane for optimal visualization of the tendon. The sagittal-oblique images are prescribed parallel to the glenoid surface. Typical sequences obtained at the authors' institution are listed in **Table 1**.

NORMAL OSSEOUS STRUCTURES

The osseous shoulder is comprised of the proximal humerus, scapula, and clavicle. Multiple components of the scapula contribute to the shoulder, including the glenoid, coracoid process, and acromion. The glenohumeral joint forms what is conventionally thought of as the shoulder joint, whereas the articulation of the other scapular components with the clavicle and the humerus gives the joint added stability and range of motion. In this section, the authors discuss the normal anatomy of the 3 bones that make up the shoulder.

Proximal Humerus

The proximal humerus consists of the humeral head, the greater and lesser tuberosities, the humeral neck, and the bicipital groove. The humeral head makes the most significant contribution to the shoulder. It is typically round, with slight flattening of the posteroinferior surface. This slight flattening should not be confused with a Hill-Sachs lesion as a sequela of anterior shoulder dislocation, which is seen at or above the level of the coracoid process (**Fig. 1**).[1] The central portion of the humeral head is spherical, whereas the peripheral contour is more elliptical. The morphology of the humeral head varies somewhat between men and women, particularly with respect to the radius of curvature, which is larger in men than women.[2] Distinction is commonly

This work was not supported by any funding agency.
The authors have nothing to disclose.
Department of Radiology, Hospital of the University of Pennsylvania, 3400 Spruce Street, 1 Silverstein, Philadelphia, PA 19104, USA
* Corresponding author.
E-mail address: tessa.cook@uphs.upenn.edu

Magn Reson Imaging Clin N Am 19 (2011) 581–594
doi:10.1016/j.mric.2011.05.005

Table 1
Standard pulse sequences for MRI examination of the shoulder

Pulse Sequence	FOV (cm)	Slice Thickness (mm)	Matrix	TR/TE
Axial T2 fat saturation	14	4	256 × 256	3500/45
Coronal oblique T1	14	4	256 × 256	560–615/11–14
Coronal oblique T2 with fat saturation	14	4	256 × 256	3500/50–54
Sagittal oblique T1	14	4	256 × 256	518–628/10–12
Sagittal oblique T2 with fat saturation	14	4	256 × 256	3500/45

Abbreviations: FOV, field of view; TE, echo time; TR, repetition time.

made between the anatomic and the surgical necks of the humerus. The anatomic neck forms the oblique circumference of the humeral head and separates the head from the tuberosities. The surgical neck forms the axial circumference of the humerus immediately inferior to the tuberosities and is often involved in fractures.[3] The cartilage overlying the humeral head is only approximately 1 mm thick. Subchondral cysts can be present within the humeral head and are normally found at the insertions of the supraspinatus and infraspinatus tendons. The cysts in these locations do not represent degenerative sequelae, whereas cysts located more anteriorly are associated with subscapularis tendon pathology.

The bicipital groove, also known as intertubercular groove, runs between the greater and lesser tuberosities and supports the long head of the biceps tendon. The transverse humeral ligament crosses the long head of the biceps tendon perpendicular to the bicipital groove. The width and depth of the groove both affect the risk of subluxation of the long head of the biceps tendon. A shallow bicipital groove predisposes to dislocation of the long head of the biceps tendon.[4]

Scapula

The scapula is composed of a spine, neck, and body, as well as the acromion, coracoid process, and glenoid. The latter three structures form articulations with the humeral head and the clavicle to become components of the shoulder joint.

The acromion is a posterior shoulder landmark, formed as a posterolateral extension of the scapular spine, superior to the glenoid. It articulates

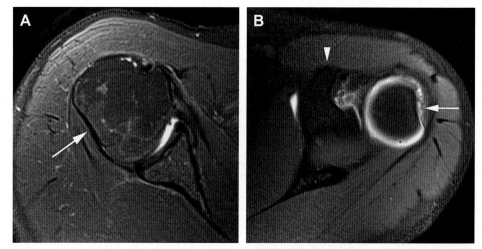

Fig. 1. Normal humeral head versus Hill-Sachs lesion. (*A*) On the axial T2-weighted with fat-saturation MR image, there is a slight flattening of the posteroinferior surface of the humeral head (*arrow*), which is a normal finding. (*B*) Axial T1-weighted with fat-saturation MR arthrogram image shows Hill-Sachs defect (*arrow*) in this patient with history of previous anterior shoulder dislocation, which is seen at the level of the coracoid process (*arrowhead*).

with the clavicle and is the origin of the deltoid and trapezius muscles. The shape of the acromion is symmetric bilaterally but can vary with gender.[5] Bigliani and colleagues'[6] classification system for acromial morphology offers three types: I (flat), II (curved), and III (hooked) (**Fig. 2**). It is hypothesized that the hooked acromion is in fact an acquired form and increases an individual's predisposition to rotator cuff pathology.[7]

The coracoid process is an anterior shoulder landmark, arising from the anterolateral aspect of the scapula, superior and medial to the glenoid fossa. It also represents the tendinous origins of a number of upper extremity and chest wall muscles, including the pectoralis minor and long head of the biceps brachii. The morphology of the coracoid is extremely variable.[8,9]

The glenoid articulates with the medial aspect of the humeral head to form the shoulder joint. The glenoid is pear shaped (also known as inverted-comma shaped) or oval shaped in the coronal plane[10] and does not vary appreciably in size between men and women; significant differences in glenoid morphology have been found among different ethnicities.[11] The glenoid cavity is retroverted by approximately 5° to 7°.[12] The postero-inferior rim of the glenoid can have various shapes, including triangular, J shaped, and deltoid. The latter two are associated with varying degrees of posterior shoulder instability (**Fig. 3**),[13,14] as is loss of tilting and concavity of the inferior glenoid.[15] At the superior aspect of the glenoid, the supraglenoid tubercle serves as the attachment for the long head of the biceps.

Clavicle

The clavicle is an S-shaped bone that forms the sternoclavicular joint medially and the acromioclavicular joint laterally. Its morphology is extremely

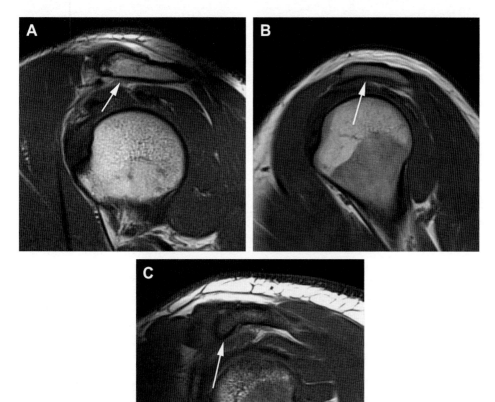

Fig. 2. Various acromion shapes. Sagittal-oblique T1-weighted MR images of the shoulder demonstrate (*A*) type I acromion with flat surface (*arrow*), (*B*) type II acromion with curved surface that parallels the superior contour of the humeral head, and (*C*) type III acromion with anterior hook that projects inferiorly.

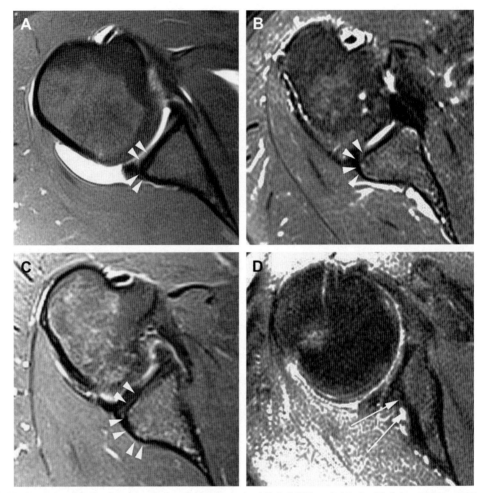

Fig. 3. Various glenoid rim shapes and glenoid hypoplasia. (*A*) Axial T1-weighted with fat-saturation MR arthrogram image demonstrates the normal triangular type glenoid rim shape (*arrowheads*). Axial T2-weighted with fat-saturation MR images show rounded J-shaped (*B*) and deltoid-shaped (*C*) posteroinferior glenoid rim (*arrowheads*). (*D*) Severe posterior glenoid dysplasia (*arrows*).

variable, ranging from flat to sharply curved. Increased thickness and curvature is seen in manual workers, and the right clavicle is often stronger than the left.[16]

NORMAL SOFT-TISSUE STRUCTURES

Several muscles, tendons, ligaments, and cartilaginous structures work in synchrony to move and support the shoulder. The normal MR imaging appearance of these structures is important to recognize in an effort to identify associated pathology.

Rotator Cuff

The rotator cuff allows for range of motion at the shoulder and protects and stabilizes the glenohumeral joint. Four muscles comprise the rotator cuff: the supraspinatus, infraspinatus, teres minor,

and subscapularis. The four fan-shaped muscles all arise from the scapula and attach to the humerus, with the subscapularis inserting on the lesser tuberosity and the other three muscles inserting on the greater tuberosity. The subscapularis lies anterior to the scapular body, whereas the supraspinatus, infraspinatus, and teres minor lie posteriorly in order from superior to inferior. The insertion pattern of the rotator cuff tendons is consistent across individuals, with the tendons arranged in a horseshoe-shaped configuration about the humeral head.[17] The subscapularis tendon is the most anterior, followed by the supraspinatus tendon at the superior aspect of the humeral head, and the infraspinatus and teres minor tendons posteriorly (**Fig. 4**).

The supraspinatus muscle arises from the supraspinous fossa along the dorsal scapula and is

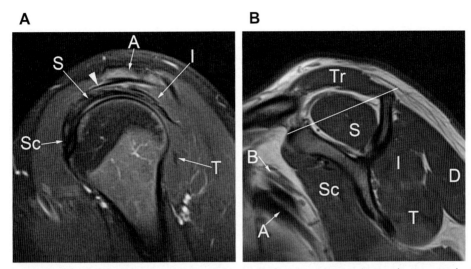

Fig. 4. Normal shoulder. (A) Sagittal-oblique T2-weighted with fat-saturation MR image shows normal subscapularis (Sc), supraspinatus (S), infraspinatus (I), and teres minor (T) tendons. Other structures are the acromion (A) and coracoacromial ligament (*arrowhead*). (B) Medial to Fig. 6 (A), sagittal-oblique T1-weighted MR image shows normal subscapularis (Sc), supraspinatus (S), infraspinatus (I), and teres minor (T) muscles. Other muscles seen are deltoid muscle (D) and trapezius muscle (Tr). Axillary artery and vein (A) and brachial plexus (B) are seen anteriorly. Presence of supraspinatus muscle bulk superior to the line drawn on top of the *Y* of the scapula is one of the useful guides for looking for the presence of muscle atrophy.

innervated by the suprascapular nerve. Its tendon passes inferior to the clavicle and inserts on the greater tuberosity of the humerus. The supraspinatus is required for normal lateral abduction of the upper extremity. The infraspinatus muscle arises from the infraspinous fossa along the dorsal scapula and is also innervated by the suprascapular nerve. Its tendon also inserts on the greater tuberosity. The infraspinatus allows for external rotation and posterior abduction of the upper extremity. The teres minor muscle arises from the dorsolateral scapula and is innervated by the axillary nerve. Its tendon unites with the posterior inferior aspect of the capsule and inserts on and just inferior to the greater tuberosity. Along with the infraspinatus, the teres minor assists in external rotation of the shoulder. Some fibers of the teres minor can fuse with those of the infraspinatus. The subscapularis arises from the subscapular fossa of the ventral scapula and is innervated by the subscapular nerves. Its tendon runs along the subscapular bursa and inserts on the lesser tuberosity. The subscapularis is responsible for internal rotation of the shoulder, as well as anterior abduction of the humerus (see **Fig. 4**; **Figs. 5** and **6**).

Biceps Tendon/Pulley System

The tendon of the long head of the biceps is intimately associated with the shoulder. It attaches to the superior glenoid rim, anterior and posterior superior labrum, and the coracoid.[18] It is secured in the bicipital groove, between the greater and lesser tuberosity, by the transverse ligament. The long head of the biceps tendon traverses through what is called the rotator interval, which is bordered superiorly by the supraspinatus, inferiorly by the subscapularis, and medially by the base of the coracoid process. The biceps pulley, also known as the biceps sling, is comprised of a combination of the coracohumeral, superior glenohumeral and transverse humeral ligaments.

Glenoid Labrum

A fibrocartilaginous layer, the glenoid labrum, covers the bony glenoid. The labrum provides points of attachment for the glenohumeral ligaments, which stabilize the shoulder joint. There is variability in the morphology and thickness of the labrum, greater at the superior aspect compared with the inferior aspect.[19] The superior labrum is closely associated with the biceps tendon.[20] The glenoid labrum contributes to several normal variants in the shoulder, which are discussed subsequently.

Glenohumeral Ligaments

The superior, middle, and inferior glenohumeral ligaments are responsible for stabilizing and strengthening the glenohumeral joint capsule. The

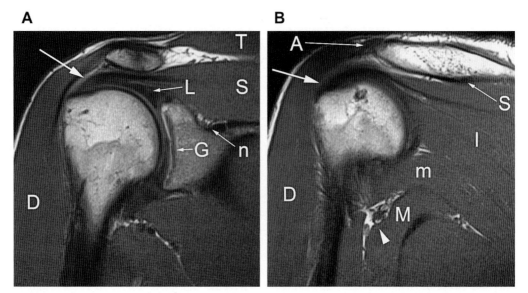

Fig. 5. Normal shoulder. Coronal-oblique T1-weighted MR image shows the normal supraspinatus and infraspinatus muscles and tendons. (*A*) Supraspinatus muscle (S) and tendon (*arrow*) take a more straight course. Other structures shown are the deltoid muscle (D), glenoid (G), superior labrum (L), suprascapular notch (n), and trapezius muscle (T). (*B*) Posterior to Fig. 4 (*A*), unlike the supraspinatus muscle and tendon, the infraspinatus muscle (I) and tendon (*arrow*) take on an oblique course. Other structures shown are the acromion (A), teres major muscle (M), teres minor muscle (m), scapula (S), and posterior circumflex vessels and axillary nerve (*arrowhead*).

origins of the glenohumeral ligaments are generally thought of with respect to their positions on a clock, superimposed on the glenoid labrum en face: 12 o'clock is defined at the superior aspect, 3 o'clock at the anterior aspect, 6 o'clock at the inferior aspect, and 9 o'clock at the posterior aspect. The superior and middle glenohumeral ligaments attach between 12 o'clock and 1 o'clock. The superior glenohumeral ligament runs from the anterior superior glenoid rim to the humeral head, just above the greater tuberosity.[21] It combines with the coracohumeral ligament and the anterosuperior aspect

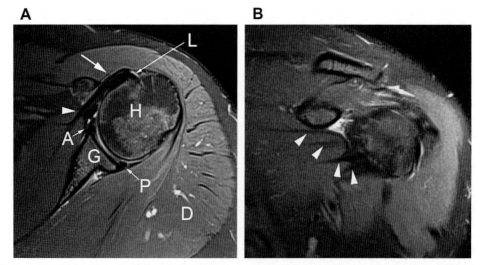

Fig. 6. Normal subscapularis tendon. (*A*) Axial T2-weighted with fat-saturation MR image of the shoulder showing the normal subscapularis tendon (*arrow*) and myotendinous junction (*arrowhead*). Other structures visualized are the deltoid muscle (D), anterior labrum (A), posterior labrum (P), glenoid (G), humeral head (H), and long head of the biceps tendon (L). (*B*) Coronal-oblique T2-weighted with fat-saturation MR image of the shoulder nicely demonstrates different tendons (*arrowheads*) arising from the subscapularis muscle.

of the glenohumeral joint capsule to form the rotator interval capsule.[22] The middle glenohumeral ligament (MGHL) runs from the anterior superior glenoid to the humerus, adjacent to the lesser tuberosity. There is a great deal of variability in the anatomy of the MGHL[23]; some of these variants are discussed later. The inferior glenohumeral ligament (IGHL) is actually a complex of anterior and posterior bands. The anterior bands attach from 2 to 4 o'clock, whereas the posterior bands attach from 7 to 9 o'clock.[24] It is responsible for stabilizing the anterior shoulder when the arm is abducted, externally rotated, and held at 90° to the body (**Fig. 7**).

Coracohumeral Ligament

The coracohumeral ligament (CHL) is not a true ligament connecting two bones, but instead represents a part of the shoulder capsule.[25] The CHL originates from the coracoid process and terminates on the humeral head, but it incorporates itself into the shoulder capsule before insertion on the greater and lesser tuberosities (**Fig. 8**). As such, it forms the main component of the rotator interval or the roof of the rotator cuff interval.[26] The CHL ensheathes the anterior aspect of the supraspinatus tendon. Its posterior attachment to the supraspinatus tendon stabilizes the tendon of the long head of the biceps in the bicipital groove.[27] On axial T2-weighted images, the CHL is low in signal, perpendicular to the SGHL, and anterior to the tendon of the long head of the biceps.

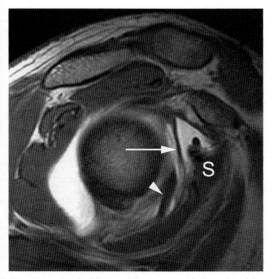

Fig. 7. Sagittal-oblique MR image of the shoulder shows middle glenohumeral ligament (*arrow*) and inferior glenohumeral ligament (*arrowhead*). Subscapularis muscle and tendon shown (S).

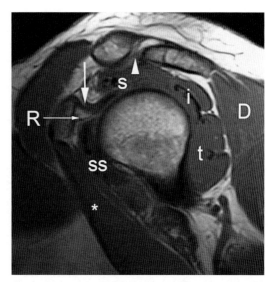

Fig. 8. Coracohumeral ligament and rotator interval. Sagittal-oblique T1-weighted MR image of the shoulder shows intact coracohumeral ligament (*arrow*). The rotator interval (R) is seen bordered superiorly by the supraspinatus (S) and inferiorly by the superior margin of the subscapularis (SS). Other structures are the infraspinatus muscle and tendon (i), teres minor muscle and tendon (t), acromioclavicular joint (*arrowhead*), deltoid muscle (D), and biceps (*short head*) muscle (*asterisk*).

Quadrilateral Space

The quadrilateral, or quadrangular, space is bounded by the humerus, teres major, teres minor, and long head of the triceps. It is an anatomic space through which the axillary nerve and the posterior humeral circumflex artery pass. Compression of either of these structures can lead to quadrilateral space syndrome, which is manifest on MR imaging by abnormal signal or T1-hyperintense fatty atrophy of the teres minor on oblique sagittal images (**Fig. 9**).[28,29]

Bursae

There are 4 important fluid-filled bursae within the shoulder: the subacromial, subdeltoid, subscapular, and subcoracoid bursae. The subacromial, subdeltoid, and subcoracoid bursae are sometimes seen as one large, continuous bursa.

The subacromial bursa is bounded superiorly by the deltoid, acromion, and coracoacromial ligament and inferiorly by the rotator cuff and, in particular, the supraspinatus.[30] In the normal shoulder, there is no communication between the subacromial bursa and the glenohumeral joint. However, in the setting of a rotator cuff tear, a communication between these two spaces can develop. The role of the subacromial bursa is to decrease frictional

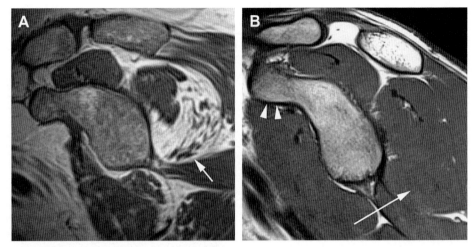

Fig. 9. Quadrilateral space syndrome. Sagittal-oblique T1-weighted MR image of the shoulder (*A*) demonstrates severe fatty atrophy of the teres minor muscle (*arrow*). (*B*) Normal muscle bulk of teres minor shown for comparison. Normal coracoid process (*arrowheads*).

forces on the supraspinatus tendon and between the deltoid and the rotator cuff.

The subdeltoid bursa either communicates with or is separated by a thin septum from the subacromial bursa. As its name indicates, it is bound superiorly by the deltoid muscle, laterally by the greater tuberosity, and inferiorly by the rotator cuff.[31] As with the subacromial bursa, the subdeltoid bursa does not communicate with the glenohumeral joint. It is surrounded by 1 to 2 mm of T1-hyperintense fat, which increases in thickness with age and increasing subcutaneous fat.

The subscapular bursa cushions the subscapularis tendon as it crosses over the scapular neck and under the coracoid process.[30] Unlike the other bursae, it communicates with the glenohumeral joint between the superior, middle, and inferior glenohumeral ligaments. Its morphology is variable, but it is best visualized using axial imaging.

The subcoracoid bursa is bound anteriorly by the tendons of the short head of the biceps and the coracobrachialis, posteriorly by the subscapularis tendon, and superiorly by the coracoid process. It communicates with the subacromial and subdeltoid bursae in a small percentage of individuals.[32] The subcoracoid bursa is best seen on oblique sagittal or coronal T2-weighted images (**Fig. 10**).

Additional smaller bursae exist within the shoulder and are not commonly visualized on MR imaging.

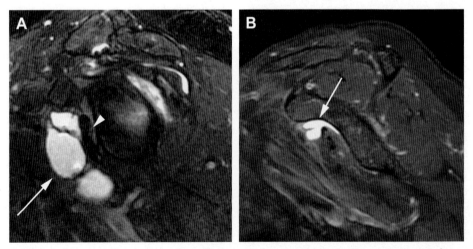

Fig. 10. Subcoracoid bursa and superior subscapularis recess. Sagittal-oblique T2-weighted with fat-saturation MR images show (*A*) markedly distended subcoracoid bursa (*arrow*) located anterior to the subscapularis muscle and tendon (*arrowhead*). (*B*) Note that more medial to (*A*), the superior subscapularis recess (*arrow*) takes on a more saddlebaglike configuration over the subscapularis.

These smaller bursae generally do not communicate with the glenohumeral joint and include the infraspinatus, teres major, and pectoralis major bursae.

NORMAL OSSEOUS VARIANTS

Normal osseous variants occur in the shoulder. A few are discussed here to distinguish them from fractures or other sequelae of trauma or hematologic disease.

Os Acromiale

Normal ossification of the acromion commences at 15 years of age and is usually completed in the early to mid 20s.[33] Incomplete ossification results in an os acromiale (**Fig. 11**). This variant has been identified in 8% to 14% of the population (7%–15%[1]). There is variation in gender and ethnicity when it comes to the morphology of the os acromiale, which is suspected to have genetic underpinnings.[34] Additionally, there appears to be an association between prior shoulder trauma or stress and subsequent development of an os acromiale; however, it is important to note that the os acromiale itself is not a fracture fragment and should not be mistaken for one.[33]

Acromial Pseudospur

The acromial or subacromial pseudospur is a normal variant that is thought to either represent prominence of the acromial angle at the attachment of the coracoacromial ligament or a slip of the attachment of the deltoid.[35] The former is commonly referred to as an acromial pseudospur.[36] The subacromial pseudospur is described when the deltoid tendon, which attaches to the undersurface of the acromion, is only partially imaged in coronal cross section (**Fig. 12**). The T1-hypointense pseudospur does not represent a true osteophyte, but rather a wisp of deltoid tendon seen in isolation.[37]

Marrow Changes

It is common for hematopoietic (red) marrow to be present in the proximal humeral metaphysis and to extend cephalad into the humeral epiphysis. The distribution of the hematopoietic marrow can be continuous or discontinuous, with a curvilinear zone of transition between red and nonhematopoietic (yellow) marrow or regional variation with focal areas of red marrow. Hematopoietic marrow will appear hypointense on T1-weighted imaging with respect to nonhematopoietic marrow, because of the latter's high fat content.[38]

Cystic Changes in the Bare Area of the Humeral Head

Cystic lesions in the posterosuperior (bare area) of the humeral head should not be mistaken for degenerative sequelae or vascular channels. Instead, they are typically pseudocysts that communicate with the joint space and represent a normal variant.[39]

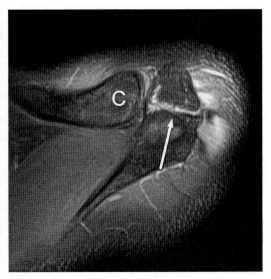

Fig. 11. Os acromiale. Axial T2-weighted MR image through the acromioclavicular joint demonstrates os acromiale (*arrow*) and clavicle (C).

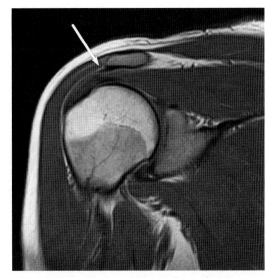

Fig. 12. Subacromial pseudospur. Coronal-oblique T1-weighted image of the shoulder shows subacromial pseudospur (*arrow*) formed by slip of the attachment of the deltoid as it attaches to the undersurface of the acromion.

NORMAL NONOSSEOUS VARIANTS

Several normal variants can be seen in the soft tissues of the shoulder. These variants can mimic degenerative changes, fractures, tendon tears, and other abnormalities and should be recognized as a normal anatomic variation instead of pathology. In particular, variant anatomy of the labrum can be misconstrued as labral pathology. However, when viewing the glenoid articular surface as a clock face, normal variants will typically be found in the 11-o'clock to 3-o'clock position, whereas pathology will be located beyond the 3-o'clock position.

Normal Thinning of Humeral Cartilage

Unlike the cartilage of the knee, which can average 4 mm in thickness, the cartilage of the humeral head is significantly thinner. The humeral cartilage is thickest in the central portion of the humeral head near the glenoid fossa, where it measures approximately 1.9 mm. Toward the periphery, the cartilage thins progressively and measures approximately 1.2 mm.[40,41] The thickness of the humeral head cartilage is essentially symmetric, with the exception of slightly greater thickness of the posterior superior humeral cartilage as compared with the anterior superior cartilage. Humeral cartilage is best assessed using MR arthrography, but it is important to recognize that the thickness of the humeral head cartilage on MR imaging can be represented by only 1 to 2 pixels when accounting for chemical shift.[42] Thus, recognition of this feature as a normal variant is essential in avoiding its misdiagnosis as posttraumatic or degenerative sequelae.

Normal Thinning of Cartilage of Tubercle of Assaki

The tubercle of Assaki is the thickest subchondral bone of the glenoid and is found at the center of the glenoid.[1] The cartilage overlying the tubercle of Assaki is often thinned and is described as a bare spot. This variant is normal and should not be mistaken for a focal cartilaginous defect (**Fig. 13**).[43]

Sublabral Recess

The sublabral recess, also known as sublabral sulcus, represents the variant configurations of the labral-bicipital complex at the 12-o'clock position: the attachment of the superior labrum to the glenoid at the insertion of the long head of the biceps tendon.[18] Three types of sublabral recess have been identified. The type I variant demonstrates close apposition of the labrum to the

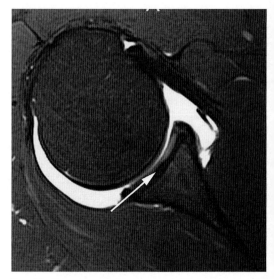

Fig. 13. Tubercle of Assaki. Axial T1-weighted with fat-saturation MR arthrogram image shows focal thickening of the subchondral bone in the mid aspect of the glenoid with thinning of overlying cartilage (*arrow*).

glenoid and the biceps tendon. Types II and III demonstrate a sulcus between the normally triangular labrum and the glenoid, into which an instrument can be inserted during arthroscopy. The sulcus is shallow in the type II variant and deep in the type III variant. The sublabral recess is best seen filling with contrast and extending medially toward the glenoid on MR arthrography with T1-weighted, fat-saturated, coronal-oblique images (**Fig. 14**).[44] It can be mistaken for a type

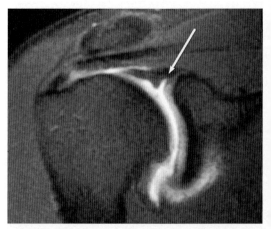

Fig. 14. Sublabral recess. Coronal T1-weighted with fat-saturation MR arthrogram image following intra-articular contrast injection with fat suppression demonstrates a smooth cleft of contrast (*arrow*) extending medially beneath the labrum at the 12-o'clock position.

II superior labrum anterior-posterior tear; however, it should be noted that this lesion often extends laterally or posteriorly.[45]

Sublabral Foramen

The sublabral foramen, also known as the sublabral hole, represents normal detachment of the anterosuperior labrum from the glenoid and typically occurs at the 2-o'clock position, anterior to the attachment of the biceps tendon.[18] This variant is seen in approximately 11% of individuals and best visualized on coronal-oblique, T1-weighted MR arthrography with fat saturation.[46] The sublabral foramen is often mistaken for an anterosuperior labral tear, an injury of high-performance throwing athletes often accompanied by clinical symptoms.[47,48] The sublabral recess can coexist and communicate with the sublabral foramen.

Buford Complex

The Buford complex represents a combination of two variants: a markedly thickened MGHL and congenital absence of the anterosuperior labrum.[49] The thickened MGHL attaches directly to the anterosuperior glenoid and can be mistaken for a displaced labral fragment.[18] Axial T1-weighted MR arthrography with fat saturation can be used to visualize the cordlike MGHL adjacent to the absent labrum (**Fig. 15**), giving the appearance of an avulsed labral fragment.[44] Sagittal-oblique images will clearly demonstrate the thickened MGHL and the normal superior and inferior glenohumeral ligaments.

PROMINENT ANTERIOR BAND OF THE INFERIOR GLENOHUMERAL LIGAMENT

The anterior band of the IGHL can be prominent or thickened (**Fig. 16**). This feature is associated with either hypoplastic or absent anterior superior labrum. It is thought that in some cases, the diagnosis of sublabral foramen may actually represent this prominent anterior band of the IGHL in the setting of absent anterior superior labrum.

Absent Middle Glenohumeral Ligament

The MGHL is the most variable of the 3 ligaments.[50] As such, its variants are often mistaken for ligamentous or labral pathology. The MGHL can vary in appearance from thickened and cordlike, as in the Buford complex, to completely absent. Complete absence of the MGHL is seen in up to 30% of individuals.[51] The MGHL is best visualized on oblique sagittal or axial MR arthrography.

Accessory Head of Biceps Tendon

Various anomalous muscles exist within the shoulder, which include accessory heads of the biceps brachii muscle, coracobrachialis brevis muscle, accessory subscapularis muscle, and the aberrant muscle bundle originating from the latissimus dorsi or pectoralis muscles. One of the

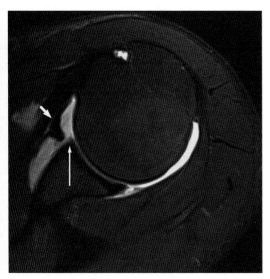

Fig. 15. Buford complex. Axial T1-weighted MR image with fat saturation following intraarticular injection demonstrates a Buford complex with thick cordlike middle glenohumeral ligament (*short arrow*) with absent anterior superior labrum (*long arrow*).

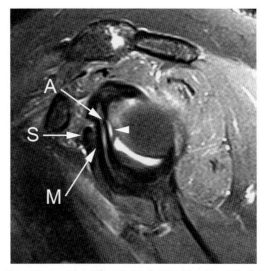

Fig. 16. Sagittal T2-weighted MR image with fat saturation demonstrates prominent anterior band of the IGHL seen attaching high at the level of the superior labrum (A). Note the absent anterior superior labrum in this patient (*arrowhead*). Other structures: subscapularis tendon (S) and middle glenohumeral ligament (M).

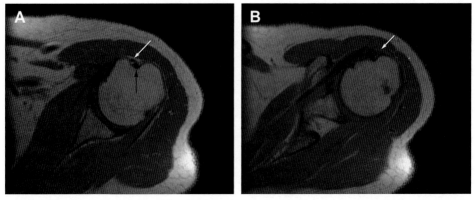

Fig. 17. Axial T1-weighted MR images of the shoulder demonstrate (*A*) an anomalous tendon (*white arrow*) adjacent and superficial to the long head of the biceps tendon (*black arrow*) within the bicipital groove. More superiorly (*B*), it is seen attaching (*arrow*) to the greater tuberosity close to the articular capsule.

most common variants is the accessory head of the biceps muscle. The supernumerary head is thought to be present in 9.1% to 22.9% of the population, where it is more commonly seen in Asians. Knowledge of this variant is important in not mistaking it for a longitudinal split tear of the long head of the biceps tendon (**Fig. 17**).[52]

Vacuum Phenomenon

Vacuum phenomenon is typically associated with degenerative changes. However, in joints, such as the hip and shoulder, it can appear during traction, particularly in children. In the shoulder, it is seen as a low-signal, curvilinear, intraarticular focus on axial gradient-echo MR imaging.[53] This appearance mimics intraarticular calcification, which may be secondary to chondrocalcinosis or loose intraarticular bodies. However, vacuum phenomenon classically appears in the superior aspect of the glenohumeral joint on only a few images and will not be accompanied by joint effusion or other abnormal findings.

SUMMARY

With the advent of new techniques in musculoskeletal imaging, MR imaging of the shoulder continues to develop as an important tool in the assessment of shoulder-joint and soft-tissue pathologies. A clear understanding of the normal anatomy of the shoulder and osseous and nonosseous variants is important in the diagnosis and management of diseases of the shoulder.

REFERENCES

1. Rudez J, Zanetti M. Normal anatomy, variants and pitfalls on shoulder MRI. Eur J Radiol 2008;68(1):25–35.
2. Iannotti JP, Gabriel JP, Schneck SL, et al. The normal glenohumeral relationships. An anatomical study of one hundred and forty shoulders. J Bone Joint Surg Am 1992;74:491–500.
3. Gray H. Anatomy of the human body. Philadelphia: Lea & Febiger; 1918. Bartleby.com, 2000. Available at: www.bartleby.com/107/. Accessed August 25, 2010.
4. Chan TW, Dalinka MK, Kneeland JB, et al. Biceps tendon dislocation: evaluation with MR imaging. Radiology 1991;179:649–52.
5. Getz JD, Recht MP, Piraino DW, et al. Acromial morphology: relation to sex, age, symmetry, and subacromial enthesophytes. Radiology 1996;199:737–42.
6. Bigliani U, Morrison DS, April EW. Morphology of the acromion and its relationship to rotator cuff tears. Orthop Trans 1986;10:459–60.
7. Schippinger G, Bailey B, McNally EG, et al. Anatomy of the normal acromion investigated using MRI. Langenbecks Arch Chir 1997;382(3):141–4.
8. Gumina S, Postacchini F, Orsina L, et al. The morphometry of the coracoid process—its aetiologic role in subcoracoid impingement syndrome. Int Orthop 1999;23(4):198–201.
9. Gallino M, Santamaria E, Doro T. Anthropometry of the scapula: clinical and surgical considerations. J Shoulder Elbow Surg 1998;7(3):284–91.
10. Prescher A, Klümpen T. The glenoid notch and its relation to the shape of the glenoid cavity of the scapula. J Anat 1997;190(3):457–60.
11. Churchill RS, Brems JJ, Kotschi H. Glenoid size, inclination, and version: an anatomic study. J Shoulder Elbow Surg 2001;10(4):327–32.
12. De Maeseneer M, Van Roy P, Shahabpour M. Normal MR imaging anatomy of the rotator cuff tendons, glenoid fossa, labrum, and ligaments of the shoulder. Radiol Clin North Am 2006;44(4):479–87.

13. Weishaupt D, Zanetti M, Nyffeler RW, et al. Posterior glenoid rim deficiency in recurrent (atraumatic) posterior shoulder instability. Skeletal Radiol 2000; 29:204–10.

14. Mulligan M, Pontius C. Posterior-inferior glenoid rim shapes by MR imaging. Surg Radiol Anat 2005; 27(4):336–9.

15. Inui H, Sugamoto K, Miyamoto T, et al. Glenoid shape in atraumatic posterior instability of the shoulder. Clin Orthop Relat Res 2002;403:87–92.

16. Moseley HF. The clavicle: its anatomy and function. Clin Orthop Relat Res 1968;58:17–28.

17. Curtis AS, Burbank KM, Tierney JJ, et al. The insertional footprint of the rotator cuff: an anatomic study. Arthroscopy 2006;22(6):603–9.

18. De Maeseneer M, Van Roy F, Lenchik L, et al. CT and MR arthrography of the normal and pathologic anterosuperior labrum and labral-bicipital complex. Radiographics 2000;20:S67–81.

19. Smith C, Funk L. The glenoid labrum. Shoulder Elbow 2010;2(2):87–93.

20. Cooper DE, Arnoczky SP, O'Brien SJ. Anatomy, histology, and vascularity of the glenoid labrum. An anatomical study. J Bone Joint Surg Am 1992;74: 46–52.

21. Ly JQ, Beall DP, Sanders TG. MR imaging of glenohumeral instability. AJR Am J Roentgenol 2003;181: 203–13.

22. Petchprapa CN, Beltran LS, Jazrawi LM, et al. The rotator interval: a review of anatomy, function, and normal and abnormal MRI appearance. AJR Am J Roentgenol 2010;195:567–76.

23. Beltran J, Bencardino J, Padron M, et al. The middle glenohumeral ligament: normal anatomy, variants and pathology. Skeletal Radiol 2002;31(5):253–62.

24. O'Brien SJ, Neves MC, Arnoczky SP, et al. The anatomy and histology of the inferior glenohumeral ligament complex of the shoulder. Am J Sports Med 1990;18:449–56.

25. Edelson JG, Grishkan A, Taitz C. The coracohumeral ligament: anatomy of a substantial but neglected structure. J Bone Joint Surg Br 1991;73:150–3.

26. Krief OP. MRI of the rotator interval capsule. Am J Roentgenol 2005;184:1490–4.

27. Werner A, Mueller T, Boehm D, et al. The stabilizing sling for the long head of the biceps tendon in the rotator interval. Am J Sports Med 2000;28(1):28–31.

28. Cothran RL Jr, Helms C. Quadrilateral space syndrome: incidence of imaging findings in a population referred for MRI of the shoulder. Am J Roentgenol 2005;184:989–92.

29. McClelland D, Paxinos A. The anatomy of the quadrilateral space with reference to quadrilateral space syndrome. J Shoulder Elbow Surg 2008; 17(1):162–4.

30. Peat M. Functional anatomy of the shoulder complex. Phys Ther 1986;66(12):1855–65.

31. Vahlensieck M. MRI of the shoulder. Eur Radiol 2000; 10(2):242–9.

32. Grainger AJ, Tirman PF, Elliott JM, et al. MR anatomy of the subcoracoid bursa and the association of subcoracoid effusion with tears of the anterior rotator cuff and the rotator interval. Am J Roentgenol 2000; 174:1377–80.

33. Hunt DR, Bullen L. The frequency of os acromiale in the Robert J. Terry collection. Int J Osteoarchaeol 2007;17(3):309–17.

34. Case DT, Burnett SE, Nielsen T. Os acromiale: population differences and their etiological significance. Homo 2006;57(1):1–18.

35. Hambly N, Fitzpatrick P, MacMahon P, et al. Rotator cuff impingement: correlation between findings on MRI and outcome after fluoroscopically guided subacromial bursography and steroid injection. AJR Am J Roentgenol 2007;189:1179–84.

36. Cone RO, Resnick D, Danzig L. Shoulder impingement syndrome: radiographic evaluation. Radiology 1984;150:29–33.

37. Kaplan PA, Bryans KC, Davick JP, et al. MR imaging of the normal shoulder: variants and pitfalls. Radiology 1992;184:519–24.

38. Mirowitz SA. Hematopoietic bone marrow within the proximal humeral epiphysis in normal adults: investigation with MR imaging. Radiology 1993;188:689–93.

39. Jin WR, Kyung N, Park YK, et al. Cystic lesions in the posterosuperior portion of the humeral head on MR arthrography: correlations with gross and histologic findings in cadavers. Am J Roentgenol 2005;184: 1211–5.

40. Fox JA, Cole BJ, Romeo AA, et al. Articular cartilage thickness of the humeral head: an anatomic study. Orthopedics 2008;31(3):1–6.

41. Yeh LR, Kwak S, Kim YS, et al. Evaluation of articular cartilage thickness of the humeral head and the glenoid fossa by MR arthrography: anatomic correlation in cadavers. Skeletal Radiol 1998;27:500–4.

42. Hodler J, Loredo RA, Longo C, et al. Assessment of articular cartilage thickness of the humeral head: MR-anatomic correlation in cadavers. Am J Roentgenol 1995;165:615–20.

43. Wilde LF, Berghs BM, Audenaert E, et al. About the variability of the shape of the glenoid cavity. Surg Radiol Anat 2004;26(1):54–9.

44. McCarthy C. Glenohumeral instability. Imaging 2003;15:174–9.

45. Bencardino JT, Beltran J, Rosenberg ZS, et al. Superior labrum anterior-posterior lesions: diagnosis with MR arthrography of the shoulder. Radiology 2000; 214:267–71.

46. Stoller DW. MR arthrography of the glenohumeral joint. Radiol Clin North Am 1997;1:97–115.

47. Grainger AJ, Elliott JM, Campbell RS, et al. Direct MR arthrography: a review of current use. Clin Radiol 2000;55:163–76.

48. Tuite MJ, Blankenbaker DG, Seifert M, et al. Sublabral foramen and Buford complex: inferior extent of the unattached or absent labrum in 50 patients. Radiology 2002;223:137–42.

49. Tirman PF, Feller JF, Palmer WE, et al. The Buford complex-a variation of normal shoulder anatomy: MR arthrographic imaging features. Am J Roentgenol 1996;166:869–73.

50. Chatterjee P, Sureka J. Normal variants of the middle glenohumeral ligament in MR imaging of the shoulder. Internet J Radiol 2009;10(1).

51. Wall MS, O'Brien SJ. Arthroscopic evaluation of the unstable shoulder. Clin Sports Med 1995; 14(4):817.

52. Gheno R, Zoner CS, Buck FM, et al. Accessory head of biceps brachii muscle: anatomy, histology, and MRI in cadavers. Am J Roentgenol 2010;194: W80–3.

53. Patten RM. Vacuum phenomenon: a potential pitfall in the interpretation of gradient-recalled-echo MR images of the shoulder. AJR Am J Roentgenol 1994;162:1383–6.

Normal and Variant Anatomy of the Wrist and Hand on MR Imaging

Joel M. Stein, MD, PhD*, Tessa S. Cook, MD, PhD, Stephanie Simonson, MD, Woojin Kim, MD

KEYWORDS

- Normal wrist and hand anatomy
- Wrist and hand magnetic resonance imaging
- Normal variants

Magnetic resonance (MR) imaging is the optimal modality for characterizing the ligaments, tendons, muscles, and neurovascular structures of the wrist and hand. Continued refinement in pulse sequence and coil design permits high-resolution examination of the many small structures and complex anatomy of this region. In this context, frequent anatomic variants and common false positives such as normal areas of high signal intensity in ligaments and tendons must be recognized to avoid misdiagnosis and improper treatment. In this article the authors discuss the osseous and soft tissue anatomy of the wrist and hand, as well as normal variants.

PROTOCOLS

The hand and wrist are best imaged using a dedicated phased-array coil to obtain high-resolution images while achieving optimal signal-to-noise ratio (**Tables 1** and **2**). High-field strength 3-Tesla magnets may be used to generate high-quality images, which can enhance evaluation of the ligaments and cartilage as well as the triangular fibrocartilage. Three imaging planes are obtained: axial, coronal, and sagittal. Axial images of the wrist should cover from the distal radius and ulna to the proximal metacarpals with the plane of imaging paralleling the distal radius. The wrist should be in

neutral position during imaging. Imaging of the thumb and fingers requires special attention to how the planes of imaging are prescribed. For the thumb, the axial images should be perpendicular to the midshaft of the proximal phalanx. Coronal images can be obtained perpendicular to the line that bisects the sesamoid bones with the sagittal imaging plane perpendicular to the coronal imaging plane. For an individual finger, axial images are obtained along the extent of the digit as prescribed by a best-fit line drawn through its center.

OSSEOUS STRUCTURES

Whereas the ulna forms the dominant articulation at the elbow, the radius is the larger bone at the wrist and provides the largest articular surface. On axial images, the distal radius forms a broad rectangle. The adjacent radial head has the shape of a circle in cross section and articulates with a slight concavity in the medial border of the radius, the sigmoid notch. On coronal images, the margins of the radial metaphysis, physis, and epiphysis are well demonstrated. The radial epiphysis is larger at the lateral aspect, where it terminates at the radial styloid process, and as a result it has a roughly triangular shape when viewed in the coronal plane. The slightly concave distal articular surface is angled medially and in

This work was not supported by any funding agency.
The authors have nothing to disclose.
Department of Radiology, Hospital of the University of Pennsylvania, 3400 Spruce Street, 1 Silverstein, Philadelphia, PA 19104, USA
* Corresponding author.
E-mail address: joel.stein@uphs.upenn.edu

Magn Reson Imaging Clin N Am 19 (2011) 595–608
doi:10.1016/j.mric.2011.05.007

Table 1
Routine wrist MR imaging protocol

Pulse Sequence	FOV (cm)	Slice Thickness (mm)	Matrix	TR/TE
Axial T1	10	3	320 × 192	480–500/19
Axial T2 FS	10	3	320 × 192	>4000/45
Coronal T1	10–12	3	256 × 256	575–625/20
Coronal T2 FS	10–12	3	320 × 192	>4500/45–57
Coronal 3D GRE	10	2	320 × 224	19/10
Sagittal T2 FS	10	3	320/192	>5000/45–49

Abbreviations: 3D GRE, 3-dimensional gradient recalled echo; FOV, field of view; FS, fast spin; TR/TE, repetition time/echo time.

the volar direction with respect to the radial shaft. Two shallow depressions along this surface articulate with the scaphoid and lunate bones. As seen on coronal images, the distal ulna is separated from the carpal bones by the triangular fibrocartilage. The central portion of the ulnar epiphysis forms the ulnar head, a rounded disk that articulates with the triangular fibrocartilage and the medial radius. The styloid process projects from the posteromedial aspect of the distal ulna and is separated from the ulnar head by a narrow groove.

The eight carpal bones are organized into proximal and distal rows that are well demonstrated on

Table 2
Routine hand MR imaging protocol

Pulse Sequence	FOV (cm)	Slice Thickness (mm)	Matrix	TR/TE
Axial T1	12–16	3	256 × 192	500–750/17–19
Axial T2 FS	12–16	3	256 × 192	>3500/55–70
Coronal T1	20	3	256 × 256	400–675/15–18
Coronal T2 FS	20	3	256 × 192	>3500/55
Coronal 2D GRE	20	2	320 × 240	180/9
Sagittal T2 FS	20	3	256 × 192	>5000/55

coronal MR images (**Fig. 1**). From lateral to medial, the proximal carpal row consists of the scaphoid, lunate, triquetrum, and pisiform bones. The trapezium, trapezoid, capitate, and hamate bones constitute the distal carpal row. In the normal wrist, a continuous line termed the proximal arc can be drawn along the base of the scaphoid, lunate, and triquetrum, separating the proximal carpal row from the radius and ulna. Similarly, a distal arc can be drawn separating the rounded base of the capitate and the adjacent somewhat triangular-shaped hamate from the cradle formed by the scaphoid, lunate, and triquetrum. The hook of the hamate, also known as the hamulus, is a hook-like process extending from the volar surface of the hamate that is best seen on axial images (**Fig. 2**). Sagittal images best reveal the normal alignment of the central column of the wrist in neutral position (**Fig. 3**). The base of the capitate sits within the crescent-shaped lunate, which itself is perpendicular to the longitudinal axis of the radius. A line drawn along the axis of the radial shaft bisects the lunate, the capitate, and the third metacarpal.

The osseous structures of the hand consist of the metacarpals and proximal, middle, and distal phalanges. The metacarpals and phalanges can be divided into a proximal base, middle shaft, and distal head. The articulations between these long bones include the metacarpophalangeal (MCP), proximal interphalangeal (PIP), and distal interphalangeal (DIP) joints. The thumb lacks a middle phalanx.

In addition to the long bones of the hand, additional sesamoid bones can be found at the palmar aspects of the MCP joints. Like other sesamoid bones, these are embedded within tendons and provide a mechanical advantage to the tendons by displacing them slightly from their joints. Most individuals have five sesamoids in the hand: at the MCP joints of the first, second, and fifth digits, as well as at the interphalangeal joint of the thumb. In the thumb, the two more proximal sesamoids are ensheathed by the adductor pollicis and the flexor pollicis brevis tendons. The number and location of the sesamoids of the hand can vary between individuals.

LIGAMENTS AND CARTILAGINOUS STRUCTURES
Wrist

The intrinsic ligaments of the wrist connect adjacent carpal bones to each other, limiting their motion and providing stability to the base of the hand. From the standpoint of stability, the most important of the intercarpal ligaments are the

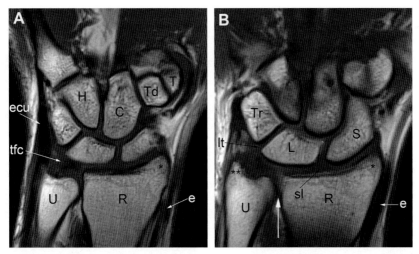

Fig. 1. Normal osseous anatomy. Coronal T1-weighted images of the wrist showing normal osseous anatomy. (*A*) Distal carpal row of trapezium (T), trapezoid (Td), capitate (C), and hamate (H) is shown. Additional structures shown: extensor pollicis brevis (e), extensor carpi ulnaris (ecu), triangular fibrocartilage complex (tfc), ulna (U), radius (R), and radial styloid (*asterisk*). (*B*) Proximal carpal row is composed of scaphoid (S), lunate (L), triquetrum (Tr), and pisiform (not shown). Other structures shown: extensor pollicis brevis (e), lunotriquetral ligament (lt), scapholunate ligament (sl), radius (R), radial styloid (*asterisk*), ulna (U), and ulnar styloid (*double asterisk*).

scapholunate and lunotriquetral ligaments (**Fig. 4**). These ligaments travel along the proximal arc, separating the radiocarpal compartment from the midcarpal compartment, and are best seen on coronal, thin-section gradient images. The scapholunate ligament connects the proximal margin of the scaphoid to that of the lunate. The lunotriquetral ligament connects the proximal aspect of the lunate to the base of the triquetrum. These ligaments are thicker at their volar and dorsal aspects and are membranous in the middle. The dorsal portion of the scapholunate ligament is thicker than the volar portion and is most important for stability. In contrast, the volar component of the lunotriquetral ligament is thicker and stronger than the corresponding dorsal component.

The extrinsic ligaments connect the distal radius and ulna to the carpal bones, and can be divided into volar and dorsal ligaments. The course of the ligaments can be appreciated on thin-section coronal gradient echo images. The extrinsic ligaments run obliquely, and are seen in cross section between the carpal bones and overlying flexor and extensor tendons on sagittal images. The volar (or palmar) extrinsic ligaments are generally thicker and stronger than the dorsal ligaments, and include the short and long radiolunate, the radioscaphocapitate, the radiolunotriquetral, the ulnotriquetral, and the ulnolunate ligaments (**Fig. 5**A). The most important of these are the radioscaphocapitate and radiolunotriquetral ligaments (see **Fig. 5**B). The radioscaphocapitate ligament arises on the

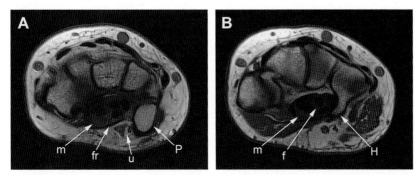

Fig. 2. Normal wrist. Axial T1-weighted images at the level of the pisiform (*A*) and hamate (*B*) more distally. The pisiform (P) articulates with the triquetrum. (*B*) The hook of the hamate (H) projects in the volar direction. As it is typically seen in only one or two images, the hook of the hamate is a very important part of one's checklist when evaluating for fractures. Other structures noted: flexor tendons (f), flexor retinaculum (fr), median nerve (m), and ulnar neurovascular bundle (u).

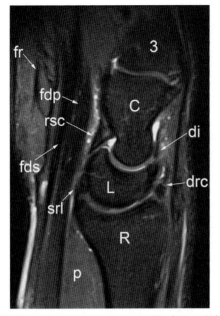

Fig. 3. Normal osseous anatomy. Sagittal T2-weighted image with fat saturation shows normal relationship between the radius (R), lunate (L), capitate (C), and the base of third metacarpal.[3] Additional structures shown: dorsal intercarpal ligament (di), dorsal radiocarpal ligament (drc), radioscaphocapitate ligament (rsc), short radiolunate ligament (srl), flexor retinaculum (fr), flexor digitorum superficialis (fds), flexor digitorum profundus (fdp), and pronator quadratus muscle (p).

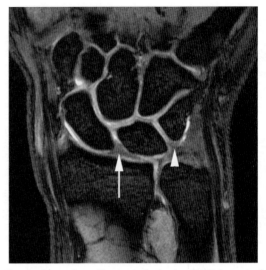

Fig. 4. Coronal gradient recalled echo (GRE) image of the wrist shows normal scapholunate (arrow) and lunotriquetral (arrowhead) ligaments.

volar surface of the radial styloid process, courses over the waist of the scaphoid, and attaches to the capitate. The radiolunotriquetral ligament originates medial to the radioscaphocapitate, invests both the lunate and triquetrum, and is the largest

ligament of the wrist. The dorsal extrinsic ligaments include the dorsal radioscaphoid, radiolunate, and radiotriquetral ligaments, in addition to other minor ligaments (Fig. 6).

The triangular fibrocartilage (TFC) complex cushions the ulnar head during axial loading and anchors it to the distal radius. The complex consists of the TFC, the volar and dorsal radioulnar ligaments, the meniscus homolog, the ulnar collateral ligament, and the sheath of the extensor carpi ulnaris tendon. The TFC or articular disk is best seen on coronal images (Fig. 7A). It sits between the ulnar head and the base of the lunate, extending from the medial margin of the distal ulna to attach between the ulnar head and styloid

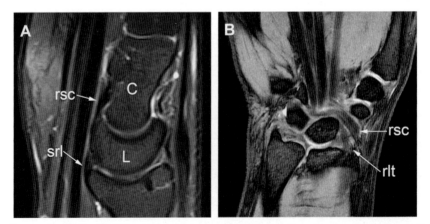

Fig. 5. Volar ligaments. (A) Sagittal T2-weighted image with fat saturation shows radioscaphocapitate (rsc) and short radiolunate (srl) ligaments. Capitate (C) and lunate (L) are labeled. (B) Coronal GRE image shows radiolunotriquetral (rlt) and radioscaphocapitate (rsc) ligaments.

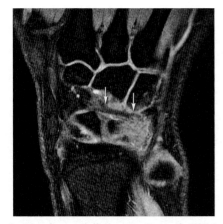

Fig. 6. Dorsal carpal ligament. Coronal GRE image showing intact dorsal intercarpal ligament (*arrows*).

process. The ulnar aspect is somewhat thicker, but at its center the TFC is biconcave, allowing for articulation with the ulnar head proximally and the lunate distally. This central area of articulation may be quite thin and even perforated. The overall thickness of the TFC is inversely proportional to the degree of ulnar variance, being thinner and more prone to tear with positive ulnar variance. The thickened margins of the TFC are called the volar and dorsal radioulnar ligaments, and extend from the medial cortex of the distal radius to that of the styloid process. The ulnar collateral ligament extends from the styloid process to the medial margin of the triquetrum. The meniscus homolog is an inconsistently present triangular-shaped fold of connective tissue found between the styloid process, ulnar collateral ligament, and triquetrum

(see **Fig. 7**B). The prestyloid recess is a fluid-filled space between the meniscus homolog and the styloid process. As best seen on axial images, the tendon of the extensor carpi ulnaris runs in a groove along the medial aspect of the ulna and eventually inserts at the base of the fifth metacarpal. The tendon sheath is a component of the TFC complex but is not well seen on MR imaging.

The flexor retinaculum (see **Fig. 2**), also known as the transverse carpal ligament, serves as the origin for several structures, including the abductor pollicis brevis, opponens pollicis, flexor pollicis brevis, palmaris brevis, flexor digiti minimi, and opponens digiti minimi muscles.[1]

Hand

Each of the five digits is supported by radial and ulnar collateral ligaments at the MCP, PIP, and DIP joints. The radial collateral ligaments extend from the metacarpal heads to the bases of the articulating proximal phalanges, along the radial aspect of the joint.[2] The ulnar collateral ligaments extend from the metacarpal heads to the bases of the articulating proximal phalanges along the ulnar aspect of the joint. A similar arrangement is found at the PIP and DIP joints. In the thumb, the radial collateral ligament of the MCP joint is weaker than its counterpart ulnar collateral ligament; in fact, the ulnar collateral ligament is responsible for stabilizing the thumb.[3] The ulnar collateral ligament of the thumb is commonly injured in a fashion referred to as gamekeeper's thumb (**Figs. 8–10**).[4]

The volar plate is a fibrocartilaginous structure found at the volar aspects of the MCP, PIP, and

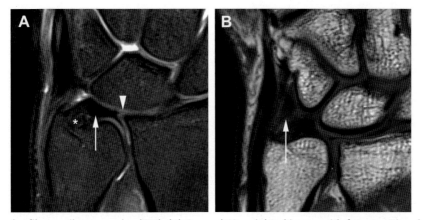

Fig. 7. Triangular fibrocartilage complex (TFC). (*A*) Coronal T2-weighted image with fat saturation shows normal intact TFC (*arrow*). Notice the focal area of increased signal at the radial attachment of the TFC (*arrowhead*); this is because the TFC attaches to the hyaline cartilage of the radius not its cortex. Therefore, this should not be mistaken for focal tear at the radial attachment. In addition, TFC attachment near the ulnar fovea can have a slightly increased signal (*asterisk*), which should not be mistaken for ulnar-sided tear of the TFC. (*B*) Coronal T1-weighted image shows the meniscus homolog (*arrow*).

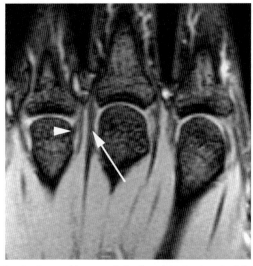

Fig. 8. Coronal image of the hand at the level of the metacarpophalangeal joints showing interosseous tendons (*arrow*) comprising the superficial layer with collateral ligaments (*arrowhead*) within the deeper layer.

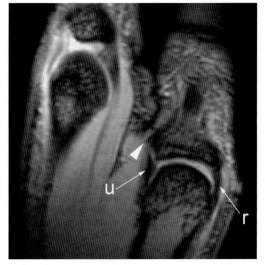

Fig. 10. Normal thumb. Coronal GRE image of the thumb shows normal radial (r) and ulnar (u) collateral ligaments at the level of the metacarpophalangeal joint with intact adductor aponeurosis superficially (*arrowhead*).

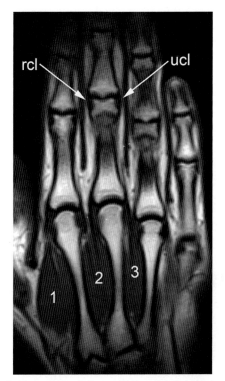

Fig. 9. Normal hand. Coronal T1-weighted MR image of the hand demonstrates normal radial (rcl) and ulnar collateral ligaments (ucl) at the proximal interphalangeal joint. First (1), second (2), and third (3) dorsal interossei are seen between the metacarpals.

DIP joints (**Fig. 11**). It serves as the point of attachment for the radial and ulnar collateral ligaments.[5] At the MCP joints, the volar plate is more fibrous and malleable, whereas the interphalangeal volar plates are more cartilaginous and rigid.[6]

The flexor tendons of the hand (see **Fig. 11**) are augmented by a pulley system that consists of focal areas of thickening of the tendon sheath (the annular pulleys) (**Fig. 12**) as well as crossing fibers between them called the cruciate ligaments.[7] The pulley system permits flexibility of the fingers while maintaining the position and alignment of the flexor tendons. The thumb has two annular pulleys and the remaining digits each have five annular pulleys. In all five fingers, the most proximal annular pulley overlies the metacarpal heads. The flexor digitorum profundus and flexor digitorum superficialis tendons enter these metacarpal pulleys and insert along the palmar surfaces of the distal phalanges. The flexor digitorum superficialis splits around the flexor digitorum profundus to insert on the palmar aspect of the neck of the middle phalanx, while the flexor digitorum profundus inserts on the palmar aspect of the base of the distal phalanx.

The extensor tendons of the hand (see **Fig. 11**) are anchored by a dorsal or extensor hood apparatus (**Fig. 13**) that overlies the MCP joints of the thumb and digits.[8] Each hood apparatus is formed from the extensor digitorum, which arises from the lateral humeral epicondyle. Each extensor hood is

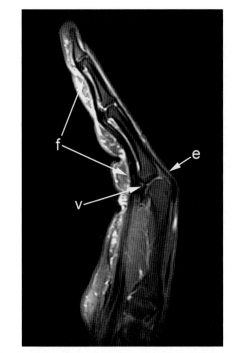

Fig. 11. Normal hand. Sagittal T2-weighted MR image of the hand with fat saturation shows normal flexor tendons (f). Extensor tendon and hood (e) and volar plate (v) are also labeled.

composed of both sagittal bands and transverse fibers. The sagittal bands arise from the MCP volar plate, lie proximal to the joint, and fuse with the deep transverse metacarpal ligament that connects the four digital metacarpals. The transverse fibers are contributed by the dorsal interossei and lumbricals, and attach at the level of the proximal and distal phalanges.[9]

MUSCLES AND TENDONS
Wrist

The flexors and extensors of the wrist have their muscle bellies along the proximal and mid forearm.

The flexor and extensor tendons travel along the volar and dorsal surface of the wrist, overlying the joint capsule, to insert on the carpal bones and phalanges. As they pass along slight grooves in the distal radius and ulna, the extensor tendons and their tendon sheaths are divided into six compartments by the overlying extensor retinaculum. The compartments are numbered from the radial to ulnar direction, and the organization is well seen on axial MR images (**Fig. 14**). Compartment I contains the abductor pollicis longus and extensor pollicis brevis, which lie along the lateral border of the radius. Compartment II lies along the dorsolateral surface of the distal radius, and contains the extensor carpi radialis longus and brevis. Compartment III contains the extensor pollicis longus, and is separated from compartment II by a bony prominence called Lister's tubercle. Compartment IV is along the dorsomedial surface of the radius, and contains the extensor digitorum and extensor indicis within a shared tendon sheath. Compartments V and VI contain the extensor digiti minimi and extensor carpi ulnaris, respectively, lying along the dorsal and medial surfaces of the ulnar head.

The flexor tendons that insert on the phalanges pass over the carpal bones within the carpal tunnel. These tendons include the four flexor digitorum profundus tendons, the four flexor digitorum superficialis tendons, and the flexor pollicis longus tendon. The trapezium and the hook of the hamate form the lateral and medial borders of the carpal tunnel. The flexor retinaculum spans from the hook of the hamate to the tuberosities of the trapezium and scaphoid to form the roof of the carpal tunnel. The flexor carpi ulnaris tendon is medial to the hook of the hamate and outside the carpal tunnel. The flexor carpi radialis courses along the trapezium between the fibers of the flexor retinaculum. The palmaris longus tendon, when present, travels over the proximal part of the flexor retinaculum and eventually blends with the central retinaculum and palmar aponeurosis.

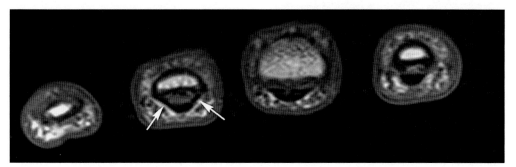

Fig. 12. Volar pulley. Axial T1-weighted image just distal to the proximal interphalangeal joint of the fourth digit demonstrates a normal annular pulley (*arrows*).

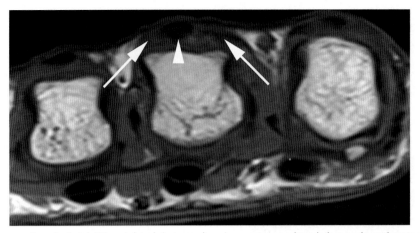

Fig. 13. Extensor hood. Axial T1-weighted image showing extensor hood (*arrows*) and extensor tendon (*arrowhead*).

Hand

The hand is controlled by extrinsic and intrinsic muscles. The extrinsic muscles include the flexor digitorum superficialis and profundus, extensor digitorum, extensor indicis, and extensor digiti minimi. There are extrinsic muscles that specifically operate the thumb; these are the flexor pollicis longus, extensor pollicis longus and brevis, and the abductor pollicis longus. The extrinsic muscles are so named because their muscle bellies lie in the forearm instead of the hand. The intrinsic

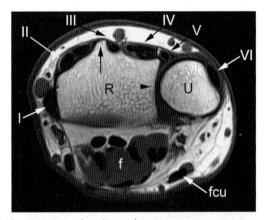

Fig. 14. Normal wrist and extensor compartments. Axial T1-weighted image through the wrist demonstrates the six extensor compartments: (I) abductor pollicis longus and extensor pollicis brevis, (II) extensor carpi radialis longus and brevis, (III) extensor pollicis longus, (IV) extensor digitorum and extensor indicis, (V) extensor digiti minimi, (VI) extensor carpi ulnaris. Lister's tubercle (*arrow*) separates the third compartment from the second compartment. Other structures seen: distal radioulnar joint (*arrowhead*), radius (R), ulna (U), flexor carpi ulnaris (fcu), and flexor tendons (f).

muscles of the hand include those of the thenar and hypothenar eminences, the interosseous muscles, and the lumbrical muscles.

The thenar eminence is found at the lateral aspect of the palmar surface of the hand. It is composed of the abductor pollicis brevis laterally, the flexor pollicis brevis medially, and the opponens pollicis dorsally (**Fig 15**).[10] Together with the adductor pollicis muscles, this group represents the intrinsic muscles of the thumb. The flexor pollicis brevis has ulnar and radial heads, between which lies the tendon of the flexor pollicis longus that originates in the forearm.

The hypothenar eminence is found at the medial aspect of the palmar surface of the hand. From medial to lateral, it is composed of the abductor digiti minimi, flexor digiti minimi, and opponens digiti minimi muscles (see **Fig 15**), which control motion of the fifth digit.[10] Together with the muscles of the thenar eminence, these comprise the intrinsic muscles of the hand.

The palmar and dorsal interosseous muscles (interossei) are so named because they are positioned between the metacarpal bones along the palmar and dorsal aspects of the hand, respectively. There are 4 dorsal interossei, each with two heads, which arise from the metacarpals of the four digits (see **Fig 15**). These muscles insert on the bases of the proximal phalanges as well as into the extensor digitorum communis, where they form the extensor hood apparatus. There are three palmar interossei, which are smaller than their dorsal counterparts. These interossei arise from the ulnar aspect of the second metacarpal, the radial aspect of the fourth metacarpal, and the radial aspect of the fifth metacarpal, and insert on the bases of the corresponding proximal phalanges. Some anatomists include the ulnar

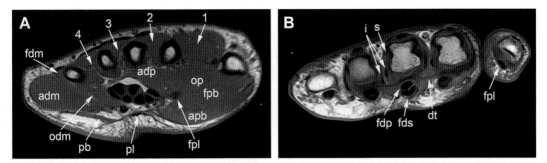

Fig. 15. Normal hand. Axial T1-weighted MR images of the hand through proximal (*A*) and distal (*B*) levels. The first through fourth interosseus muscles are noted (1, 2, 3, 4), with the arrows pointing at dorsal interossei. Labeled structures: (*A*) Adductor pollicis (adp), opponens pollicis (op), flexor pollicis brevis (fpb), abductor pollicis brevis (apb), flexor pollicis longus tendon (fpl), palmaris longus insertion (pl), palmaris brevis (pb), opponens digiti minimi (odm), abductor digiti minimi (adm), and flexor digiti minimi (fdm). (*B*) Flexor pollicis longus (fpl), deep transverse metacarpal ligaments (dt), flexor digitorum superficialis (fds), flexor digitorum profundus (fdp), interosseous tendons (i), and sagittal band (s).

head of the flexor pollicis brevis in this group, bringing the total to four. There is a great deal of variability in the anatomy and arrangement of the interosseous muscles.[11]

The lumbrical muscles are intrinsic to the fingers, and aid in flexion of the MCP joints and extension of the interphalangeal joints.[12] Unlike other muscles, the lumbricals attach to tendons of the flexor digitorum profundus proximally and to the extensor hoods distally. Each lumbrical muscle runs along the radial aspects of one of the four digits.

The palmar aponeurosis is the fascia of the palmar muscles, and is composed of central, lateral, and medial components. The fan-shaped central component originates from the palmaris longus tendon, and gives rise to the palmaris brevis tendon. It covers the flexor tendons and branches of the median and ulnar nerves.[13] The lateral and medial components overlie the muscles of the thumb and fifth digit.

Nerves

The median and ulnar nerves are most easily identified on axial images. The median nerve passes through the superficial and lateral part of the carpal tunnel just deep to the flexor retinaculum. It is intermediate to high in signal on all pulse sequences, in contrast to the adjacent tendons. The ulnar nerve travels with the ulnar artery and vein along the anterolateral aspect of the wrist within the ulnar tunnel, also known as Guyon's canal (**Fig. 16**). This fibro-osseous tunnel is bordered by the flexor retinaculum, the pisiform and hook of the hamate, the hypothenar musculature, and overlying fascia.

NORMAL OSSEOUS VARIANTS
Lunotriquetral Coalition

Congenital fusions of the carpal bones occur because of incomplete segmentation of a common

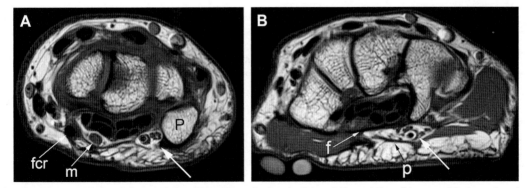

Fig. 16. Guyon's canal. Axial T1-weighted images at the level of the pisiform (*A*) and hamate (*B*) show the ulnar neurovascular bundle traversing through Guyon's canal (*arrow*). Other structures noted: flexor carpi radialis (fcr), median nerve (m), pisiform bone (P), flexor retinaculum (f), and palmaris longus tendon (p).

cartilaginous carpal precursor. The most common of these anomalies is lunotriquetral coalition (**Fig. 17**), which has a reported prevalence of 0.1% in the Caucasian population[14] but may be seen in up to 10% of African Americans,[15] and is more common in women. Lunotriquetral coalition is bilateral in 60% of cases.[16] Carpal coalitions may be complete or partial and may be osseous, fibrous, or cartilaginous. Widening of the scapho-lunate joint is frequently seen in conjunction with lunotriquetral coalition, but seems to reflect a normal variant rather than ligamentous injury.[17] Lunotriquetral coalition is usually an incidental finding, but has been reported as a cause of wrist pain in rare cases where there is associated degenerative arthritis,[18] incomplete cartilaginous coalition,[19,20] or traumatic disruption of a fibrocar-tilaginous coalition.[21]

Type II Lunate

A type I lunate bone has classical anatomy; it artic-ulates with the radius proximally, the triquetrum medially, the scaphoid laterally, and the capitate distally. The type II lunate has an additional facet that articulates with the hamate (**Fig. 18**). The type II lunate is at least as common as type I, being present in 50% to 65% of specimens or subjects in cadaveric and imaging studies depending on the criteria used.[22–25] Of note, type II lunate is frequently associated with degenerative changes at the proximal pole of the hamate and can be a cause of ulnar-sided wrist pain. In dissected specimens, Viegas and colleagues[22] found carti-lage erosion with exposed subchondral bone in

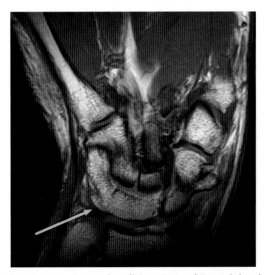

Fig. 17. Lunotriquetral coalition. Coronal T1-weighted image of the wrist shows an osseous coalition between the lunate and the triquetrum (*arrow*).

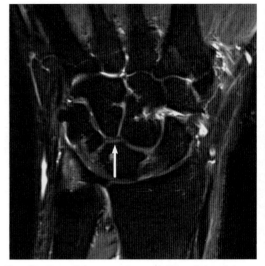

Fig. 18. Type II lunate. Coronal T2-weighted image with fat saturation of the wrist shows a type II lunate characterized by the presence of a facet that articu-lates with the hamate distally (*arrow*).

44% of type II lunates and none of the type I lunates examined. Marrow edema and chondral lesions at the proximal pole of the hamate associ-ated with type II lunate may be seen on MR images.[24,25]

Carpal Boss and Os Styloideum

The carpal boss is the clinical finding of a bony protuberance along the dorsum of the wrist between the base of the second and third metacar-pals, which may be associated with pain or limited wrist mobility. The carpal boss may be attributable to degenerative osteophytes or may reflect the presence of an os styloideum, one of many acces-sory ossicles in the wrist. The os styloideum is most easily recognized on sagittal images as a round osseous density adjacent to the dorsal base of the second and third metacarpals and the distal aspects of the capitate and trapezoid, and should not be mistaken for a fracture (**Fig. 19**). Pain related to os styloideum may be caused by associated osteoarthritis, overlying ganglion, bursitis, or ex-tensor tendon subluxation.[26]

NORMAL LIGAMENT VARIANTS
High Signal Intensity in Ligaments

The ligaments of the wrist are normally hypointense on all pulse sequences. Higher than normal focal signal intensity in a ligament may reflect a tear but can be a normal finding, particularly at attach-ment sites. The radial and ulnar attachments of the triangular fibrocartilage frequently show such focal

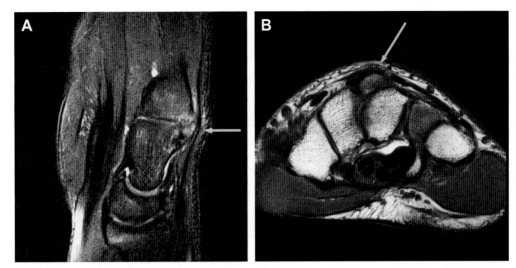

Fig. 19. Os styloideum. Sagittal T2-weighted image with fat saturation (*A*) and axial T1-weighted (*B*) images demonstrate the presence of an accessory ossicle, known as os styloideum (*arrow*), along the dorsal aspect of the wrist between the bases of the second and third metacarpals.

intermediate to high signal. In the case of the ulnar attachment, intermediate signal is seen as a result of different fiber bundles coming together. At the radial attachment, hyaline cartilage may result in curvilinear high signal intensity that could be misinterpreted as a tear (see **Fig. 7**).[27] Intermediate to high signal at attachment points of the intercarpal ligaments that is less than that of fluid can also be a normal finding.[28] Intermediate signal within the substance of the lunotriquetral or scapholunate ligaments can be seen in normal individuals, and ligament tears should not be suspected unless the signal intensity is equivalent to fluid.[28] The TFC may also have intermediate signal intensity centrally, due to myxoid degeneration.[28]

Perforations in Ligaments

Defects in the TFC and in the membranous central portions of the lunotriquetral and scapholunate ligaments are also frequently seen with aging.[27] In a study of anatomic specimens, Viegas and Ballantyne[29] detected no such lesions in subjects 45 years of age or younger but found perforations in the scapholunate ligament, lunotriquetral ligament, or triangular fibrocartilage in about one-third of subjects older than 60 years. Asymptomatic defects and communications in the TFC are most common at the radial aspect.[30]

NORMAL VARIANTS OF MUSCLES AND TENDONS
Accessory Abductor Digiti Minimi

Multiple variants of muscle anatomy at the wrist may be incidentally identified by MR imaging.[31,32]

The most common of these is the accessory abductor digiti minimi muscle, which may be found in as many as 24% of normal wrists.[31] It may originate from the palmar carpal ligament, the tendon of the palmaris longus muscle, or the forearm fascia. The accessory abductor digiti minimi travels along the radial aspect of the abductor digiti minimi proper, and the two muscles insert together on the medial aspect of the base of the fifth proximal phalanx.

Proximal Origin of the Lumbricals

The four lumbrical muscles arise from the medial aspects of the corresponding tendons of the flexor digitorum profundus. The origin is typically just distal to the carpal tunnel with the fingers in extension; however, one or more lumbrical muscles may originate within the carpal tunnel (**Fig. 20**) in up to 22% of individuals, or may be pulled into the tunnel with finger flexion.[33] Anomalous proximal origin of the lumbrical muscles within the carpal tunnel may be a cause of carpal tunnel syndrome, particularly when associated with muscle belly hypertrophy, hematoma, or lipoma.

Palmaris Longus Variants

The normal palmaris longus muscle originates from the common flexor tendon at the medial epicondyle of the humerus, has its muscle belly with the other flexors at the proximal forearm, and sends a long tendon that eventually blends with the fibers of the palmar aponeurosis. However, the palmaris longus may be absent in 2% to 20% of individuals. In addition, because of variant configurations of the

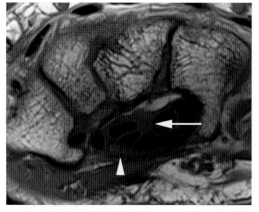

Fig. 20. Anomalous proximal origin of the lumbrical muscle (*arrow*) seen to arise within the carpal tunnel. Arrowhead indicates the median nerve.

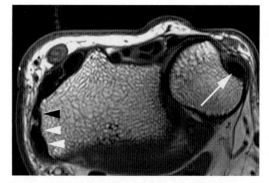

Fig. 21. Axial T1-weighted image of the wrist at the level of the distal radioulnar joint demonstrates focal increased signal within the central portion of the extensor carpi ulnaris tendon (*arrow*), which is often a normal finding and should not be confused with tendinosis. There are multiple bundles of the abductor pollicis longus (*white arrowheads*), which should not be confused with partial tears. Black arrowhead indicates extensor pollicis brevis.

tendinous and muscular components, the palmaris longus can have different appearances at the wrist or be confused with a soft tissue mass. The palmaris longus may be muscular throughout its length, tendinous proximally and muscular distally, digastric with proximal and distal muscular portions, or bifid distally.[32]

High Signal Intensity in Tendons

The normal tendons of the wrist are seen as round or oval structures on axial images and, like ligaments, have low signal intensity on all pulse sequences. As in other parts of the musculoskeletal system, high signal within tendons may reflect degeneration or tear, but focal signal abnormalities can also be caused by the fusing of multiple tendon layers, changes in the fibrous components particularly at insertion sites, or the magic angle phenomenon. Specific pseudolesions have been well recognized. High signal intensity within the tendon of the extensor carpi ulnaris is a frequent normal finding (**Fig. 21**). In this case, centrally increased signal at the level of the distal radioulnar joint may be related to interdigitation of tendinous slips coming together from proximal and distal muscle bellies of the extensor carpi ulnaris.[34-] Similarly, the normal abductor pollicis longus tendon may have a striated appearance that can be misinterpreted as a longitudinal tear but reflects the fusion of multiple tendinous bundles with interposed fat. High signal within the extensor pollicis longus tendon distal to Lister's tubercle is frequently seen as a result of the magic angle phenomenon.[34] As it takes an oblique course distal to the carpal tunnel, the flexor pollicis longus tendon also frequently has relatively high signal due to the magic angle phenomenon, such that it

may appear isointense to the surrounding thenar muscles.[27]

Extensor Digitorum Brevis Manus

The extensor digitorum brevis manus is an accessory muscle that is rarely found in the fourth extensor compartment of the wrist. It often mimics inflammatory or neoplastic processes in the dorsum of the wrist. When present, it may be solely responsible for independent extension of the second digit, and is thus important to recognize for surgical planning.[35]

Variant Interosseous Muscles

Studies have shown a great deal of variety in the number and attachment of the dorsal and palmar interossei.[12] The insertion sites of the palmar interossei can sometimes include the volar plate in addition to the extensor apparatus. In some individuals, the palmar interossei can also have multiple heads like the dorsal interossei, sometimes as many as three.

NORMAL VARIANTS OF NERVES
Bifurcation of the Median Nerve

Variations in the anatomy of the median nerve at the wrist have been extensively studied in the surgical literature. As it exits the carpal tunnel the median nerve typically splits into multiple branches, including the common and proper palmar digital branches and the recurrent branch of the median nerve. A bifid median nerve occurs when the median nerve splits either before entering or within the carpal tunnel (**Fig. 22**). A

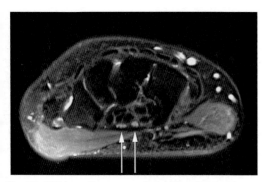

Fig. 22. Bifid median nerve. Axial T2-weighted image with fat saturation shows bifid median nerve (*arrows*).

recent MR imaging study of 194 wrists revealed bifurcation of the median nerve proximal to the carpal tunnel in 6%, whereas bifurcation within the carpal tunnel was even more common, being present in 18% of wrists.[36] In an ultrasound study of 170 patients with carpal tunnel syndrome and 120 controls, Bayrak and colleagues[37] found a significantly higher percentage of bifid median nerves in patients with carpal tunnel syndrome compared with controls (19% vs 9%). Independent of whether or a not a bifid median nerve is a cause of pathology, knowledge of its presence is important prior to carpal release surgery to avoid nerve injury.[38]

SUMMARY

An understanding of the normal MR imaging appearance of the wrist and hand, as well as variations in the normal anatomy, is important for radiologists in light of the increasing use of MR imaging in the evaluation of wrist and hand pathology.

REFERENCES

1. Kline SC, Moore JR. The transverse carpal ligament. An important component of the digital flexor pulley system. J Bone Joint Surg Am 1992;74:1478–85.
2. Edelstein DM, Kardashian G, Lee SK. Radial collateral ligament injuries of the thumb. J Hand Surg Am 2008;33:760–70.
3. Wessely MA, Grenier J-M. MR imaging of the wrist and hand. Clinical Chiropractic 2007;10:156–64.
4. Hinke DH, Erickson SJ, Chamoy L, et al. Ulnar collateral ligament of the thumb: MR findings in cadavers, volunteers, and patients with ligamentous injury (gamekeeper's thumb). Am J Roentgenol 1994; 163:1431–4.
5. Bowers WH, Wolf JW, Nehil JL, et al. The proximal interphalangeal joint volar plate. I. An anatomical and biomechanical study. J Hand Surg Am 1980;5: 79–88.
6. Bowers WH. The proximal interphalangeal joint volar plate II. A clinical study of hyperextension injury. J Hand Surg Am 1981;6:77–81.
7. Hauger O, Chung CB, Lektrakul N, et al. Pulley system in the fingers: normal anatomy and simulated lesions in cadavers at MR imaging, CT, and US with and without contrast material distention of the tendon sheath. Radiology 2000;217:201–12.
8. Clavero JA, Golano P, Farinas O, et al. Extensor mechanism of the fingers: MR imaging—anatomic correlation. Radiographics 2003;23:593–611.
9. Littler JW. The finger extensor mechanism. Surg Clin North Am 1967;47:415–32.
10. Wheeless CR III. Wheeless' textbook of orthopedics. Available at: http://www.wheelessonline.com. Accessed September 30, 2010.
11. Eladoumikdachi F, Valkov PL, Thomas J, et al. Anatomy of the intrinsic hand muscles revisited: part I. Interossei. Plast Reconstr Surg 2002;110: 1211–24.
12. Mehta HJ, Gardner WU. A study of lumbrical muscles in the human hand. Am J Anat 1961;109: 227–38.
13. Bojsen-Moller F, Schmidt L. The palmar aponeurosis and the central spaces of the hand. J Anat 1974; 117:55–68.
14. Carlson DH. Coalition of the carpal bones. Skeletal Radiol 1981;7:125–7.
15. Delaney TJ, Eswar S. Carpal coalitions. J Hand Surg Am 1992;17:28–31.
16. Cockshott WP. Carpal fusions. Am J Roentgenol 1963;89:1260–71.
17. Metz VM, Schimmerl SM, Gilula LA, et al. Wide scapholunate joint space in lunotriquetral coalition: a normal variant? Radiology 1993;188:557–9.
18. Marburger R, Burgess RC. Symptomatic lunate-triquetral coalition. J South Orthop Assoc 1995;4: 307–10.
19. Simmons BP, McKenzie WD. Symptomatic carpal coalition. J Hand Surg Am 1985;10:190–3.
20. Ritt MJ, Maas M, Bos KE. Minaar type 1 symptomatic lunotriquetral coalition: a report of nine patients. J Hand Surg Am 2001;26:261–70.
21. van Schoonhoven J, Prommersberger KJ, Schmitt R. Traumatic disruption of a fibrocartilage lunate-triquetral coalition—a case report and review of the literature. Hand Surg 2001;6:103–8.
22. Viegas SF, Wagner K, Patterson R, et al. Medial (hamate) facet of the lunate. J Hand Surg Am 1990;15:564–71.
23. Yazaki N, Burns ST, Morris RP, et al. Variations of capitate morphology in the wrist. J Hand Surg Am 2008;33:660–6.
24. Malik AM, Schweitzer ME, Culp RW, et al. MR imaging of the type II lunate bone: frequency, extent, and associated findings. AJR Am J Roentgenol 1999;173:335–8.

25. Pfirrmann CW, Theumann NH, Chung CB, et al. The hamatolunate facet: characterization and association with cartilage lesions—magnetic resonance arthrography and anatomic correlation in cadaveric wrists. Skeletal Radiol 2002;31:451–6.

26. Conway WF, Destouet JM, Gillula LA, et al. The carpal boss: an overview of radiographic evaluation. Radiology 1985;156:29–31.

27. Pfirrmann CW, Zanetti M. Variants, pitfalls and asymptomatic findings in wrist and hand imaging. Eur J Radiol 2005;56:286–95.

28. Wrist and hand. In: Helms CA, Major NM, Anderson MW, et al, editors. Musculoskeletal MRI. 2nd edition. Philadelphia: Saunders Elsevier; 2009. p. 247–50.

29. Viegas SF, Ballantyne G. Attritional lesions of the wrist joint. J Hand Surg Am 1987;12:1025–9.

30. Zanetti M, Linkous MD, Gilula LA, et al. Characteristics of triangular fibrocartilage defects in symptomatic and contralateral asymptomatic wrists. Radiology 2000;216:840–5.

31. Zeiss J, Guilliam-Hadet L. MR demonstration of anomalous muscles about the volar aspect of the wrist and forearm. Clin Imaging 1996;20:219–21.

32. Timins ME. Muscular anatomic variants of the wrist and hand: finding on MR imaging. AJR 1999;172:1397–401.

33. Middleton WD, Kneeland JB, Kellman GM. MR imaging of the carpal tunnel: normal anatomy and preliminary findings in carpal tunnel syndrome. AJR 1987;148:307–16.

34. Timins ME, O'Connell SE, Erickson SJ, et al. MR imaging of the wrist: normal findings that my simulate disease. Radiographics 1996;16:987–95.

35. Ranade AV, Rai R, Prabhu LV, et al. Incidence of extensor digitorum brevis manus muscle. Hand 2008;3:320–3.

36. Pierre-Jerome C, Smitson RD Jr, Shah RK, et al. MRI of the median nerve and median artery in the carpal tunnel: prevalence of their anatomical variations and clinical significance. Surg Radiol Anat 2010;32:315–22.

37. Bayrak IK, Bayrak AO, Kale M, et al. Bifid median nerve in patients with carpal tunnel syndrome. J Ultrasound Med 2008;27:1129–36.

38. Propeck T, Quinn TJ, Jacobson JA, et al. Sonography and MR imaging of bifid median nerve with anatomic and histologic correlation. AJR 2000;175:1721–5.

Normal and Variant Anatomy of the Elbow on Magnetic Resonance Imaging

Joel M. Stein, MD, PhD*, Tessa S. Cook, MD, PhD,
Stephanie Simonson, MD, Woojin Kim, MD

KEYWORDS

- Normal elbow anatomy
- Elbow magnetic resonance imaging • Normal variants

Magnetic resonance imaging (MRI) provides excellent delineation of the bones of the elbow and the surrounding soft tissue structures. The components of the elbow can be divided into osseous structures, the joint capsule and ligaments, muscles and tendons, and nerves. In this article, the authors review the normal anatomy and the appearance of these structures on MRI as well as the anatomic variants that should be recognized and distinguished from pathologic entities.

PROTOCOL

Axial, coronal, and sagittal images are acquired using T1- and T2-weighted images (**Table 1**). The axial images must include the radial tuberosity where the biceps tendon attaches. Typically, patients are placed in supine position with the arm to their side, and as a result, excellent field homogeneity is required for off-center fat suppression. Although the patient can alternatively be positioned prone with the arm extended overhead, this position is less well tolerated and can also introduce motion degradation artifact. The distal biceps brachii tendon takes an oblique course and is therefore susceptible to partial volume-average effects and difficult to visualize on a single image. The extent of the tendon can be better imaged with the flexed abducted supinated view, whereby the elbow is flexed with the shoulder abducted and the forearm in supination (**Fig. 1**).[1]

OSSEOUS STRUCTURES

The elbow joint is composed of three bones (humerus, radius, and ulna) that form three articulations (ulnohumeral, radiohumeral, and radioulnar) within a common joint capsule. The ulnohumeral and radiohumeral articulations allow for flexion and extension of the forearm. The radiohumeral and radioulnar articulations permit pronation and supination of the forearm.

The tubular shaft of the humerus flares distally to form the medial and lateral condyles. As the condyles sweep outward, they form paired bony protuberances, the medial and lateral epicondyles, that serve as attachment sites for ligaments and tendons. The most distal aspects of the condyles are the articular surfaces, the medial trochlea and lateral capitellum. The trochlea is the more central and larger of the two and is shaped like a pulley with central concavity and flared margins. The trochlea articulates within the crescent trochlear notch along the anterior surface of the proximal ulna, forming a hinge joint that permits flexion and extension. The proximal aspect of the trochlear notch is formed by the olecranon, whereas the distal aspect is the coronoid process.

This work was not supported by any funding agency.
Department of Radiology, Hospital of the University of Pennsylvania, 3400 Spruce Street, 1 Silverstein, Philadelphia, PA 19104, USA
* Corresponding author.
E-mail address: joel.stein@uphs.upenn.edu

Magn Reson Imaging Clin N Am 19 (2011) 609–619
doi:10.1016/j.mric.2011.05.002
1064-9689/11/$ – see front matter © 2011 Elsevier Inc. All rights reserved.

Table 1
Standard pulse sequences for MRI examination of the elbow

Pulse Sequence	Field of View (cm)	Slice Thickness (mm)	Matrix	TR/TE
Coronal T1	14	3	256 × 192	500–700/12–14
Coronal T2 FS	14	3	256 × 256	>4000/54
Axial T1	12–14	3	256 × 256	400–750/10–11
Axial T2 FS	12–14	3	256 × 256	>3500/47
Sagittal T2 FS	14–16	3	256 × 256	>3500/47–52

Abbreviations: FS, fat saturation; TE, echo time; TR, repetition time.

Dorsal and ventral indentations above the trochlea, which are the olecranon fossa and coronoid fossa, receive these processes when the elbow is in maximal extension or flexion, respectively. The capitellum is a nearly spherical eminence at the distal aspect of the lateral condyle that articulates with the slightly cup-shaped end of the radial head, permitting both flexion and extension and rotation of the radius with respect to the humerus. The radial head has the form of a disk attached to the tapered neck of the proximal radius. This disk articulates with the radial notch of the proximal ulna on the lateral surface of the coronoid process, allowing for axial rotation of the radius with respect to the ulna. The radial fossa is an indentation above the capitellum that accepts the head of the radius when the elbow is in maximal flexion. The relationships between the various osseous structures of the elbow are well depicted on coronal and sagittal magnetic resonance images (**Fig. 2**).

JOINT CAPSULE AND LIGAMENTS

A common joint capsule surrounds all three joints of the elbow. The capsule is composed of a more superficial fibrous layer and a deeper synovial layer. There are three fat pads between these two layers (**Fig. 3**). The two anterior fat pads are situated within the coronoid fossa and radial fossa, whereas the posterior fat pad sits within the olecranon fossa. The ligaments of the elbow range from focal areas of thickening of the capsule to more discrete fibers visible on MRI. As the primary motion of the elbow is flexion and extension, the anterior and posterior aspects of the joint capsule are thin. The major stabilizers of the elbow are the

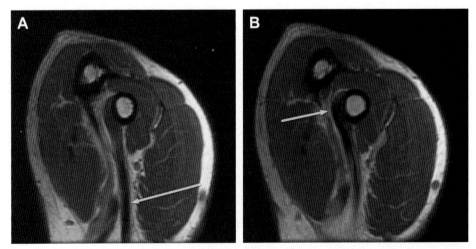

Fig. 1. Proton density–weighted magnetic resonance image of a normal distal biceps brachii tendon using the flexed abducted supinated view, which images the distal biceps brachii tendon in its long axis, demonstrating (*A*) straight course of the tendon (*arrow*) to its (*B*) insertion on the radial tuberosity (*arrow*). With this technique, the entire course of the distal biceps brachii tendon from the myotendinous junction to its attachment on the radial tuberosity can be imaged in one or two images.

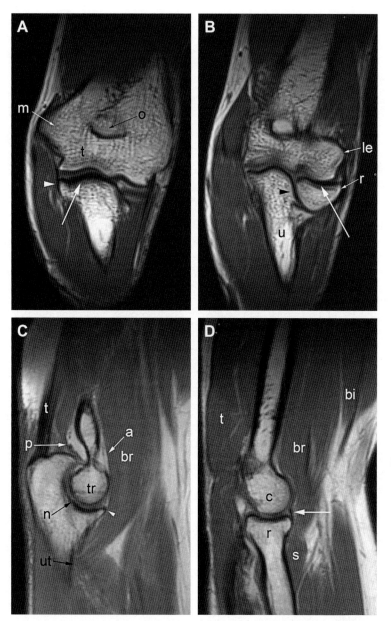

Fig. 2. Normal osseous anatomy of the elbow. Coronal (*A*, *B*) and sagittal (*C*, *D*) T1-weighted magnetic resonance images of the normal elbow show normal osseous anatomy and surrounding soft tissue structures. (*A*) The trochlea of the distal humerus (t) articulates with the proximal ulna forming the ulnohumeral joint (*arrow*). The sublime tubercle (*arrowhead*) of the proximal ulna is the most medial part of the medial ulna and serves as the attachment site for the ulnar collateral ligament; it is a useful landmark for identifying the ulnar collateral ligament. The other structures are the olecranon fossa (o) and medial epicondyle (m). (*B*) On the lateral side, the radiohumeral articulation (*arrow*) is formed by the capitellum and the radial head (r), and the lateral epicondyle (le) is seen just superiorly. Black arrowhead denotes the proximal radioulnar joint. The ulnar shaft (u) is partially seen more distally. (*C*) Normal ulnohumeral articulation between the trochlea (tr) of the distal humerus with the trochlear notch (n) of the proximal ulna is shown. The brachialis muscle (br) attaches distally onto the ulnar tuberosity (ut). The coronoid process of the proximal ulna (*arrowhead*) is seen more anteriorly. Other visualized structures include the anterior (a) and posterior (p) fat pads and triceps muscle and tendon (t). (*D*) More laterally, the radiohumeral articulation (*arrow*) between the capitellum (c) and the radial head (r) is seen. Other structures are the triceps muscle (t), biceps brachii muscle (bi), brachialis muscle (br), and supinator muscle (s).

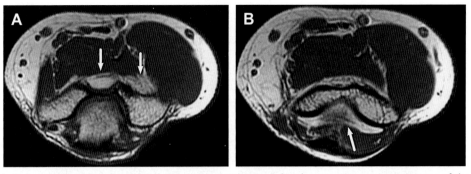

Fig. 3. Anterior and posterior fat pads of the elbow. Axial T1-weighted magnetic resonance images of the elbow showing (A) anterior (*arrows*) and (B) posterior (*arrow*) fat pads.

medial (ulnar) and lateral (radial) collateral ligament complexes.

The ulnar collateral ligament, also known as the medial collateral ligament, consists of three ligamentous bundles, the anterior, posterior, and transverse bundles. The anterior bundle is the major medial stabilizer of the elbow and is the only component of the ulnar collateral ligament seen as a discrete ligament on MRI. As best demonstrated on coronal images (**Fig. 4**), the anterior bundle arises from the inferior margin of the medial epicondyle and attaches to the medial aspect of the coronoid process at the sublime

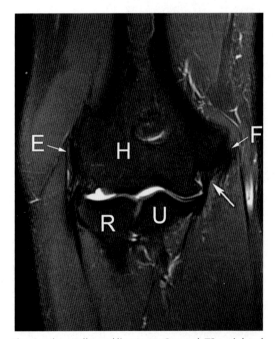

Fig. 4. Ulnar collateral ligament. Coronal, T2-weighted, fat-saturated image of the elbow demonstrates normal ulnar collateral ligament (*arrow*) with its distal attachment on the sublime tubercle. Other structures: humerus (H), radial head (R), proximal ulna (U), common extensor tendon (E), and common flexor tendon (F).

tubercle. The posterior bundle is a thickening of the joint capsule that extends from below the medial epicondyle to the medial olecranon. The transverse bundle consists of fibers extending from the inferior aspects of the anterior and posterior bundles, that is, from the olecranon to the coronoid process, and does not contribute to elbow stability.

The radial collateral ligament, also known as the lateral collateral ligament, complex consists of the annular ligament, radial collateral ligament, and lateral ulnar collateral ligament. The annular ligament is the primary stabilizer of the proximal radioulnar joint and is best seen on axial images wrapping around the side of the radial head from one side of the radial notch to the other. An accessory collateral ligament is variably present and extends from the annular ligament to the supinator crest of the lateral ulna. The radial collateral ligament arises from the anterior margin of the lateral epicondyle, inserts onto the annular ligament and fascia of the supinator muscle, and is best seen on coronal images (**Fig. 5**). The lateral ulnar collateral ligament is the major posterolateral stabilizer of the elbow and can be seen on coronal or sagittal images (**Fig. 6**), arising more posteriorly and superficially from the lateral epicondyle and inserting at the supinator crest.

MUSCLES AND TENDONS

The muscles and tendons about the elbow can be divided into anterior, posterior, medial, and lateral compartments. The anterior and posterior compartments contain the flexors and extensors of the forearm, respectively. The medial compartment contains the flexors of the wrist and fingers and the pronator teres. The lateral compartment contains the extensors of the wrist and fingers and the supinator. Axial images through the elbow best demonstrate the various muscles within these compartments. Sagittal images depict the longitudinal extent of the muscles of the anterior and posterior compartments, whereas coronal images show the extent of muscles of the medial and lateral compartments.

The anterior compartment consists of the brachialis and biceps muscles. The brachialis muscle arises from the distal humerus, courses over the anterior joint capsule, and inserts on the ulnar tuberosity (**Fig. 7**). The biceps muscle is superficial to the brachialis and has a long tendon that inserts at the radial tuberosity (**Fig. 8**). The bicipital aponeurosis, also known as the lacertus fibrosus, arises from the distal biceps tendon and courses medially, blending with the fascia overlying the muscles of the medial compartment (**Fig. 9**).

The posterior compartment contains the triceps and anconeus muscles. The triceps tendon inserts on the posterior olecranon (see **Fig. 8**). The anconeus arises at the posterior edge of the lateral epicondyle and inserts at the lateral aspect of the olecranon. Thus, the anconeus provides a good landmark for laterality on axial images (see **Fig. 9**).

The common flexor tendon originates at the medial epicondyle, providing attachment for three flexors of the wrist. From anterior to posterior, these are the flexor carpi radialis, the palmaris longus, and the flexor carpi ulnaris (see **Fig. 4**). The flexor digitorum superficialis attaches to the common flexor tendon as well as the lateral margin of the coronoid process and travels deep to the wrist flexors. Deeper still is the flexor digitorum profundus, which arises along the anterior and lateral aspects of the proximal ulnar shaft and

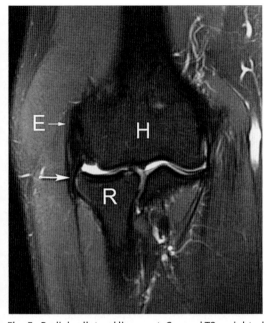

Fig. 5. Radial collateral ligament. Coronal T2-weighted fat-saturated image of the elbow shows normal radial collateral ligament (*white arrow*). Other structures: humerus (H), radial head (R), and common extensor tendon (E).

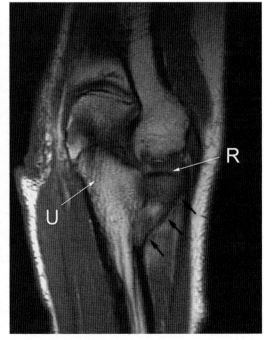

Fig. 6. Lateral ulnar collateral ligament. Coronal T1-weighted image of the elbow showing normal lateral ulnar collateral ligament (*small black arrows*) attaching to the supinator crest of the proximal ulna. Other structures: radial head (R) and proximal ulna (U).

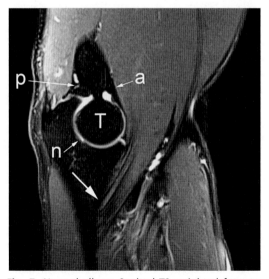

Fig. 7. Normal elbow. Sagittal T2-weighted fat-saturated image of the elbow shows the brachialis muscle and tendon (*arrow*). Other structures: anterior (a) and posterior (p) fat pads, trochlea (T), and trochlear notch of ulna (n).

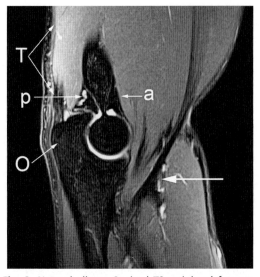

Fig. 8. Normal elbow. Sagittal T2-weighted fat-saturated image of the elbow shows the biceps tendon (*arrow*) and the triceps muscle and tendon (T), which is seen attaching to the posterior olecranon (O). Other structures: anterior (a) and posterior (p) fat pads.

travels closest to the ulna. The pronator teres has origins at the medial epicondyle and medial aspect of the coronoid process, travels deep to the flexor carpi radialis, and inserts on the lateral aspect of the radial shaft.

The common extensor tendon originates at the lateral epicondyle and divides from medial to lateral to form the extensor carpi ulnaris, extensor digiti minimi, extensor digitorum, and extensor carpi radialis brevis (see **Figs. 4** and **5**). The supinator originates at the lateral epicondyle and the supinator crest of the ulna, envelopes the radius beneath the extensors, and terminates along the anterolateral aspect of proximal third of the radius (**Fig. 10**).

NERVES

The three major nerves of the elbow are the radial, median, and ulnar nerves. Like peripheral nerves elsewhere in the body, these nerves demonstrate intermediate signal on T1-weighted images, appearing nearly isointense to surrounding muscle, and exhibit slightly higher signal intensity on T2-weighted images. Their delineation is partly dependent on the amount of surrounding fat. These nerves are most easily identified within their respective neurovascular bundles and in relation to surrounding muscles on axial images through the distal humerus. The ulnar nerve is particularly well seen at the level of the medial epicondyle as it passes through the cubital tunnel.

The radial nerve travels in the upper arm along the spiral groove of the humeral shaft, underlying the triceps, and courses anterolaterally past the elbow between the brachialis and brachioradialis muscles. The common radial nerve splits around the proximal aspect of the supinator to give

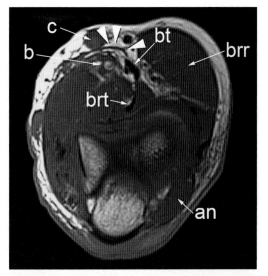

Fig. 9. Bicipital aponeurosis. Axial T1-weighted image of the elbow at the level of the bicipital aponeurosis (*arrowheads*). Deeper biceps (bt) and brachialis (brt) tendons are noted. The anconeus muscle (an) is a useful landmark for the lateral side of the elbow on axial images. Other structures: brachioradialis (brr), brachial artery (b), and cephalic vein (c).

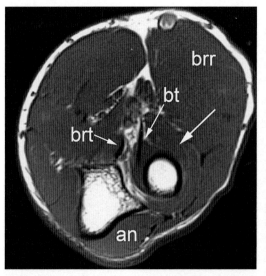

Fig. 10. Supinator muscle. Axial T1-weighted image at the level of the radial neck shows supinator muscle (*arrow*), one of the deep dorsal muscles seen wrapping around the neck. Other structures: anconeus muscle (an), brachioradialis muscle (brr), brachialis tendon (brt), and biceps tendon (bt).

superficial and deep branches. The deep branch travels between deep and superficial layers of the supinator muscle. The deep branch continues as the posterior interosseous nerve.

The median nerve courses along the inner aspect of the upper arm medial to the brachial artery and biceps tendon as it approaches the elbow joint. The brachial artery bifurcates to form the radial and ulnar arteries at the proximal margin of the pronator teres. The median nerve travels onward between the humeral and ulnar heads of the pronator teres, whereas the ulnar artery travels deep to the ulnar head. The median nerve then continues along the midline of the forearm, deep to the flexor digitorum superficialis, and eventually gives rise to the anterior interosseous nerve.

The ulnar nerve is located posterior to the medial epicondyle within the cubital tunnel, which is a fibro-osseous tunnel formed by the medial epicondyle and the cubital retinaculum, also known as the arcuate ligament of Osborne (**Fig. 11**). The nerve courses distally through the flexor carpi ulnaris muscle and supplies the flexor carpi ulnaris and medial half of flexor digitorum profundus muscle.

NORMAL OSSEOUS VARIANTS
Pseudodefect of the Capitellum

A groove between the posterolateral aspect of the capitellum and the lateral epicondyle can cause apparent irregularity of the otherwise-smooth capitellum that may be mistaken for an osteochondral defect.[2] This pseudodefect can be seen on coronal magnetic resonance images and more-lateral sagittal images (**Fig. 12**). Knowledge of the characteristic location and appearance of the pseudodefect allows it to be distinguished from osteochondral lesions of the capitellum, which typically are located more anteriorly and, in the case of unstable lesions, are surrounded by edema or cystic changes on T2-weighted images.[3]

Pseudolesion of the Trochlear Notch

Within the crescent trochlear notch of the ulna, a focal area devoid of cartilage may exist between the coronoid articular surface and the olecranon articular surface, which is known as the trochlear groove (**Fig. 13**). The trochlear groove is a normal anatomic variant and should not be mistaken for an osteochondral lesion, particularly on sagittal images. The characteristic location of this structure and the absence of bone marrow edema should enable the recognition of this pseudodefect.[4]

Supracondylar Process

The supracondylar process is a bony spur found in 0.2% to 3% of individuals,[5] arising from the anteromedial aspect of the distal humeral shaft, approximately 5 to 7 cm above the medial epicondyle (**Fig. 14**). This horn-shaped excrescence projects toward the elbow and should not be

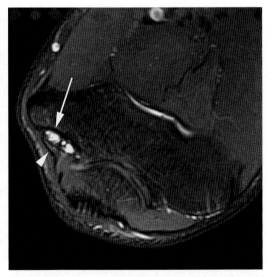

Fig. 11. Ulnar nerve. Axial T2-weighted fat-saturated image shows ulnar nerve (*arrow*) adjacent to posterior recurrent ulnar artery within the cubital tunnel, which is formed by the medial epicondyle and the cubital retinaculum, also known as the arcuate ligament of Osborne (*arrowhead*).

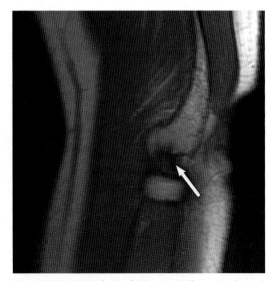

Fig. 12. Pseudodefect of the capitellum. Far-lateral, sagittal, T1-weighted image of the elbow shows irregularity of the posterior aspect of the capitellum (*arrow*). This irregularity represents a normal anatomic variant called the pseudodefect of the capitellum, which should not be mistaken for an osteochondral lesion.

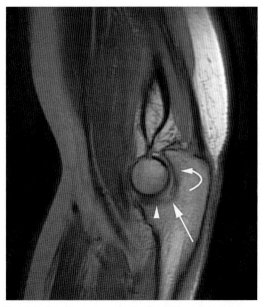

Fig. 13. Trochlear groove. Sagittal T1-weighted magnetic resonance image of the elbow shows a focal area without overlying cartilage (*arrow*) between the articular surface of the coronoid (*arrowhead*) and olecranon (*curved arrow*). The trochlear groove is a normal anatomic variant and should not be confused with an osteochondral lesion.

confused with osteochondromas of the humeral metaphysis that project away from the elbow. A fibrous band called the ligament of Struthers runs from the tip of the supracondylar process to the medial epicondyle, forming a fibro-osseous tunnel around the medial neurovascular bundle of the forearm. This band may cause symptomatic compression of the median nerve, which has been diagnosed on MRI,[6] or, more rarely, the brachial artery or ulnar nerve.

NORMAL NONOSSEOUS VARIANTS
Synovial Folds

Synovial folds or plicae are thin projections from the synovial membrane, the inner layer of the joint capsule, into the joint space. Like the joint capsule, these projections have low signal intensity on conventional pulse sequences. Synovial folds may be confused with intra-articular loose bodies, particularly on sections in which a connection to the synovial membrane is not demonstrated. The common joint capsule of the elbow is formed by fusion of embryologic radiohumeral, ulnohumeral, and radioulnar cavities, and synovial folds represent the membranous remnants of this process.[7] Thus, synovial folds can be found in multiple characteristic locations about the elbow joint. The most common synovial fold is the so-called lateral synovial fold or synovial fringe, which was present in 43 of 50 (86%) of elbow specimens in a cadaver study.[8] On MRI, the lateral synovial fold can be seen as a tongue of synovial tissue extending from the lateral capsule between the radial head and the capitellum (**Fig. 15**). The lateral synovial fold can cause pain when pinched between the capitellum and radial head, but this usually reflects incompetence of the ulnar collateral ligament.[9]

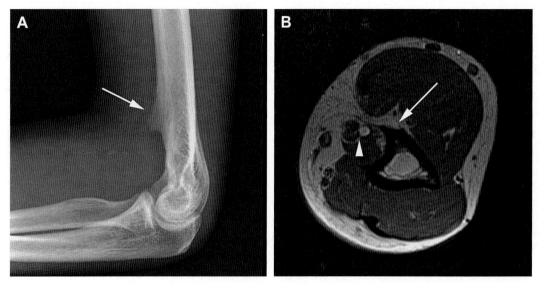

Fig. 14. Supracondylar process. (*A*) Lateral radiograph of the elbow shows a bony spur arising from the anterior aspect of the distal humeral shaft (*arrow*). (*B*) Axial T1-weighted magnetic resonance image of the elbow proximally shows the horn-shaped bony excrescence projecting anteriorly (*arrow*); notice its close proximity to the median nerve and the brachial artery (*arrowhead*). This entity should not be confused with osteochondroma.

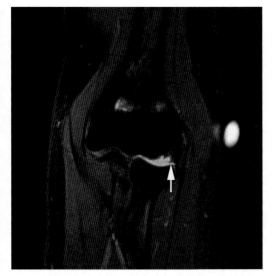

Fig. 15. Synovial fringe. Coronal T2-weighted magnetic resonance image of the elbow with fat-saturation demonstrates a small tongue of synovial tissue (*arrow*), representing the synovial fringe.

Synovial folds are also commonly seen in the posterior olecranon fossa extending from near the posterior fat pad. When thickened, such folds may be a cause of a locking elbow, but there is considerable overlap in thickness between locking synovial folds and those incidentally discovered in asymptomatic individuals.[10]

Ligaments

Several ligamentous variants exist. Beckett and colleagues[11] identified four different groups of variants involving the ulnar collateral ligament complex. About 23% of their specimens contained an accessory ligament, also known as an extra band, that passed from the posterior aspect of the capsule to insert on the transverse bundle. The lateral collateral ligament complex consists of the radial collateral ligament, the lateral ulnar collateral ligament, and the annular ligament, also known as the orbicular ligament. A fourth ligament, called the accessory lateral collateral ligament, may extend from the annular ligament to the supinator crest; this variant was observed in one-third of the specimens evaluated by Beckett and colleagues. The lateral ulnar collateral ligament may be absent. Alternatively, it may have an anomalous insertion where it inserts more distally onto the ulnar shaft beyond the supinator crest.

Variants of the Palmaris Longus Muscle

The palmaris longus muscle is among the most variable in the musculoskeletal system. This muscle has been extensively studied in the orthopedic literature, primarily because it is commonly used for reconstructive surgery and also because certain variants may be associated with median nerve compression. The palmaris longus is ideal as a donor graft because of its long tendon and the lack of functional implications of its absence. Indeed, absence of the palmaris longus is the most common variant encountered and has been observed in 2% to 20% of individuals. The prevalence varies among ethnic groups, being most common in Caucasians. Additional variants include reversed, duplicated, bifid, or hypertrophied palmaris longus muscles.[12]

Anconeus Epitrochlearis

The anconeus epitrochlearis is an accessory muscle that arises from the medial epicondyle, passes over the ulnar nerve, and inserts on the olecranon (**Fig. 16**). When present, this muscle replaces the cubital tunnel retinaculum, which is considered a remnant of the anconeus epitrochlearis.[13] The anconeus epitrochlearis can be a cause of ulnar nerve compression when prominent or edematous[14] but is also frequently encountered in asymptomatic elbows. The anconeus epitrochlearis has been identified in 3% to 28% of specimens in cadaver studies[13] and was recently reported in 23% of asymptomatic subjects on MRI.[15] A portion of the medial head of the triceps may rarely insert on the medial epicondyle, and this can also be a cause of ulnar nerve compression.[16]

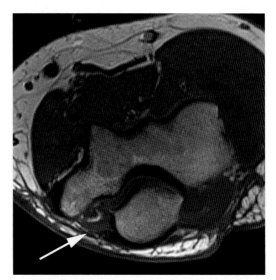

Fig. 16. Anconeus epitrochlearis. Axial T1-weighted magnetic resonance image of the elbow shows an accessory muscle (*arrow*) superficial to the ulnar nerve, representing the anconeus epitrochlearis muscle. This muscle can cause ulnar neuropathy.

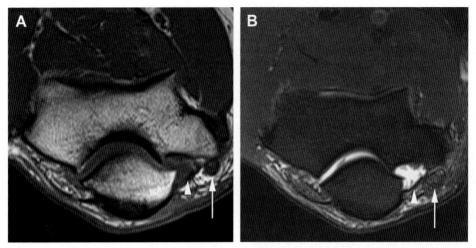

Fig. 17. Ulnar nerve subluxation. Axial T1-weighted (*A*) and axial T2-weighted fat-saturated (*B*) images through the cubital tunnel show subluxation of the ulnar nerve (*arrow*). Note intact cubital retinaculum (*arrowhead*). Because subluxation can occur in healthy asymptomatic individuals, clinical correlation for ulnar neuropathy is necessary.

Nerves

In addition to the anconeus epitrochlearis muscle already described, anatomic variants of the cubital tunnel retinaculum may lead to ulnar neuropathy, but these variants can also be incidentally detected in asymptomatic individuals. Thickening of the cubital tunnel retinaculum may lead to dynamic compression of the ulnar nerve during elbow flexion but can be seen in 22% of normal subjects.[13] Absence of the retinaculum is seen in up to 23% of the population[17] and may allow for anterior subluxation or dislocation of the ulnar nerve and possible development of friction neuritis.[13] However, ulnar nerve subluxation may occur with an intact cubital tunnel retinaculum (**Fig. 17**) and can be found incidentally in 10% to 16% of asymptomatic subjects.[18] Thus, clinical correlation for ulnar neuropathy is required when interpreting these findings in the cubital tunnel region.

MRI findings of neuropathy include increased signal in the affected nerve on fluid-sensitive sequences, focal or diffuse thickening of the nerve, and edema or fatty atrophy in acute or chronically affected muscles. The ulnar nerve is the most frequently injured nerve at the elbow because it is relatively exposed while coursing through the cubital tunnel. In addition to trauma, ulnar neuropathy may arise from osteophytes and loose bodies as well as the anconeus epitrochlearis and retinaculum variants already described. However, it is important to recognize that high signal intensity in the ulnar nerve on fluid-sensitive sequences is actually common in asymptomatic individuals, encountered in 60% in a recent study by Husarik and colleagues.[15] Thus, additional findings, such

as changes in ulnar nerve diameter, should be used in conjunction with signal abnormality to avoid overestimating ulnar neuropathy. Husarik and colleagues did not report abnormal signal in the median or radial nerves in their study of asymptomatic individuals. The investigators did encounter a fairly frequent anomalous course of the median nerve. The median nerve typically courses between the pronator teres and brachialis muscles alongside the brachial or ulnar artery. An anomalous intermuscular course of the median nerve between these two muscles, but deep to and separate from the brachial and ulnar arteries, was seen in 17% of subjects.

SUMMARY

The elbow is a joint consisting of three separate articulations with various structures providing stability in which the anterior bundle of the ulnar collateral ligament on the medial side and lateral ulnar collateral ligament on the lateral side play important roles. With its superior evaluation of soft tissues, MRI provides excellent evaluation of the osseous and neuromuscular structures. Precise understanding of the imaging anatomy of the elbow and its normal variants is important in the diagnosis and management of diseases of the elbow joint.

REFERENCES

1. Giuffrè BM, Moss MJ. Optimal positioning for MRI of the distal biceps brachii tendon: flexed abducted supinated view. AJR Am J Roentgenol 2004;182: 944–6.

2. Rosenberg ZS, Bletran J, Cheung YY. Pseudodefect of the capitellum: potential MR imaging pitfall. Radiology 1994;191:821–3.

3. Kijowski R, De Smet AA. MRI findings of osteochondritis dissecans with surgical correlation. AJR Am J Roentgenol 2005;185:1453–9.

4. Fowler KA, Chung CB. Normal MR imaging anatomy of the elbow. Radiol Clin North Am 2006;44:553–67.

5. Natsis K. Supracondylar process of the humerus: study on 375 Caucasian subjects in Cologne, Germany. Clin Anat 2008;21:138–41.

6. Pecina M, Boric I, Anticevic D. Intraoperatively proven anomalous Struthers' ligament diagnosed by MRI. Skeletal Radiol 2002;31:532–5.

7. Clarke RP. Symptomatic, lateral synovial fringe (plica) of the elbow joint. Arthroscopy 1988;4:112–6.

8. Duparc F, Putz R, Michot C, et al. The synovial fold of the humeroradial joint: anatomical and histological features, and clinical relevance in lateral epicondylalgia of the elbow. Surg Radiol Anat 2002;24:302–7.

9. Helms CA, Major NM, Anderson MW, et al. Elbow. In: Musculoskeletal MRI. 2nd edition. Philadelphia: Saunders Elsevier; 2009. p. 232.

10. Awaya H, Schweitzer ME, Feng SA, et al. Elbow synovial fold syndrome: MR imaging findings. AJR Am J Roentgenol 2001;177:1377–81.

11. Beckett KS, McConnell P, Lagopoulos M, et al. Variations in the normal anatomy of the collateral ligaments of the human elbow joint. J Anat 2000; 197:507–11.

12. Park MJ, Namdari S, Yao J. Anatomic variations of the palmaris longus muscle. Am J Orthop 2010;39: 89–94.

13. O'Driscoll SW, Horii E, Carmichael SW, et al. The cubital tunnel and ulnar neuropathy. J Bone Joint Surg Br 1991;73:613–7.

14. Jeon IH, Fairbairn KJ, Wallace WA. MR imaging of edematous anconeus epitrochlearis: another cause of medial elbow pain? Skeletal Radiol 2005;34: 103–7.

15. Husarik DB, Saupe N, Pfirrmann CW, et al. Elbow nerves: MR findings in 60 asymptomatic subjects—normal anatomy, variants, and pitfalls. Radiology 2009;252:148–56.

16. O'Hara JJ, Stone JH. Ulnar nerve compression at the elbow caused by a prominent medial head of the triceps and an anconeus epitrochlearis muscle. J Hand Surg Br 1996;21:133–5.

17. Dellon AL. Musculotendinous variations about the humeral epicondyle. J Hand Surg Br 1986;11:175–81.

18. Bozentka DJ. Cubital tunnel syndrome pathophysiology. Clin Orthop 1998;351:90–4.

Normal MR Imaging Anatomy of the Thigh and Leg

Saifuddin Vohra, DO, George Arnold, MD,
Shashin Doshi, MD, David Marcantonio, MD*

KEYWORDS

• Anatomy • Thigh • Leg • MR imaging • Pitfalls

Developing a solid understanding of basic magnetic resonance imaging (MR imaging) principles and musculoskeletal imaging protocols, as well as the appearance of normal imaging anatomy, is crucial to interpret musculoskeletal MR imaging examinations at a diagnostic level. This knowledge can then be applied to one's understanding of pathology commonly encountered in the area of interest. Careful attention should be focused on awareness of commonly encountered anatomic variants and diagnostic pitfalls to improve diagnostic accuracy and avoid misinterpretation.

In this article, focus is placed on depicting normal anatomy at representative levels throughout the thigh and leg, describing and providing rationale for routine imaging protocols, and discussing frequently encountered anatomical variants and imaging pitfalls. This will serve as a basic foundation for accurate evaluation of the many pathologic processes that may involve the thigh and leg.

MR imaging of a healthy volunteer was performed on a 3T MR imaging unit (Siemens, Erlangen, Germany). Select axial T1-weighted (T1W) images are displayed to depict anatomical structures to best advantage, and allow the reader to conceptualize relevant anatomy while emphasizing compartmental organization.

PROTOCOLS

Routine thigh and leg MR imaging protocols at our institution include a combination of T1W, T2W, and short tau inversion recovery (STIR) sequences. T1W sequences provide excellent depiction of anatomic detail, bone marrow signal alteration, fat within mass lesions, identification of subacute blood products, and presence of enhancing tissue after gadolinium contrast administration. T2W sequences identify tissues with increased water content that can be seen in the setting of a broad range of pathology, including neoplastic, infectious, inflammatory, and traumatic processes. Acquisition of T2W sequences is performed using the fast spin-echo (FSE) technique to reduce scan time and minimize susceptibility artifact from field inhomogeneity. Frequency selective fat suppression is used on T2W sequences to accentuate pathologic abnormalities. STIR sequences allow for a more sensitive evaluation of soft tissue and bone marrow edema, and offer more reliable uniform fat suppression; however, currently, in many institutions, FSE T2W and STIR sequences are used similarly.[1] Intravenous gadolinium contrast administration allows differentiation of cystic versus solid masses, and detection of hyperemic tissues related to viable tumor as opposed to necrosis, and phlegmonous/inflammatory tissue as opposed to abscess formation.[1] The axial plane of imaging is preferred for a compartmental approach to evaluation and in assessing the neurovascular structures, muscles, and fascial layers. The coronal plane provides a general overview of the region of interest, and the sagittal plane aids in better depicting the cranial-caudal extent of muscle disease and myotendinous junction involvement.[1,2] The field strength, coil (volume

The authors having nothing to disclose.
Division of Musculoskeletal Radiology, Department of Diagnostic Radiology-Imaging Center, William Beaumont Hospital, 3601 West 13 Mile Road, Royal Oak, MI 48073, USA
* Corresponding author.
E-mail address: David.Marcantonio@beaumont.edu

Magn Reson Imaging Clin N Am 19 (2011) 621–636
doi:10.1016/j.mric.2011.05.011

surface phased array), slice thickness, field of view, matrix size, and other select imaging parameters are optimized with the goal of increasing the signal-to-noise ratio and decreasing scan time, thereby decreasing motion artifact. Patient-specific factors including body habitus and ability to cooperate, desired region of coverage, and presence of metallic hardware or foreign bodies must also be considered.

Specifically, our routine protocol for both the thigh and leg (**Table 1**) includes an axial T2W sequence with fat saturation, at least 2 planes of T1W sequences without fat saturation, and coronal and sagittal STIR sequences. If gadolinium contrast is indicated, at minimum, precontrast and postcontrast fat-suppressed axial T1W sequences are obtained. At least one additional postcontrast fat-suppressed T1W sequence is acquired, either in the sagittal or coronal orientation; however, both are preferable. Ultimately, the final imaging protocol is tailored to patient-specific factors with the desired intention of obtaining the best image quality to answer the clinical question.

IMAGING ANATOMY
Thigh

The thigh is best described in terms of compartmental anatomy, and is composed of anterior, posterior, and medial (adductor) compartments. In terms of spread of pathologic processes, such as tumor and infection, other delineated compartments include the skin and subcutaneous fat, bone bounded by periosteum and cortex, and parosteal space (between the bone and overlying soft tissues).[3] The thigh extends from the superior margin of the subtrochanteric region through the distal femoral metadiaphysis. Each compartment is composed of muscles, neurovascular structures, and intermuscular fascia. Muscles are of intermediate signal intensity to fat on T1W and T2W FSE sequences.[1] Peripheral nerves are round or oval and have a fascicular appearance, best depicted on T2W sequences. They are isointense to muscle on T1W sequences with intermixed increased signal intensity similar to fat. On T2W sequences, they are isointense to slightly hyperintense relative

Table 1
Thigh (femur) and leg (tibia/fibula) routine imaging protocols: flex surface coil set up: Patient placed feet first, supine, with leg at the center of the bore of the magnet. Area of interest/concern bracketed with vitamin E capsules. 3T MR imaging unit (Siemens, Erlangen, Germany)

| Thigh | | | | | | |
Sequence	Fat Saturation	FOV, cm	Matrix	Slice Thickness/Gap, mm	TR/TI, ms	TE, ms
Coronal T1	N	40	256 × 256	5/2.5	750	9.5
Axial T1	N	20	256 × 256	4/2.0	750	9.6
Sagittal T1	N	40	256 × 256	5/2.5	750	9.5
Axial T2	Y	20	256 × 256	4/1.2	5250	81
Coronal STIR	N/A	40	184 × 384	3/0.9	7380/210	27
Sagittal STIR	N/A	40	184 × 384	3/0.9	7380/210	27
[a]Axial T1 Pre.	Y	20	256 × 256	4/2.0	750	9.6
Leg						
Sequence	Fat Saturation	FOV, cm	Matrix	Slick Thickness/Gap, mm	TR/TI, ms	TE, ms
Coronal T1	N	35	256 × 256	5/1.5	750	9.5
Axial T1	N	20	256 × 256	5/1.5	750	9.6
Sagittal T1	N	40	256 × 256	5/2.5	750	9.5
Axial T2	Y	20	256 × 256	5/1.5	5250	81
Coronal STIR	N/A	35	184 × 384	3/0.9	7380/210	27
Sagittal STIR	N/A	40	184 × 384	3/0.9	7380/210	27
[a]Axial T1 Pre.	Y	20	256 × 256	5/1.5	750	9.6

Abbreviations: FOV, field of view; N, no; N/A, not applicable; STIR, short tau inversion recovery; Y, yes.
[a] Optional, if intravenous contrast is indicated. Post–gadolinium contrast T1W sequences are obtained in at least 2 orthogonal planes with fat suppression.

to muscle.[1] In general, arteries should be hypointense to muscle on all sequences.[1] Veins have variable signal intensity on T1W and T2W sequences.

The iliotibial tract, tensor muscle of fascia lata, quadriceps femoris (vastus medialis, vastus lateralis, vastus intermedius, and rectus femoris), and sartorius muscles are located within the anterior compartment. The sartorius muscle is long, thin, and bandlike, originating from the anterior superior iliac spine, obliquely coursing over the proximal thigh along the inner margin of the quadriceps muscles, and extending to the posteromedial aspect of the knee. Its tendon extends anteriorly and attaches to the anteromedial surface of the proximal tibia superficial to the gracilis and semitendinosus tendons. Together, these 3 tendons comprise the pes anserinus tendon complex. The rectus femoris muscle originates from the anterior inferior iliac spine as 2 tendons: the straight and reflected heads. The vastus lateralis muscle arises from the anterior superior aspect of the femoral shaft and the lateral facet of the linea aspera; the vastus medialis muscle originates from the intertrochanteric line and medial aspect of linea aspera; the vastus intermedius muscle arises between these 2 muscles and subjacent to the rectus femoris muscle, along the anterior aspect of the femoral shaft. Differentiation of these muscles is sometimes difficult as they may be partially fused at their origins and insertions. Distally, these 4 muscles form the quadriceps tendon, which contains the patella, the largest sesamoid in the body.[4]

The posterior compartment contains the semimembranosus, semitendinosus, and long and short heads of the biceps femoris muscles. The major innervation of the lower extremity, the sciatic nerve, is also located in this compartment. The semitendinosus and long head of the biceps femoris muscles originate from a common tendon along the medial facet and distal margin of the ischial tuberosity. The semitendinosus muscle, fusiform in shape, is more tendinous distally, and inserts along the medial aspect of the proximal tibia deep to the sartorius tendon. The short head of the biceps femoris muscle originates from the linea aspera in the mid to distal thigh and joins the long head of the biceps femoris muscle to insert on the fibular head laterally. The semimembranosus tendon arises from the lateral facet of the ischial tuberosity and has a broad insertion along the proximal posteromedial tibia.

The medial compartment contains the adductor brevis, longus, and magnus muscles as well as gracilis, pectineus, and obturator externus musculature. The gracilis muscle is the most superficial and medial, and originates from the inferior ischiopubic ramus and inserts deep to the sartorius tendon along the proximal medial tibia after curving anteriorly around the posteromedial femoral condyle. The pectineus muscle is triangular in shape and originates at the superior pubic ramus along with the adductor longus muscle more medially. It inserts onto the pectineal line of the femoral shaft, whereas the adductor longus muscle inserts onto the middle third of the linea aspera. The adductor brevis muscle is also triangular in shape, and originates from the inferior pubic ramus and inserts along the upper third of the linea aspera. The adductor magnus muscle, the largest of the adductor muscle group, originates along the inferior pubic ramus and ischial tuberosity, and inserts along the entire linea aspera as well as the adductor tubercle of the distal femur. The obturator externus muscle, the deepest of the muscles in the medial compartment, originates from the anterior two-thirds of the obturator foramen (formed by the lateral surface of the ischiopubic ramus) and inserts into the trochanteric fossa of the proximal femur. The neurovascular bundle, including the saphenous nerve, is located in this compartment.[5]

Leg

The leg extends from the proximal tibial metaphysis through the distal metaphysis. The soft tissues are similarly organized in a compartmental fashion, and are supported by the tibia and fibula. The lower leg is composed of 4 compartments: anterior, superficial posterior, deep posterior, and lateral. The interosseous membrane separates the anterior and deep posterior compartments. The transverse septum separates the superficial and deep posterior compartments.

The anterior compartment contains the tibialis anterior, extensor digitorum longus, and extensor hallucis longus muscles, and the anterior neurovascular bundle, including the anterior tibial artery and vein, and deep peroneal nerve. The tibialis anterior muscle originates from the lateral surface of the tibia and neighboring interosseous membrane in the upper leg, and extends distally over the anterior tibia to insert upon the dorsal aspect of the first metatarsal. The extensor digitorum longus muscle originates from the anterior surface of the interosseous membrane and fibula, courses inferiorly along the anterior tibia, and gives rise to tendons that insert upon the distal phalanges of the second through fifth toes. The peroneus tertius muscle, when variably present, is closely associated with the extensor digitorum longus muscle, coursing in the same synovial sheath; however, its tendon attaches to the dorsal aspect of the base of the fifth metatarsal.[4] The extensor hallucis longus muscle originates from the distal aspect of the fibula and interosseous membrane, and extends distally across the ankle and foot to insert upon the distal phalanx of the first toe. At the level of the ankle, the tendons in this compartment are stabilized by the superior and inferior extensor retinacula.

The deep posterior compartment contains the popliteus, tibialis posterior, flexor digitorum, and flexor hallucis longus muscles, as well as the posterior tibial and peroneal arteries and the posterior tibial nerve. The popliteus muscle originates from the lateral femoral condyle and inserts upon the popliteal line of the tibia. The flexor digitorum longus muscle originates from the popliteal line and posterior aspect of the tibia. Its tendon passes posterior and around the medial malleolus, and gives rise to 4 tendinous slips that insert upon the bases of the distal phalanges of the second through fourth toes. The flexor hallucis longus muscle originates from the distal two-thirds of the fibula, and its tendon courses around the medial malleolus, posterior to the flexor digitorum longus tendon, and between the medial and lateral tubercles of the posterior process of the talus to insert upon the distal phalynx of the first toe. The tibialis posterior muscle originates from the lateral aspect of the tibia and adjacent interosseous membrane. It courses around the medial malleolus, anterior to the flexor digitorum longus tendon, and has a broad insertion upon multiple structures along the plantar surface of the foot, predominantly inserting upon the navicular and, to a lesser degree, the cuneiform bones.

The plantaris, soleus, and medial and lateral heads of the gastrocnemius muscles, along with the sural nerve, are located within the superficial posterior compartment. The medial and lateral heads of the gastrocnemius musculature originate from immediately superior to the medial and lateral femoral condyles, respectively, and insert upon the deep aspect of the Achilles tendon at mid leg. The soleus muscle originates from the tibia and fibula, deep to the gastrocnemius musculature, and inserts upon the deep aspect of the Achilles tendon at a variable level. The plantaris muscle belly is short and originates from the distal lateral linea aspera in close association with the lateral head of gastrocnemius muscle. Its long tendon courses inferiorly between the soleus muscle and the medial head of gastrocnemius muscle, and inserts upon the posterior superior aspect of the calcaneus along the medial margin of the Achilles tendon.

The lateral compartment contains the peroneus longus and peroneus brevis muscles as well as the common and superficial peroneal nerves. It is separated from the anterior and posterior compartments by intermuscular septa. The peroneus longus muscle arises from the upper half of the lateral surface of the fibula and adjacent structures, descends lateral and then posterior to the peroneus brevis muscle, and inserts along the plantar surface of the base of the first metatarsal.[4,5] It lies posterior to the lateral malleolus and lateral to the calcaneus at these respective levels. Along the plantar surface of the foot, the tendon courses adjacent to the cuboid (cuboid tunnel) and tarsometatarsal articulations. The peroneus brevis muscle originates from the middle one-third of the lateral aspect of the fibula and inserts upon the dorsolateral aspect of the base of the fifth metatarsal. Both peroneal tendons are stabilized by the superior and inferior peroneal retinacula.

Anatomic variants occur most commonly within the mid to distal leg, and with less frequency within the thigh. Accessory muscles comprise most of the variant anatomy. The peroneus tertius, a common anatomic variant located within the anterior compartment, originates from the anterior aspect of the distal fibula and extensor digitorum longus muscle as discussed previously. Accessory soleus musculature is most commonly unilateral, and arises from the fibula, soleal line of the tibia, and anterior aspect of the soleus. There are 5 types related to insertion location.[6] The peroneus quartus muscle is located within the lateral compartment. It originates from and is situated medial and posterior to the peroneus brevis and longus musculature. Several types exist and are further classified based on their insertions. The peroneus calcaneus internus muscle is a rare anatomic variant that is usually asymptomatic; however, it has been clinically associated with posterior ankle impingement and flexor hallucis longus tenosynovitis. Flexor digitorum accessorius longus is an uncommon variant that has been associated with tarsal tunnel syndrome.[6]

Variations, including accessory slips and anomalous origins of the gastrocnemius and popliteus musculature, some of which may lead to popliteal artery entrapment syndrome depending on their effect upon the underlying popliteal vasculature, are also not infrequently encountered. An uncommon accessory popliteus shares a common origin with the lateral head of the gastrocnemius and courses inferomedially within the deep popliteal fossa, situated anterior to the popliteal vessels. It inserts onto the posteromedial joint capsule of the knee, and may potentially have a compressive effect upon the overlying popliteal neurovascular bundle.

Tensor fasciae suralis, a very rare accessory muscle, can arise from any hamstring muscle; however, it most commonly originates from the distal semitendinosus muscle. It can insert onto the medial head of the gastrocnemius, posterior fascia of the leg, or onto the superficial aspect of the Achilles tendon by means of a long, thin tendon. Tensor fasciae suralis is superficial within the popliteal fossa, situated lateral to the semimembranosus and semitendinosus muscles and medial to the biceps femoris muscle.

SUMMARY

Familiarity with normal MR imaging anatomy, commonly encountered anatomic variants, and awareness of diagnostic pitfalls are crucial to accurately detect disease, communicate relevant findings, and plan and perform musculoskeletal interventional procedures. See the Appendix for illustrative figures.

ACKNOWLEDGMENTS

Mike Tenzer, MD, our healthy imaging volunteer, provided many of the images used in this section.

APPENDIX

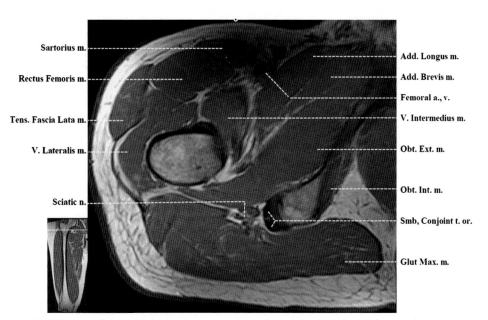

Fig. 1. Axial T1W image. Upper thigh. Compartmental muscle anatomy. Add., Adductor; a., artery; Glut Max., gluteus maximus; m., muscle; n., nerve; Obt. Ext./Int., obturator externus/internus; Smb, semimembranosus; t., tendon; Tens., tensor; v., vein; V., vastus.

Key Points

- The biceps femoris long head muscle originates from the medial facet of the ischial tuberosity and the semitendinosus muscle originates from the medial facet and distal margin. They originate as a conjoint tendon posteromedially, whereas the semimembranosus muscle arises from the lateral facet more anteriorly.
- In the proximal thigh, the anterior and medial compartments are divided by the iliopsoas muscle (which inserts upon the lesser trochanter) and neurovascular bundle. The posterior and anterior compartments are separated by the gluteus maximus muscle.
- The vastus intermedius muscle arises along the anterolateral femur deep to the vastus lateralis muscle.
- The sciatic nerve is immediately lateral to the common hamstring tendon origin along the ischial tuberosity, and deep to the gluteus maximus muscle.
- The adductor longus, brevis, and magnus (not seen) muscles, maintain this relationship from anterior to posterior until the adductor brevis muscle inserts upon the upper aspect of the linea aspera and the distal pectineal line.

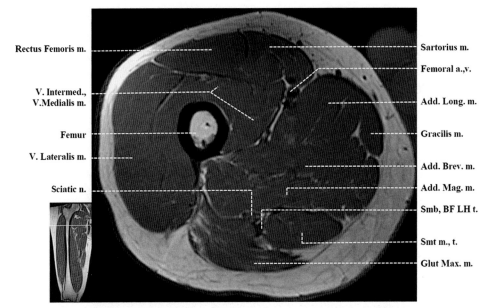

Fig. 2. Axial T1W image. Upper thigh. Compartmental muscle anatomy. Add., Adductor; a., artery; BF LH, biceps femoris long head; Interm., intermedius; Long., longus; m., muscle; n., nerve; Smb, semimembranosus; Smt, semitendinosus; t., tendon; v., vein; V., vastus.

Key Points

- Most medially the gracilis muscle is seen, which originates from the inferior pubic ramus.
- The deep (profunda) femoral artery and vein are the major femoral branch vessels positioned between the vastus medialis muscle and the adductor magnus muscle.
- The sciatic nerve is adjacent to the posterior aspect of the adductor magnus muscle, deep to the gluteus maximus muscle.

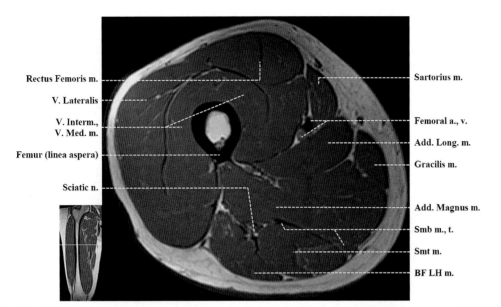

Rectus Femoris m.
V. Lateralis
V. Interm.,
V. Med. m.
Femur (linea aspera)
Sciatic n.

Sartorius m.
Femoral a., v.
Add. Long. m.
Gracilis m.
Add. Magnus m.
Smb m., t.
Smt m.
BF LH m.

Fig. 3. Axial T1W image. Mid thigh. Compartmental muscle anatomy. Add., Adductor; a., artery; BF LH, biceps femoris long head; Lat. Intmsclr. Sptm., lateral intermuscular septum; m., muscle; n., nerve; Smb, semimembranosus; Smt, semitendinosus; t., tendon; v., vein; V., vastus.

Key Points

- The sciatic nerve is adjacent to the posterior aspect of the adductor magnus muscle.
- The gracilis muscle is seen most medially.

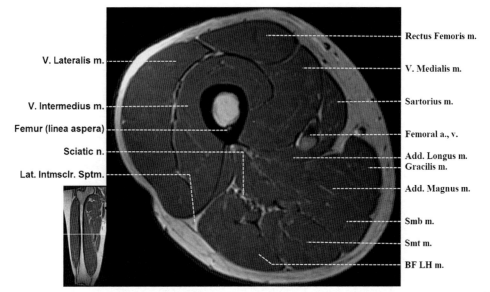

Fig. 4. Axial T1W image. Mid thigh. Compartmental muscle anatomy. Add., Adductor; a., artery; BF LH, biceps femoris long head; Lat. Intmsclr. Sptm., lateral intermuscular septum; m., muscle; n., nerve; Smb., semimembranosus; Smt., semitendinosus; v., vein; V., vastus.

Key Points

- The femoral artery and vein are within the adductor canal of Hunter (floor formed by the adductor longus muscle).
- The sciatic nerve is interposed between the adductor magnus muscle and the biceps femoris long head muscle.
- The anterior and posterior compartments are separated by the lateral intermuscular septum.
- The semitendinosus, semimembranosus, and biceps femoris long head are entirely muscular at this level, and have flipped medial-lateral orientation relative to their origin.

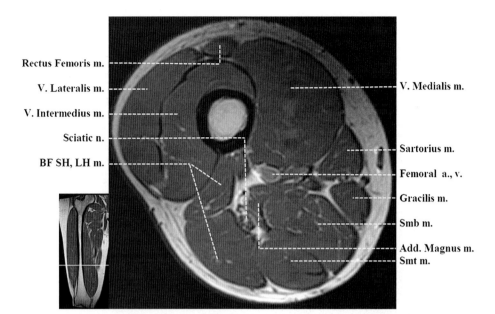

Rectus Femoris m.
V. Lateralis m.
V. Intermedius m.
Sciatic n.
BF SH, LH m.

V. Medialis m.
Sartorius m.
Femoral a., v.
Gracilis m.
Smb m.
Add. Magnus m.
Smt m.

Fig. 5. Axial T1W image. Lower thigh. Compartmental muscle anatomy. Add., Adductor; a., artery; BF SH, LH, biceps femoris short head, long head; m., muscle; n., nerve; Smb, semimembranosus; Smt, semitendinosus; v., vein; V., vastus.

Key Points

- A small portion of the adductor magnus muscle remains.
- The femoral artery and vein become the popliteal vessels below this level after exiting the adductor canal of Hunter via the adductor hiatus.
- The sciatic nerve is between the adductor magnus muscle and biceps femoris long head muscle.

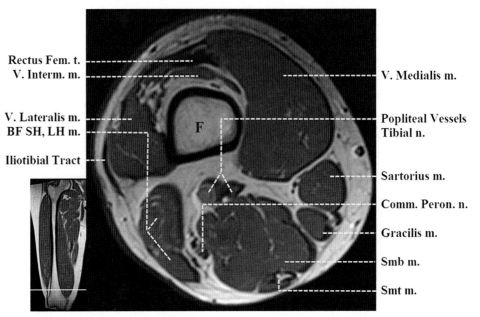

Fig. 6. Axial T1W image. Lower thigh. Compartmental muscle anatomy. BF SH, LH, biceps femoris short head, long head; Comm. Peron., common peroneal; F, femur; Fem., femoris; Interm., intermedius; m., muscle; n., nerve; Smb, semimembranosus; Smt, semitendinosus; t., tendon; V., vastus.

Key Points

- The sciatic nerve has divided into the common peroneal nerve and the tibial nerve.
- The adductor magnus muscle is no longer well seen.
- The gracilis muscle is immediately posterior to the sartorius muscle.

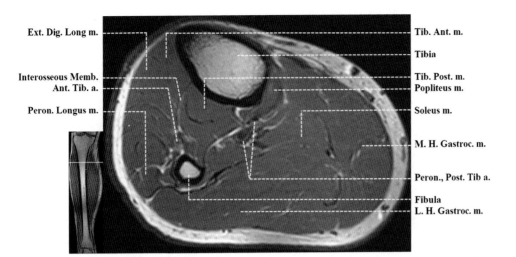

Fig. 7. Axial T1W image. Upper leg. Compartmental muscle anatomy. a., artery; Ant. Tib., anterior tibial; Ext. Dig. Long, extensor digitorum longus; Memb., membrane; M.H./L.H. Gastroc., gastrocnemius, medial and lateral heads; m., muscle; Peron. Longus, peroneus longus; Peron., peroneal; Post. Tib, posterior tibialis; Tib. Ant., tibialis anterior; Tib. Post., tibialis posterior.

Key Points

- The anterior compartment is separated from the deep posterior compartment by the interosseous membrane.
- The peroneus brevis muscle is not seen at this level.
- The peroneal artery and posterior tibial artery are situated between the deep and superficial posterior compartments.
- The plantaris tendon (not well seen) courses between the soleus muscle and medial head of gastrocnemius muscle at this level.
- The common peroneal nerve has not yet bifurcated into its superficial (lateral compartment) and deep (anterior compartment) branches.

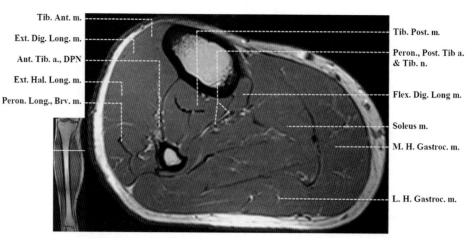

Fig. 8. Axial T1W image. Upper leg. Compartmental muscle anatomy. a., artery; Ant. Tib., anterior tibial; DPN, deep peroneal nerve; Ext. Dig. Long., extensor digitorum longus; Ext. Hal. Long., extensor hallucis longus; Flex. Dig. Long, flexor digitorum longus; M.H./L.H. Gastroc., gastrocnemius, medial and lateral heads; m., muscle; n., nerve; Peron. Longus., Brv., peroneus longus, brevis; Peron., peroneal; Post. Tib, posterior tibialis; Tib. Ant., tibialis anterior; Tib. Post., tibialis posterior; Tib., tibial.

Key Points

- The posterior tibial artery and the tibial nerve maintain a constant relationship in this region.
- The plantaris tendon is flattened and not clearly defined.
- The medial head gastrocnemius muscle extends more inferiorly than the lateral head gastrocnemius muscle creating asymmetry in the posterior calf.
- The intermuscular septa are not as well seen as in the thigh.

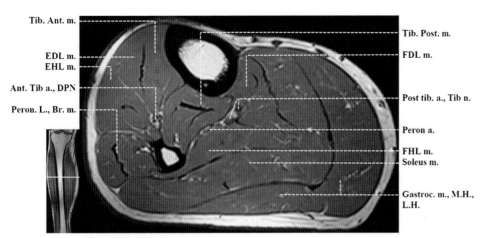

Fig. 9. Axial T1W image. Mid leg. Compartmental muscle anatomy. a., artery; Ant. Tib., anterior tibial; DPN, deep peroneal nerve; EDL, extensor digitorum longus; EHL, extensor hallucis longus; FDL, flexor digitorum longus; FHL, flexor hallucis longus; Gastroc. M.H./L.H., gastrocnemius, medial and lateral heads; m., muscle; n., nerve; Peron. L., Br., peroneus longus, brevis; Peron., peroneal; Post. tib., posterior tibialis; Tib. Ant., tibialis anterior; Tib. Post., tibialis posterior; Tib., tibial.

Key Points

- The anterior tibial artery and the deep peroneal nerve course inferiorly adjacent to the anterior aspect of the interosseous membrane.
- The posterior tibial artery and the tibial nerve maintain a constant relationship in this region, which continues inferiorly to the level of the ankle, interposed between the flexor hallucis longus and flexor digitorum longus muscles.
- Nutrient vessel can be seen within the posterior cortex of the tibia.

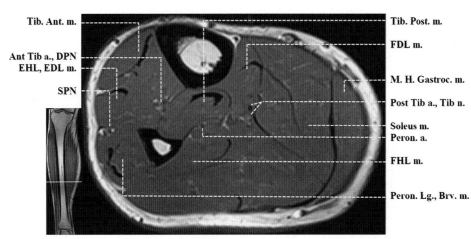

Fig. 10. Axial T1W image. Mid leg. Compartmental muscle anatomy. a., artery; Ant. Tib., anterior tibial; DPN, deep peroneal nerve; EDL, extensor digitorum longus; EHL, extensor hallucis longus; FDL, flexor digitorum longus; FHL, flexor hallucis longus; M.H. Gastroc., gastrocnemius, medial head; m., muscle; n., nerve; Peron. Lg., Brv., peroneus longus, brevis; Peron., peroneal; Post Tib, posterior tibialis; SPN, superficial peroneal nerve; Tib. Ant., tibialis anterior; Tib. Post., tibialis posterior; Tib., tibial.

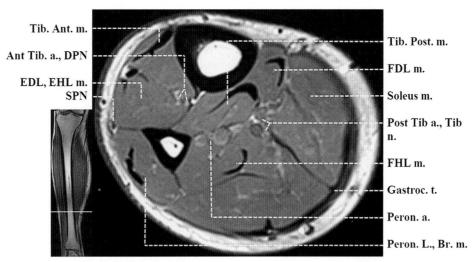

Fig. 11. Axial T1W image. Lower leg. Compartmental muscle anatomy. a., artery; Ant Tib., anterior tibial; DPN, deep peroneal nerve; EDL, extensor digitorum longus; EHL, extensor hallucis longus; FDL, flexor digitorum longus; FHL, flexor hallucis longus; Gastroc., gastrocnemius; m., muscle; n., nerve; Peron. L., Br., peroneus longus, brevis; Peron., peroneal; Post Tib, posterior tibialis; SPN, superficial peroneal nerve; t., tendon; Tib. Ant., tibialis anterior; Tib. Post., tibialis posterior; Tib., tibial.

Key Point

- The peroneal artery is situated near the fibula between the tibialis posterior muscle and flexor hallucis longus muscle.

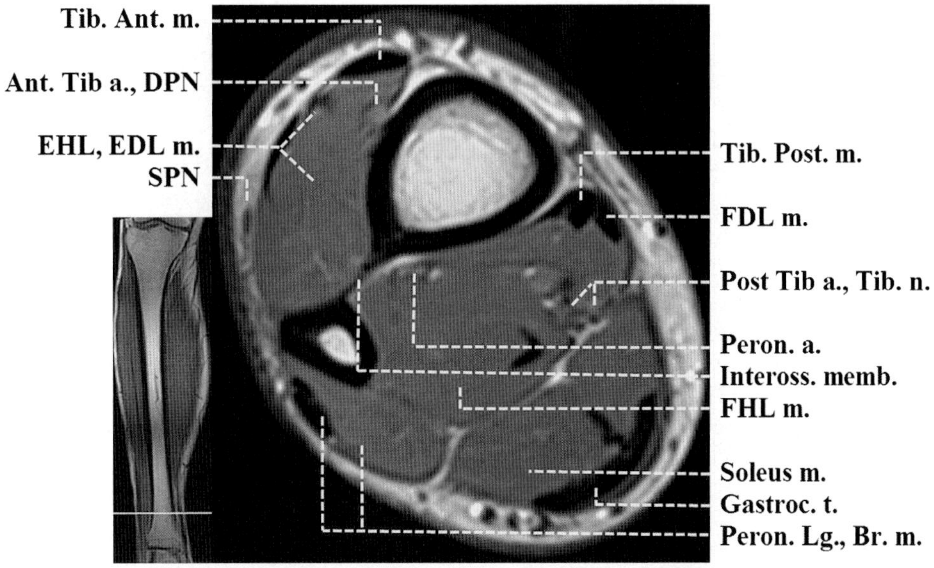

Fig. 12. Axial T1W image. Lower leg. Compartmental muscle anatomy. a., artery; Ant Tib., anterior tibial; DPN, deep peroneal nerve; EDL, extensor digitorum longus; EHL, extensor hallucis longus; FDL, flexor digitorum longus; FHL, flexor hallucis longus; Gastroc., gastrocnemius; m., muscle; n., nerve; Peron. Lg., Br., peroneus longus, brevis; Peron., peroneal; Post Tib, posterior tibialis; SPN, superficial peroneal nerve; t., tendon; Tib. Ant., tibialis anterior; Tib. Post., tibialis posterior; Tib., tibial.

Key Points

- The extensor hallucis longus muscle is almost entirely tendinous.
- The posterior tibial artery and the tibial nerve are interposed between the flexor hallucis longus muscle and the tibialis posterior muscle. As the soleus muscle belly decreases in size, the gastrocnemius tendon thickens.

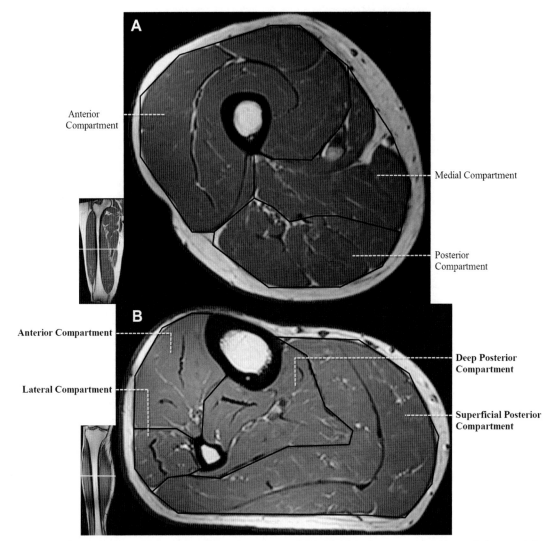

Fig. 13. Axial T1W images. Compartmental muscle anatomy. (*A*) Mid thigh. Compartmental boundaries are delineated by solid black lines. (*B*) Mid leg. Compartmental boundaries are delineated by solid black lines.

REFERENCES

1. Kaplan PA, Helms CA, Dussault R, et al. Basic principles of musculoskeletal MRI. Musculoskeletal MRI. 1st edition. Philadelphia: WB Saunders; 1995. p. 1–22.
2. Farber JM, Buckwalter KA. MR imaging in nonneoplastic muscle disorders of the lower extremity. Radiol Clin North Am 2002;40:1013–31.
3. Anderson MW, Temple TH, Dussault RG, et al. Compartmental anatomy: relevance to staging and biopsy of musculoskeletal tumors. AJR Am J Roentgenol 1999;173:1663–71.
4. El-Khoury GY, Bergman RA, Montgomery WJ. Hip and thigh, leg. In: Whitten CG, Walker CW, Montgomery WJ, editors. Sectional anatomy by MRI. 2nd edition. Philadelphia: Churchill Livingstone Inc.; 1995. p. 555–602, 669–722.
5. Bancroft LW, Peterson JJ, Kransdorf MJ, et al. Compartmental anatomy relevant to biopsy planning. Semin Musculoskelet Radiol 2007;11:16–27.
6. Sookur PA, Naraghi AM, Bleakney RR, et al. Accessory muscles: anatomy, symptoms, and radiologic evaluation. Radiographics 2008;28:481–99.

Normal MR Imaging Anatomy of the Knee

Saifuddin Vohra, DO, George Arnold, MD,
Shashin Doshi, MD, David Marcantonio, MD*

KEYWORDS

• Anatomy • Knee • MR imaging • Pitfalls

There are several keys to successfully interpreting MR imaging examinations. Initially, constructing a solid foundation consisting of a good understanding of basic MR imaging principles and imaging protocols as well as the appearance of normal imaging anatomy is crucial. This knowledge can be then applied to one's understanding of pathology commonly encountered in the area of interest. Careful attention should be focused on awareness of commonly encountered normal variants and diagnostic pitfalls to improve accuracy and avoid misinterpretation. In this article, MR imaging of a healthy volunteer was performed on a 3-T MR imaging unit (Siemens, Munich, Germany). Normal anatomy is depicted at representative levels throughout the knee, and descriptions of frequently encountered anatomic variants are provided.

PROTOCOLS

At the authors' institution, a combination of intermediate-weighted proton density (PD) and T2-weighted fast spin echo sequences with and without fat suppression are used to provide excellent anatomic detail and localize pathology. Fat suppression accentuates bone marrow and soft tissue edema on fluid-sensitive sequences, and non–fat-suppressed images increase conspicuity of bone marrow abnormalities on short echo time (TE) sequences. Furthermore, fast spin echo PD sequences employing fat saturation are accurate and sensitive for evaluation of meniscal tears and articular cartilage disruption.

In general, optimal evaluation is achieved when the imaging planes are oriented perpendicular to and parallel to the long axis of the structure in question. The multiplanar capability of MR imaging allows for oblique sagittal image acquisition oriented parallel to the lateral femoral condyle, which optimizes evaluation of the anterior cruciate ligament (ACL), horns of the menisci, femorotibial joint and femoral trochlear articular cartilage, cruciate ligaments, and extensor mechanism. The coronal plane of imaging is preferred for evaluation of the body of the menisci, and medial and lateral stabilizing structures. The axial plane is used to evaluate the patellar articular cartilage, quadriceps tendon, and medial and lateral stabilizing structures.

The routine knee MR imaging protocol at the authors' institution (**Table 1**) consists of axial intermediate PD with fat saturation, PD sagittal oblique without fat saturation, PD coronal without fat saturation, intermediate T2 coronal with fat saturation, and intermediate T2 sagittal oblique with fat saturation sequences. When indicated, intravenous gadolinium contrast may help to further characterize neoplastic, infectious, and inflammatory processes. Prior to gadolinium contrast administration, an axial T1-weighted sequence with fat suppression is obtained as a control sequence. Following intravenous gadolinium contrast administration, T1-weighted fat-suppressed sequences are obtained in the axial plane, and at least one additional orthogonal plane. Indications for intra-articular dilute gadolinium contrast administration include suspected

The authors having nothing to disclose.
Division of Musculoskeletal Radiology, Department of Diagnostic Radiology-Imaging Center, William Beaumont Hospital, 3601 West 13 Mile Road, Royal Oak, MI 48073, USA
* Corresponding author.
E-mail address: David.Marcantonio@beaumont.edu

Magn Reson Imaging Clin N Am 19 (2011) 637–653
doi:10.1016/j.mric.2011.05.012

Table 1
Routine MR imaging protocol: knee (volume surface phased array) coil

Sequence	Fat Saturation	FOV (cm)	Matrix	TR (ms)	TE (ms)	Slice Thickness/Gap (mm)
Intermediate PD axial	Y	14	313 × 384	4430	11	3/0.6
Intermediate T2 sagittal oblique	Y	14	200 × 256	2920	56	3/0.6
Intermediate T2 coronal	Y	14	200 × 256	4050	56	3/0.6
PD coronal	N	14	314 × 448	1200	15	3/0.6
PD sagittal oblique	N	14	314 × 448	1200	15	3/0.6

Setup: Feet first, supine, knee minimally flexed, neutral to slightly externally rotated; 3-T MR unit (Siemens, Germany). Post-gadolinium contrast T1-weighted sequences are obtained in at least 2 orthogonal planes with fat suppression.
Abbreviations: FOV, field of view; PD, proton density; TE, echo time; TR, repetition time.

meniscal retear after meniscectomy, and evaluation for instability of an osteochondral lesion.

The field strength, coil (volume surface phased array), slice thickness, field of view, matrix size, and other select imaging parameters are optimized with the goal of increasing the signal to noise ratio and decreasing scan time, thereby decreasing motion artifact. Metal artifact reduction can be achieved by orienting the long axis of metallic prosthesis parallel to both magnetic field and frequency encoding axis, employing fast spin echo techniques with increased echo train length, increasing receiver band width, decreasing field of view, and increasing the matrix size in the direction of the frequency encoding gradient.[1]

IMAGING ANATOMY

The knee, a hinge-type joint, is primarily composed of 3 articulating compartments: patellofemoral, medial femorotibial, and lateral femorotibial. A combination of muscles, tendons, ligaments, and extensions of the joint capsule collectively help to offer multidirectional stability to the knee, while allowing for necessary mobility. Numerous bursae about the knee allow for ease of motion of the stabilizing structures in relation to one another.

The medial femorotibial compartment is formed by the medial femoral condyle and medial tibial plateau articulation, and houses the medial meniscus and articular cartilage. Major medial stabilizers include the deep (coronary ligaments) and superficial portions of the medial collateral ligament (MCL), medial tendons (sartorius, gracilis, semitendinosus, and semimembranosus), and deep crural fascia of vastus medialis, which helps to form the medial patellar retinaculum anteriorly. Posteriorly, the deep portion of the MCL, with contributing fibers from the semimembranosus tendon and synovial sheath, form the posterior

oblique ligament, a major stabilizer of the posteromedial knee. The MCL bursa is located along the middle third of the medial knee joint between the superficial and deep components of the MCL.[2]

The lateral femorotibial compartment is formed by the lateral femoral condyle and lateral tibial plateau articulation, and houses the lateral meniscus and articular cartilage. It can communicate with the proximal tibiofibular joint in a minority of individuals. Lateral joint stabilizers are composed of muscles, tendons, and ligaments. The anterolateral joint is stabilized by the joint capsule and the iliotibial tract, which inserts on Gerdy's tubercle along the anterolateral tibia, and is a fascial extension of the tensor fascia lata. The posterolateral corner is a complex anatomic area providing stabilization, achieved by several structures including the fibular (lateral) collateral ligament (FCL), biceps femoris tendon, popliteus muscle and tendon, popliteal fibular and popliteal meniscal ligaments, oblique popliteal, arcuate, and fabellofibular ligaments, and lateral gastrocnemius muscle. These structures are collectively referred to as the arcuate ligament complex. The major stabilizers of the posterolateral corner are adequately visualized on routine knee MR imaging examinations. The FCL has an oblique course from the lateral femoral condyle, immediately anterior to the origin of the lateral head of the gastrocnemius muscle, to the fibular head. The biceps femoris common tendon, directly posterior to the iliotibial tract at the level of the femoral condyles, joins the FCL to form the conjoint tendon before inserting upon the fibular head. The intra-articular segment of the popliteus tendon originates just below and passes beneath the FCL (through the popliteus hiatus), and then the arcuate ligament. The extra-articular segment of the tendon quickly joins its muscle belly, which in turn attaches to the posteromedial proximal tibial surface.

The menisci are C-shaped structures composed of relatively small anterior and larger posterior horns and a central body. The menisci are divided into an inner avascular or white-white zone (>5 mm from the capsule), middle hypovascular or red-white zone (3–5 mm from the capsule), and outer vascular or red-red zone (<3 mm from the capsule).[3,4]

Several potential diagnostic pitfalls exist involving the menisci, and awareness of anatomic variants related to these structures is essential to avoid misinterpretation. The most common meniscomeniscal ligament is the anterior transverse meniscal ligament, which can be a potential diagnostic pitfall because the junction of the ligament and meniscus can mimic a tear if not properly followed through its entirety.[5,6] The meniscofemoral ligaments of Humphrey and Wrisberg, located anterior and posterior to the posterior cruciate ligament (PCL), respectively, can similarly be mistaken for pseudotears or meniscal fragments of the posterior horn of the lateral meniscus at their meniscal attachment.[6] A rare variant, the oblique meniscomeniscal ligament, courses obliquely from the posterior horn of either meniscus through the intercondylar notch between the cruciate ligaments to the anterior horn of the opposite meniscus, and can be mistaken for a flipped meniscal fragment.[5] Physiologic small fluid within the popliteus tendon sheath can simulate a lateral meniscal tear at the body-posterior horn junction. Meniscal flounce is an unusual normal variant characterized by a single fold along the inner margin of the meniscus.[3] It more commonly involves the medial meniscus and can be mistaken for a tear, especially on coronal images.

Imaging artifacts generated by patient motion, magic angle, arterial pulsation, susceptibility artifact/field inhomogeneity (eg, chondrocalcinosis), and the concave morphology of the menisci (edge artifact) all can create a diagnostic dilemma, and this can be avoided with improved understanding of MR imaging physics and by paying special attention to imaging technique. Hemosiderin-vacuum phenomenon from fracture or osteoarthrosis can mimic a meniscal fragment, and will be more conspicuous on gradient echo sequences.[4]

The cruciate ligaments are situated in the intercondylar notch between the medial and lateral compartments. The ACL courses from the posteromedial aspect of the lateral femoral condyle to insert anterolateral to the anterior tibial spine. The normal ACL has a fan-shaped striated appearance on both T1-weighted and T2-weighted sequences whereas, in contrast, the PCL appears homogeneously hypointense on all sequences. The PCL has a broad origin along the mid aspect of the medial femoral condyle and tapers as it inserts along the posterior mid tibia approximately 1 cm below the joint line.[7] Both cruciate ligaments have two distinct components, an anterolateral and posteromedial bundle. A normal recess, which can accumulate fluid, is located posterior to the PCL.[8]

The extensor mechanism of the knee is composed of the quadriceps tendon, prepatellar quadriceps continuation, and patellar tendon.[9] The quadriceps tendon is striated in appearance, due to interspersed fat between 4 contributing muscles: vastus lateralis, vastus intermedius (deep), rectus femoris (superficial), and vastus medialis. The patellar tendon is a hypointense band arising from the inferior pole of the patella and attaching to the tibial tuberosity. The prepatellar quadriceps continuation is a thin sliver of hypointense signal comprising superficial fibers from the rectus femoris tendon.

Numerous bursae are present around the knee joint, and allow for smooth motion of various stabilizing structures in relation to one another. Visualization of these potential spaces is commonly due to pathologic fluid accumulation (bursitis). The semimembranosus-gastrocnemius bursa, located within the posteromedial aspect of the knee, communicates with the knee joint in a majority of individuals, and is referred to as a popliteal (Baker's) cyst.[10] The neck of the cyst is formed by the tendon of the medial head of the gastrocnemius muscle laterally and semimembranosus tendon medially. Anteriorly, 4 bursae are commonly visualized and include the suprapatellar, prepatellar, and superficial and deep infrapatellar bursae. The anterior and posterior bursae are best seen on axial or sagittal sequences.

Medially, the pes anserine, tibial collateral ligament, and semimembranosus-tibial collateral ligament bursae are seen. The pes anserine bursa is located between the distal tibial collateral ligament and the pesanserinus, which is composed of the sartorius, gracilis, and semitendinosus tendons at their tibial insertion. The tibial collateral ligament (MCL) bursa is located at the level of the knee joint line between the superficial and deep components of the MCL, and is elongated in a vertical fashion. The semimembranosus-tibial collateral ligament bursa, an inverted U-shaped structure, does not communicate with the joint, and is positioned between the semimembranosus tendon and tibial collateral ligament at the level of the medial tibial plateau.[11] Laterally, the iliotibial band and fibular collateral ligament (FCL)-biceps femoris bursae are found. The iliotibial band bursa is situated between the tibia and distal iliotibial band immediately proximal to its insertion on Gerdy's tubercle.

The FCL-biceps femoris bursa is found lateral to the distal FCL, and insinuates anterior and anteromedial in relation to this ligament. Superiorly, it extends to the level of the crossing of the biceps femoris tendon, and remains superficial to FCL in this location.[10]

Knowledge of normal locations of bursae is important in order to distinguish these from pathologic processes. One example exists within the soft tissues deep to the distal iliotibial tract at the level of the lateral femoral condyle. As a normal bursa does not exist in this location, fluid accumulation is likely pathologic and related to iliotibial band friction syndrome; however, it must be differentiated from joint fluid within the lateral parapatellar recess.[6]

The popliteal fossa is located posterior to the knee and contains several neurovascular structures that course between the thigh and leg. The popliteal artery most commonly bifurcates at the caudal aspect of the popliteus muscle into the posterior and anterior tibial arteries. A rare but important variant branching pattern, termed the aberrant anterior tibial artery, occurs when there is high (early) division of the popliteal artery, and the anterior tibial artery courses inferiorly along the anterior surface of the popliteal muscle. This vessel is at high risk of injury during orthopedic operations involving posterior knee soft tissue manipulation, drilling through the posterior tibial cortex, and proximal tibial osteomoties.[12]

SUMMARY

It is essential to develop an understanding of basic MR imaging principles and anatomy, as well as musculoskeletal imaging protocols, prior to interpreting MR imaging examinations of the knee. Learning normal MR imaging anatomy, commonly encountered anatomic variants, and imaging pitfalls is crucial for improving radiologists' ability to accurately detect disease. (See Appendix for illustrative figures.)

ACKNOWLEDGMENTS

We thank Mike Tenzer MD, our healthy imaging volunteer, who provided many of the images used in this article.

APPENDIX

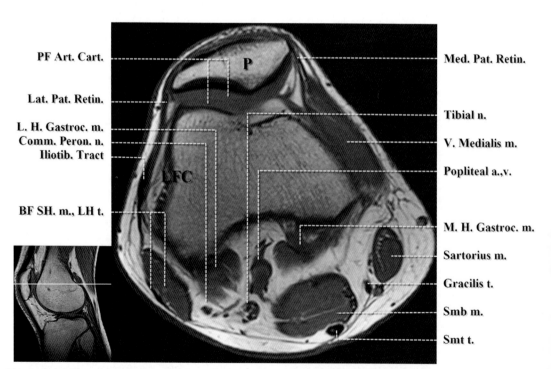

Fig. 1. Axial T1-weighted image. Mid patellofemoral compartment. a., artery; BF SH. m., LH t., biceps femoris short head muscle, long head tendon; Comm. Peron. n., common peroneal nerve; m, muscle; n, nerve; M.H./L.H. Gastroc., medial and lateral heads of gastrocnemius; Iliotib., iliotibial; Med./Lat. Pat. Retin., medial and lateral patellar retinacula; PF Art. Cart., patellofemoral articular cartilage; Smb, semimembranosus; Smt, semitendinosus; t., tendon; v., vein; V., vastus.

Key Points

- The semimembranosus muscle is the largest of the posteromedial muscles continuing inferiorly to this level. The semitendinosus tendon can be seen immediately posterior to the semimembranosus muscle. The smaller sartorius muscle is seen more medially with the gracilis tendon interposed. The vastus medialis isobliquus muscle is draped over the medial femoral condyle.
- The adductor tubercle (not seen), along the superior medial femoral condyle, is the insertion site of the adductor magnus muscle.
- The medial and lateral heads of gastrocnemius muscles originate from immediately superior to their respective femoral condyles.
- The popliteal artery is anterior to the popliteal vein within the superior aspect of the popliteal fossa.
- The common peroneal nerve follows the course of the biceps femoris musculature.
- The patellar articular cartilage is located slightly superior to the femoral trochlear articular cartilage during knee extension.

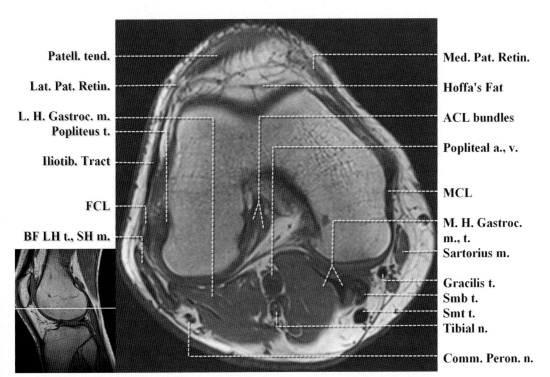

Fig. 2. Axial T1-weighted image. Inferior patellofemoral compartment. a., artery; ACL, anterior cruciate ligament; BF LH. t., SH m., biceps femoris short head muscle, long head tendon; Comm. Peron. n., common peroneal nerve; FCL, fibular collateral ligament; Iliotib., iliotibial; m., muscle; MCL, medial collateral ligament; M.H./L.H. Gastroc., medial and lateral heads of gastrocnemius; Med./Lat. Pat. Retin., medial and lateral patellar retinacula; n., nerve; Patell. tend., patellar tendon; Smb, semimembranosus; Smt, semitendinosus; t., tendon; v., vein.

Key Points

- The semimembranosus muscle forms a crescentic tendon, and together with the medial head gastrocnemius tendon, creates the neck of the semimembranosus-gastrocnemius bursae (also known as Baker's cyst).
- The femoral attachment of the tibial collateral ligament (MCL) can be seen.
- The patellar retinacula and iliotibial tract (laterally) attach the patella to the collateral ligaments.[13]
- The medial and lateral heads of gastrocnemius muscles border the popliteal artery and vein on either side. The tibial nerve is positioned immediately posterior to the popliteal vessels.
- The femoral attachment of the two bundles of the ACL is seen within the posterolateral superior aspect of the intercondylar notch just above the level of the femoral attachment of the PCL.
- The origin of the popliteus tendon is immediately inferior and posterior to the femoral attachment of the fibular collateral ligament (FCL). The inferior lateral genicular artery courses between the FCL and the popliteus tendon.

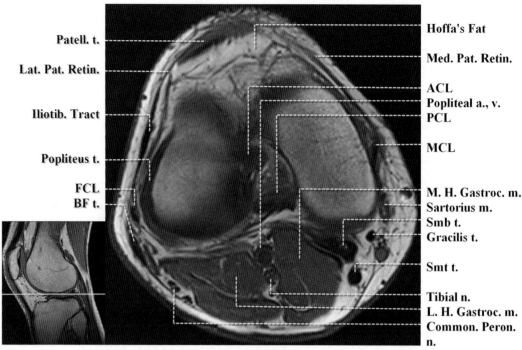

Patell. t.
Lat. Pat. Retin.
Iliotib. Tract
Popliteus t.
FCL
BF t.

Hoffa's Fat
Med. Pat. Retin.
ACL
Popliteal a., v.
PCL
MCL
M. H. Gastroc. m.
Sartorius m.
Smb t.
Gracilis t.
Smt t.
Tibial n.
L. H. Gastroc. m.
Common. Peron. n.

Fig. 3. Axial T1-weighted image. Femorotibial joint space. a., artery; ACL, anterior cruciate ligament; BF LH. t., SH m., biceps femoris short head muscle, long head tendon; Comm. Peron. n., common peroneal nerve; FCL, fibular collateral ligament; Iliotib., iliotibial; m., muscle; MCL, medial collateral ligament; M.H./L.H. Gastroc., medial and lateral heads of gastrocnemius; Med./Lat. Pat. Retin., medial and lateral patellar retinacula; n., nerve; Patell. tend., patellar tendon; Smb, semimembranosus; Smt, semitendinosus; t., tendon; v., vein.

Key Points

- The tibial nerve is positioned immediately posterior to the popliteal vessels.
- The proximal ACL is coursing toward the anteromedial aspect of the intercondylar notch. The PCL is posterior and courses toward its posterior tibial attachment 1 cm below the joint line.
- The biceps femoris tendon is seen proximal to forming the conjoint tendon with the fibular collateral ligament.
- The proximal popliteus tendon is intracapsular and closely apposed to the posterolateral knee joint. Magic angle artifact is seen to cause intermediate signal intensity alteration of the visualized proximal popliteus tendon. In general, it affects curving tendons, ligaments, and menisci about the knee when they are oriented 55° relative to the main magnetic field, and is more prominent on low TE sequences; however, it does not commonly hinder diagnostic interpretation in the knee. Artifact is considerably diminished on higher TE sequences (not shown).

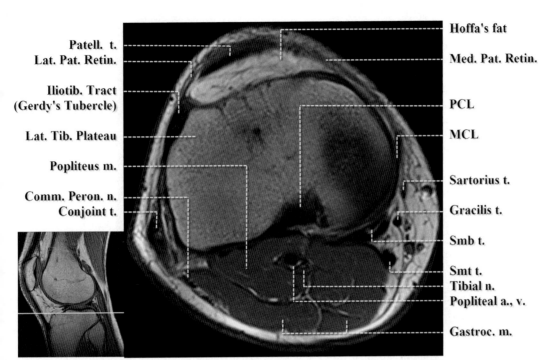

Labels on the image:

Patell. t.
Lat. Pat. Retin.
Iliotib. Tract
(Gerdy's Tubercle)
Lat. Tib. Plateau
Popliteus m.
Comm. Peron. n.
Conjoint t.

Hoffa's fat
Med. Pat. Retin.
PCL
MCL
Sartorius t.
Gracilis t.
Smb t.
Smt t.
Tibial n.
Popliteal a., v.
Gastroc. m.

Fig. 4. Axial T1-weighted image. Proximal tibia immediately below femorotibial joint line. a., artery; Comm. Peron. n., common peroneal nerve; Gastroc., gastrocnemius; Iliotib., iliotibial; Lat. Tib., lateral tibia; m., muscle; MCL, medial collateral ligament; Med./Lat. Pat. Retin., medial and lateral patellar retinacula; n, nerve; Patell., patellar; PCL, posterior cruciate ligament; Smb, semimembranosus; Smt, semitendinosus; t., tendon; v., vein.

Key Points

- The semimembranosus tendon has multiple arms that insert along the posterior and medial proximal tibia.
- The sartorius, gracilis, and semitendinosus tendons (anterior to posterior) compose the pesanserinus (goose foot complex; not seen) and course inferiorly to insert upon the proximal medial tibia. The tibial attachment of the medial collateral ligament is superior to the pesanserinus attachment.
- The conjoint tendon is formed at this level by the union of the common biceps femoris tendon and FCL, which will attach upon the fibular head. The common peroneal nerve is posteromedial to the conjoint tendon, and has given rise to the lateral sural cutaneous nerve located posteromedial.
- The iliotibial tract inserts upon Gerdy's tubercle along the anterolateral proximal tibia.

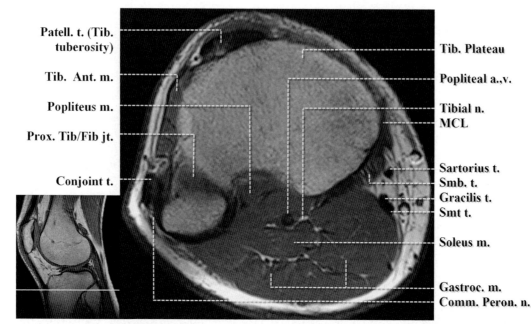

Fig. 5. Axial T1-weighted image. Proximal tibia/fibula. a., artery; Comm. Peron. n., common peroneal nerve; Gastroc., gastrocnemius; Iliotib., iliotibial; m., muscle; MCL, medial collateral ligament; n., nerve; Patell., patellar; Prox. Tib/Fib jt., proximal tibiofibular joint; Smb, semimembranosus; Smt, semitendinosus; t, tendon; Tib. Ant, tibialis anterior; Tib, tibia; v, vein.

Key Points

- The soleus muscle originates from the posterior aspect of the proximal fibula.
- The conjoint tendon is formed at this level by the union of the common biceps femoris tendon and FCL, and inserts upon the fibular head.
- The superiormost muscle fibers of the tibialis anterior muscle originate posterolateral to Gerdy's tubercle (slightly superior to the level shown). The common peroneal nerve is lateral to the fibula at this level.
- The patellar tendon inserts upon the tibial tuberosity lateral to midline.

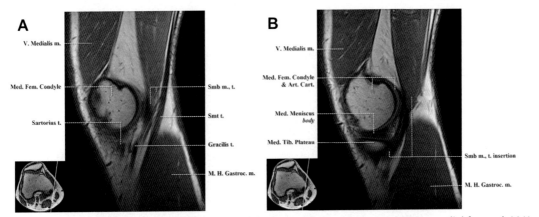

Fig. 6. Sagittal T1-weighted images. Medial aspect of the knee. (*A*) m., muscle; Med. Fem., medial femoral; M.H. Gastroc., medial head gastrocnemius; Smb, semimembranosus; Smt, semitendinosus; t., tendon; V., vastus. (*B*) Art. Cart., articular cartilage; m., muscle; Med, medial; Med. Fem., medial femoral; Med. Tib., medial tibial; M.H. Gastroc., medial head gastrocnemius; Smb, semimembranosus; Smt, semitendinosus; t., tendon; V., vastus.

Key Points

- The sartorius, gracilis, and semitendinosus tendons (anterior to posterior) course inferiorly and anteriorly to form the pesanserinus (goose foot complex). The distal medial collateral ligament (not seen) also sends a small contribution to this complex.
- The semimembranosus muscle and myotendinous junction are subjacent to the pesanserinus complex, and the tendon has a broad insertion upon the posteromedial aspect of the proximal tibia.

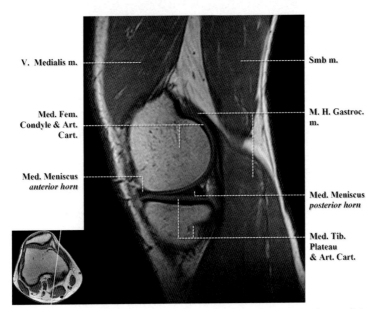

Fig. 7. Sagittal T1-weighted image. Medial aspect of the knee through posterior horn of the medial meniscus. Art. Cart., articular cartilage; m., muscle; Med., medial; Med. Fem., medial femoral; Med. Tib., medial tibial; M.H. Gastroc., medial head gastrocnemius; Smb, semimembranosus; V., vastus.

Key Points

- The medial tibial plateau has a more wedge-shaped appearance as opposed to a more polygonal-shaped lateral tibial plateau (not seen).
- The adductor magnus inserts upon the adductor tubercle (not seen) immediately posterior to the insertion of the vastus medialis muscle.
- The medial head gastrocnemius muscle originates along the superior aspect of the medial femoral condyle.

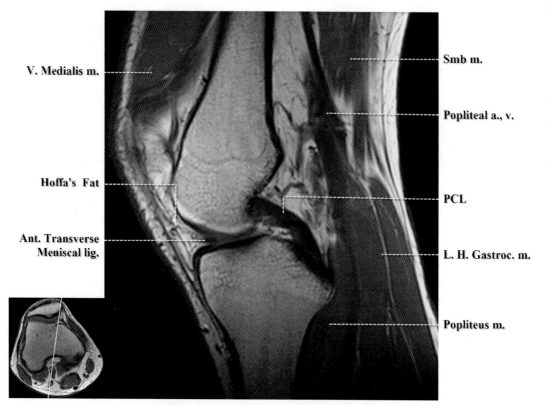

Fig. 8. Sagittal T1-weighted image. Intercondylar notch. a., artery; Ant., anterior; m., muscle; L.H. Gastroc., lateral head gastrocnemius; lig., ligament; PCL, posterior cruciate ligament; Smb, semimembranosus; V., vastus; v., vein.

Key Points

- The PCL is curved in appearance during knee extension and becomes taut with knee flexion. The intercondylar eminence is anterior to the tibial attachment of the PCL (1 cm below the joint line) within the posterior intercondylar fossa.
- The lateral meniscofemoral ligaments of Humphrey and Wrisberg, variably present, attach the lateral meniscus to the medial femoral condyle. In relation to the PCL, the ligament of Humphrey courses anterior, and the ligament of Wrisberg courses posterior.

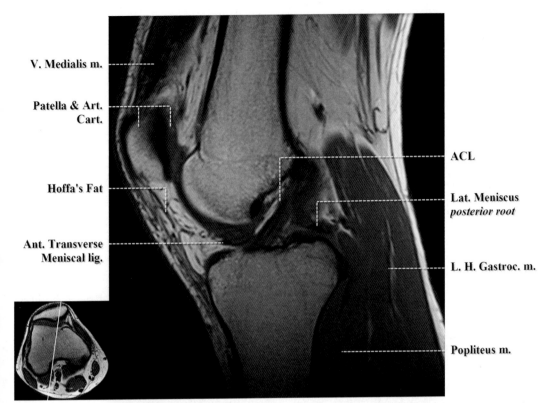

V. Medialis m.

Patella & Art. Cart.

Hoffa's Fat

Ant. Transverse Meniscal lig.

ACL

Lat. Meniscus *posterior root*

L. H. Gastroc. m.

Popliteus m.

Fig. 9. Sagittal T1-weighted image. Intercondylar notch. a., artery; ACL, anterior cruciate ligament; Art. Cart., articular cartilage; Ant., anterior; m., muscle; L.H. Gastroc., lateral head gastrocnemius; Lat., lateral; lig., ligament; V., vastus.

Key Points

- The ACL has a striated but taut appearance and is oriented slightly more vertical than Blumenstat's line (tangent to the intercondylar roof). The ACL is more heterogeneous in appearance and smaller in diameter than the PCL.
- The anterior transverse meniscal ligament courses through the infrapatellar (Hoffa's) fat pad.
- The patella is the largest true sesamoid bone in the body.

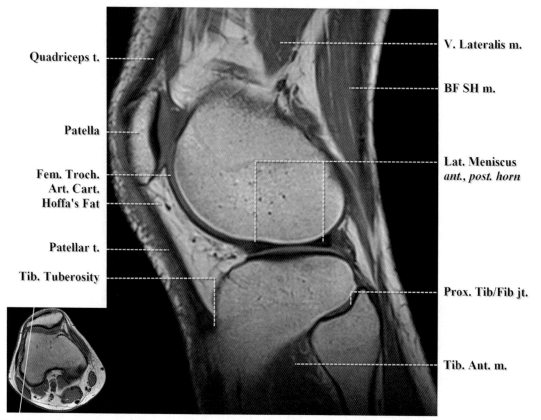

Fig. 10. Sagittal T1-weighted image. Lateral femorotibial compartment. ant., anterior; Art. Cart., articular carti-lage; BF SH, biceps femoris short head; Fem. Troch., femoral trochlear; m., muscle; Lat., lateral; post., posterior; Prox. Tib/Fib jt., proximal tibiofibular joint; Tib., tibia; Tib. Ant., tibialis anterior; t., tendon; V., vastus.

Key Points

- The anterior transverse meniscal ligament has just attached to the anterior horn.
- The intracapsular popliteus tendon is adjacent to the posterior horn.
- The biceps femoris short head muscle and biceps femoris long head tendon (not well seen) course inferiorly to form a common tendon before uniting with the FCL.
- The lateral head of gastrocnemius muscle is partially visualized inferiorly.
- The lateral tibial plateau has a polygonal shape and the medial tibial plateau (not seen) has a more wedge-shaped appearance.
- The quadriceps fat pad is just deep to the quadriceps tendon, superior to the patella, and anterior to the suprapatellar recess.

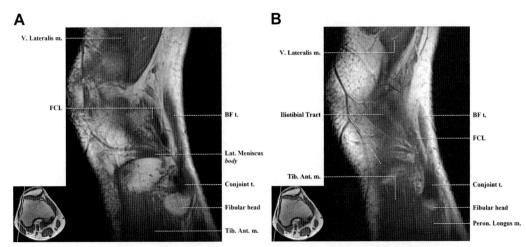

Fig. 11. Sagittal T1-weighted image. Lateralmost aspect of the knee. (*A*) BF, biceps femoris; FCL, fibular collateral ligament; m., muscle; Lat., lateral; Tib. Ant., tibialis anterior; t., tendon; V., vastus. (*B*) BF, biceps femoris; FCL, fibular collateral ligament; m., muscle; Peron., peroneus; Tib. Ant., tibialis anterior; t., tendon; V., vastus.

Key Points

- The fibular head (faintly seen) serves as the insertion of the conjoint tendon formed by the union of the FCL and the common tendon of the biceps femoris musculature.
- The iliotibial tract will insert along Gerdy's tubercle (faintly visualized).
- The common peroneal nerve (not seen) courses around the fibular neck and then divides into the superficial (lateral compartment) and deep (anterior compartment) peroneal nerves.

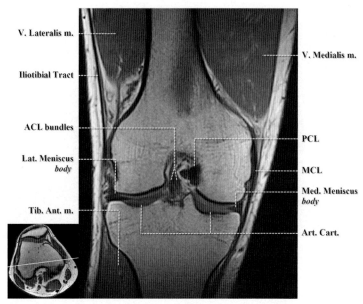

Fig. 12. Coronal T1-weighted image. Mid coronal plane. ACL, anterior cruciate ligament; Art. Cart., articular cartilage; Med., medial; MCL, medial collateral ligament; m., muscle; Lat., lateral; PCL, posterior cruciate ligament; Tib. Ant., tibialis anterior; V., vastus.

Key Points

- The PCL is ovoid in shape in the coronal plane, due to the extended knee position, resulting in an almost horizontal orientation.
- The body of medial and lateral menisci are hypointense triangles.
- The medial meniscofemoral (coronary) ligaments comprise the deep component of the MCL. The MCL is closely opposed to the body of the medial meniscus. Distally the pesanserinus tendon crosses over the tibial attachment of the MCL (not seen) and inserts upon the anteromedial proximal tibia.
- The FCL cannot been seen on a single coronal slice normally as it angles posteriorly toward its attachment along the fibular head.
- The iliotibial tract becomes more prominent on more anterior sections.
- The vastus medialis muscle is much larger than the vastus lateralis muscle at this level. The superior genicular vessel branches are located between these muscles and the adjacent femoral cortex.
- The medial femoral condyle and medial tibial plateau are more rounded whereas their lateral counterparts are more flattened in appearance. The medial femoral condyle also extends more inferiorly.

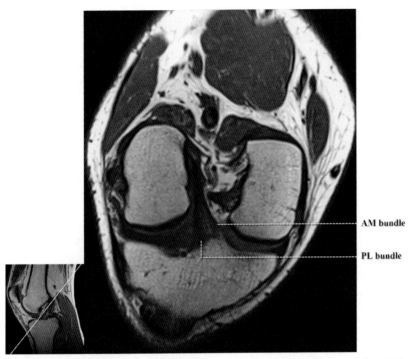

AM bundle

PL bundle

Fig. 13. Double oblique T1-weighted image. Intercondylar notch parallel to Blumenstat's line. AM, anteromedial; PL, posterolateral.

Key Point

- The ACL is composed of an anteromedial and posterolateral bundle, and attaches to the posterome-dial lateral femoral condyle, within the posterolateral aspect of the intercondylar notch, and to the medial tibial plateau, just anterolateral to the anterior tibial spine.

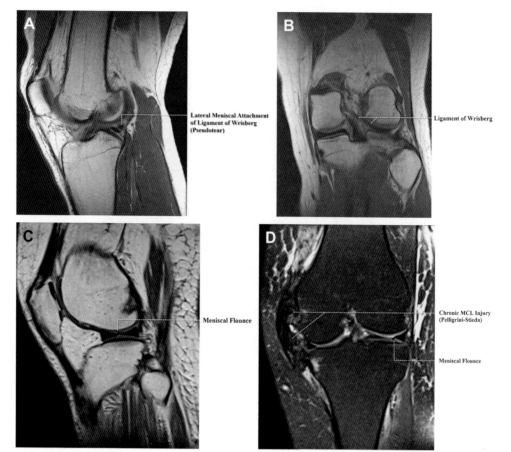

Fig. 14. Normal variants and imaging pitfalls. (*A*) Sagittal proton density–weighted (PDW) image. Lateral aspect intercondylar notch. "Pseudotear" at lateral meniscal attachment of meniscofemoral ligament of Wrisberg. (*B*) Coronal PDW image. Immediately posterior to PCL. Meniscofemoral ligament of Wrisberg (in a different patient) extends from the posterior horn of the lateral meniscus to the medial femoral condyle, immediately posterior to the PCL. (*C*) Sagittal PDW image. Lateral femorotibial compartment. Meniscal flounce, characterized by single symmetric fold along inner margin of the meniscus, more commonly seen in the medial meniscus. (*D*) Coronal intermediate T2-weighted image with fat suppression. Mid coronal plane. Irregularity and folding (meniscal flounce, in same patient) of inner margin of lateral meniscus can be mistaken for a tear on coronal images. Incidental note is made of severe chronic injury to the MCL (Pelligrini-Stieda).

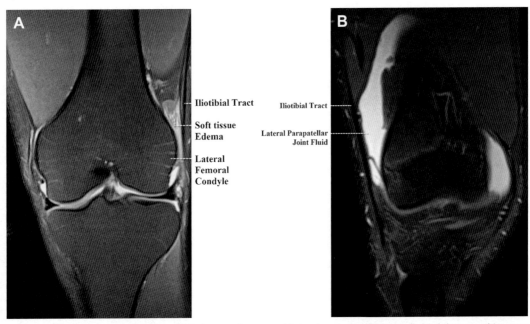

Fig. 15. Differentiating iliotibial band friction syndrome and lateral parapatellar joint fluid. (*A*) Coronal interme-diate T2-weighted image with fat suppression. Mid coronal plane. Edema is seen within the soft tissues between the iliotibial band (tract) and lateral femoral condyle in this patient with iliotibial band friction syndrome. (*B*) Coronal intermediate T2-weighted image with fat suppression. Mid coronal plane. Fluid is seen within the lateral parapatellar recess in this patient with a moderate joint effusion. Fluid is continuous with the joint effusion in all imaging planes.

REFERENCES

1. Stoller DW, Lejay H, Holland BA. Technical advances in musculoskeletal imaging. In: Barrett K, editor. Magnetic resonance imaging in orthopaedics and sports medicine, vol. 1. 3rd edition. Philadelphia: Lippincott Williams & Wilkins; 2007. p. 1–28.

2. De Maeseneer M, Van Roy F, Lenchik L, et al. Three layers of the medial capsular and supporting struc-tures of the knee: MRI imaging-anatomic correlation. Radiographics 2000;20:S83–9.

3. Stoller DW, Li AE, Anderson LJ, et al. The knee. In: Barrett K, editor. Magnetic resonance imaging in orthopaedics and sports medicine, vol. 1. 3rd edition. Philadelphia: Lippincott Williams & Wilkins; 2007. p. 305–732.

4. Anderson MW. MR imaging of the meniscus. Radiol Clin North Am 2002;40:1081–94.

5. Sanders TG, Linares RC, Lawhorn KW, et al. Oblique meniscomeniscal ligament: another potential pitfall for a meniscal tear- anatomic description and appearance at MR imaging in three cases. Radi-ology 1999;213:213–6.

6. Pfirrmann CW, Zanetti M, Hodler J. Joint magnetic resonance imaging; normal variants and pitfalls related to sports injury. Radiol Clin North Am 2002;40:167–80.

7. Manaster BJ, Andrews CL, Petersilge CA, et al. Hip & pelvis: thigh overview. In: McAllister L, editor. Diagnostic

and surgical imaging anatomy musculoskeletal. 1st edition. Salt Lake City: Amirsys Inc; 2006. p. V190–279.

8. De Abreu MR, Kim HJ, Chung CB, et al. Posterior cruciate ligament recess and normal posterior capsular insertional anatomy: MR imaging of cadav-eric knees. Radiology 2005;236:968–78.

9. Wangwinyuvirat M, Dirim B, Pastore D, et al. Prepa-tellar quadriceps continuation: MRI of cadavers with gross anatomic and histologic correlation. AJR Am J Roentgenol 2009;192:W111–6.

10. Beaman FD, Peterson JJ. MR imaging of cysts, ganglia, and bursae about the knee. Radiol Clin North Am 2007;45:969–82.

11. Hennigan SP, Schneck CD, Mesgarzadeh M, et al. The semimembranosus-tibial collateral liga-ment bursa. Anatomical study and magnetic reso-nance imaging. J Bone Joint Surg Am 1994;76(9): 1322–7.

12. Klecker RJ, Winalski CS, Aliabadi P, et al. The aber-rant anterior tibial artery: magnetic resonance appearance, prevalence, and surgical implications. Am J Sports Med 2008;36:720–8.

13. El-Khoury GY, Bergman RA, Montgomery WJ. Knee. In: Pope CF, Montgomery WJ, editors. Sectional anatomy by MRI. 2nd edition. Philadelphia: Churchill Livingstone Inc; 1995. p. 603–68.

Normal Magnetic Resonance Imaging Anatomy of the Ankle & Foot

George Arnold, MD, Saifuddin Vohra, DO,
David Marcantonio, MD, Shashin Doshi, MD*

KEYWORDS

- Anatomy • Ankle • Foot • Magnetic resonance imaged
- Pitfalls

Radiologic evaluation of the foot and ankle is often a complex task given the relatively small size of structures, detailed intricacy of anatomy, multifaceted relationships and mechanism of the anatomic structures, and wide range of pathologic entities.[1–9] In addition to a proper clinical examination, imaging is routinely used for a complete evaluation of the foot and ankle. In fact, a multimodality approach is often necessary for complete radiologic assessment. Radiography, sonography, and computed tomography all play important roles in the radiologic assessment of the foot and ankle. However, magnetic resonance imaging (MRI) is often the imaging modality of choice attributable to the superior soft tissue contrast resolution, multiplanar capability, lack of ionizing radiation, and ability to do postcontrast imaging.

The keys to optimizing MRI evaluation of the foot and ankle include: obtaining good MR images in ideal imaging planes, understanding the anatomy and relationship of the anatomic structures, and learning the more and less common pathologic entities that may affect this region. Careful attention should also be given to avoid misinterpretation or diagnostic pitfalls by understanding the appearance and significance of anatomic variants.

This article discusses anatomic relationships, anatomic variants, and MRI protocols that pertain to the foot and ankle. MR images with detailed anatomic description form the cornerstone of this article. The superb image quality will facilitate learning normal imaging anatomy, as well as conceptualizing spatial relationships of anatomic structures. MRI of a healthy volunteer was performed on a 3 Tesla magnet (Siemens Medical, Erlangen, Germany). Representative images of normal anatomy are depicted primarily using a T1 weighted sequence in the axial (short axis) plane for the ankle and the coronal (short axis) plane for the foot.

PROTOCOL

Obtaining MR images in ideal planes using specific sequences is crucial for the evaluation of anatomy and assessment of pathology. Obtaining MR images in ideal planes using specific sequences is crucial for the evaluation of anatomy and

The authors having nothing to disclose.
Division of Musculoskeletal Radiology, Department of Diagnostic Radiology-Imaging Center, William Beaumont Hospital, 3601 West 13 Mile Road, Royal Oak, MI 48073, USA
* Corresponding author.
E-mail address: Shashin.Doshi@beaumont.edu

Magn Reson Imaging Clin N Am 19 (2011) 655–679
doi:10.1016/j.mric.2011.05.010

Table 1
Ankle protocol (3 Tesla)

Sequence#	1	2	3	4	5	6	7	8
Sequence	T1NFS	T2 FS	STIR	Int PDFS	T1NFS	T1NFS	T1FS Pre	T1FS Post
Plane	Axial	Axial	Sagittal	Coronal	Sagittal	Coronal	axial	3 planes
TR/TI (mc)	780	7000	7380/130	3500	860	700	650	450–650
TE (mc)	10	70	35	55	10	10	10	10
Slice thickness (mm)/gap	3/30	3/30	3/30	3/30	3/30	3/30	3/20	3/20
FOV (cm)	14 × 9	14 × 9	17 × 10	19 × 8	17 × 10	19 × 8	14 × 9	14 × 9
Matrix	232 × 256	232 × 256	232 × 256	204 × 256	256 × 256	204 × 256	259 × 320	259 × 320
Contrast	No	No	No	No	No	No	No	Yes

Table 2
Foot protocol (3 Tesla)

Sequence#	1	2	3	4	5	6	7	8
Sequence	T1NFS	T2FS	STIR	Int PDFS	T1NFS	T1NFS	T1FS Pre	T1FS Post
Plane	Short axis (cor)	Short axis (cor)	sagittal	Long axis (axial)	Long axis (axial)	sagittal	short axis (cor)	3 planes
TR/TI (mc)	750	5000	7300/130	3500	750	750	650	450–650
TE (mc)	10	80	30	55	10	10	10	10
Slice thickness (mm)	3/30	3/30	3/30	3/30	3/30	3/30	3/20	3/20
FOV (cm)	Smallest possible (<12)	Smallest possible (<12)	Smallest possible (<12)	Smallest possible (<12)	Smallest possible (<12)	Smallest possible (<12)	Smallest possible (<12)	Smallest possible (<12)
Matrix	256 × 256	180 × 256	230 × 384	152 × 256	256 × 256	180 × 256	259 × 320	259 × 320
Contrast	No	No	No	No	No	No	No	Yes

assessment of pathology. In the foot and ankle particularly, musculoskeletal MRI technique is as important as understanding the complex anatomy. The wide range of possible pathologies that can affect this region necessitates the availability and understanding of various imaging protocols.

Several factors may contribute to the selection and customization of the appropriate MRI protocol. Of all the possible factors, the indication for the examination is the most critical. Communication with the ordering physician, the MRI technologist, and the patient is important for designing an

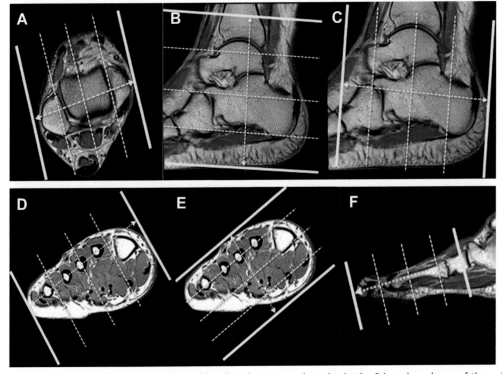

Fig. 1. Foot and ankle coil. *(A–C)* Examples of localizer images used to obtain the 3 imaging planes of the ankle. FOV should ideally include entire ankle/hindfoot to level of the metatarsal bases. *(A)* Axial localizer at level of tibiotalar joint for obtaining sagittal ankle images. Images obtained perpendicular to transmalleolar line. Cover from the medial malleolar to the lateral malleolar soft tissues. *(B)* Sagittal localizer for obtaining axial ankle images. Images obtained parallel to long axis of calcaneus. Cover from the distal tibial metaphysis to the plantar soft tissues. *(C)* Sagittal localizer for obtaining coronal ankle images. Images obtained perpendicular to long axis of calcaneus. Cover from the posterior soft tissues to the metatarsal bases. *(D-F)* Examples of localizer images used to obtain the 3 imaging planes of the midfoot/forefoot. *(D)* Short-axis (coronal) localizer at level of mid-metatarsals for obtaining sagittal midfoot/forefoot images. Images obtained perpendicular to a best-fit transmetatarsal line. Cover from the medial to the lateral soft tissues, or a smaller FOV for better resolution if focal area of interest. *(E)* Short-axis (coronal) at level of mid-metatarsals for obtaining long axis (axial) images. Images obtained parallel to a best-fit transmetatarsal line. Cover from the dorsal to the plantar soft tissues. *(F)* Sagittal localizer (ideally at level of second or third metatarsal) for obtaining short-axis (coronal) images of forefoot. Images obtained perpendicular to a line parallel to second or third metatarsals. Cover from the naviculocuneiform articulation through the toes.

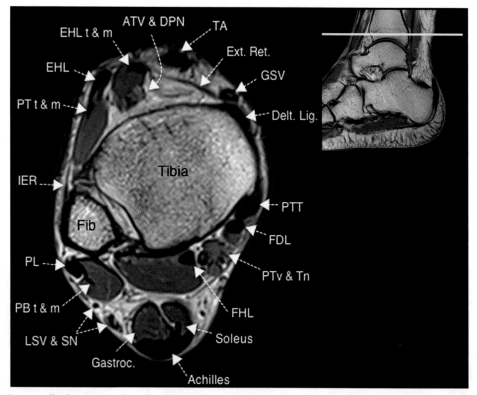

Fig. 2. Supramalleolar. Anteriorly at this level, situated from medial to lateral, the greater saphenous vein (GSV), tibialis anterior tendon (TA), extensor hallucis longus (EHL) tendon and muscle, anterior tibial vessels (ATV), deep peroneal nerves (DPN), extensor digitorum longus tendon (EDL), and peroneus tertius (PT) tendon and muscle can be seen on T1NFS axial images as low signal intensity ovoid structures. Of these, the GSV and TA lie superficial to the extensor retinculum, which can be seen at this level attaching to the lateral malleolus. Laterally, the distal fibula sits within the concavity of the fibular–tibial notch. The peroneus longus tendon (PL) is seen laterally to the peroneus brevis (PB) tendon and muscle, which course along the posterolateral aspect of the fibula. Not uncommonly, an accessory peroneus quartus tendon is present posteromedial to these tendons, surrounded by its peroneus quartus muscle, which can simulate a peroneus brevis tendon split tear. The lesser saphenous vein (LSV) can be seen within the soft tissues superficially between the peroneal tendons and the Achilles tendon. The Achilles tendon is seen most posteriorly in the midline as a low signal intensity crescent-shaped structure with a flat or concave deep surface. It is most frequently formed by equal contribution from the gastrocnemius and soles tendons. The plantaris tendon may be visualized as a 2 to 3 mm hypointense dot-like structure on axial images anteromedial to the Achilles tendon, before inserting onto the posteromedial calcaneus, or merging with the Achilles tendon or flexor retinaculum. Seen from anterior to posterior along the posteromedial aspect of the ankle, are the posterior tibialis tendon (PTT), flexor digitorum longus tendon (FDL), posterior tibial vessels (PTv) and tibial nerve (Tn), and flexor hallucis longus (FHL) tendon and muscle. The PTT and FDL are closely approximated posterior to the medial malleolus along the malleolar tibial sulcus. The PTT can be normally up to twice as large as the other flexor tendons. The flexor hallucis longus muscle (FHLm) is a large ovoid structure along the posterior malleolus. The deltoid ligament is visible at its attachment along the anteromedial aspect of the medial malleolus.

appropriate MRI protocol. Additionally, reviewing prior imaging and medical records can often be instrumental. Other factors that should be considered include the patient's clinical status, ability to cooperate with the MRI examination, availability of specific MRI coils, and availability of higher field strength magnets.

Due to the complex anatomy and wide range of possible pathology, MRI of the foot and ankle can be performed and customized with various imaging planes using a variety of imaging sequences. The authors protocol cases of the foot and ankle based primarily on the clinical indication. Typically, 1 of 3 anatomic regions of interest is selected: ankle/hindfoot, hindfoot/midfoot,

or midfoot/forefoot. Six standard imaging planes and sequences are used regardless of the indication for nonarthrogram examinations including T1 nonfat-suppressed in axial, sagittal, and coronal planes, T2 fat-suppressed short axis, short tau inversion recovery (STIR) sagittal, and intermediate proton density long axis. The terms short axis and long axis are routinely used at the authors' institution to avoid any discrepancy, which can occur with the terms coronal and axial when discussing the foot and ankle. Standard field of view (FOV) of 14 cm or smaller is routinely used for the ankle. Standard FOV of 12 cm or smaller is routinely used for the foot. Smaller fields of view are often used to improve spatial resolution and

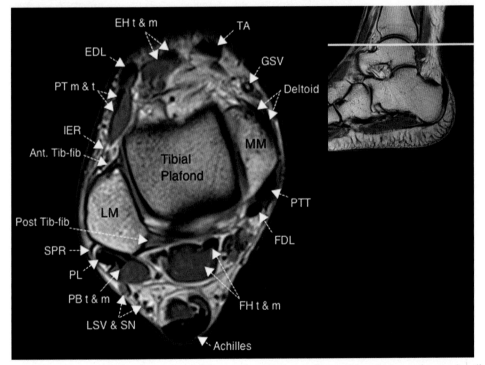

Fig. 3. Tibiotalar joint space/talar dome. In addition to the structures above, the anterior and posterior tibiofibular (tib-fib) ligaments are visible at the level of the joint space. Both can appear striated. The tibial surface at the level of the joint is referred to as the plafond, which is bordered by the medial malleolus (MM) and the lateral malleolus (LM) of the tibia. The peroneus tertius (PT) tendon becomes prominent as a separately visible structure from the remainder of the extensor digitorum longus tendon. The lateral aspect of the extensor retinaculum becomes visible as a fine band contiguous with the peroneus tertius tendon. The superior peroneal retinaculum (SPR) can be seen as a fine band circumscribing the peroneal tendons. A smaller portion of the FHL muscle remains visible.

anatomic detail, while remaining large enough to also allow for an adjacent control structure or anatomic reference point. Indications for a routine ankle protocol include, but are not limited to, ligament injury, tendon pathology, impingement, plantar fasciitis, os trigonum or sinus tarsi syndrome, occult fracture, osteochondral defect, or osteonecrosis. Indications for routine foot protocols (with attention to either the forefoot or hindfoot and including the midfoot) include ligament injury, tendon pathology, plantar fasciitis, plantar plate injury, occult fracture, degenerative disease, osteonecrosis, or Lisfranc joint or ligament instability.

In addition to demonstrating exquisite anatomic detail, the T1 non-fat-saturation (NFS) sequences are useful for the evaluation of a radiographically occult fracture, or for focal or regional bone marrow signal abnormality that may relate to

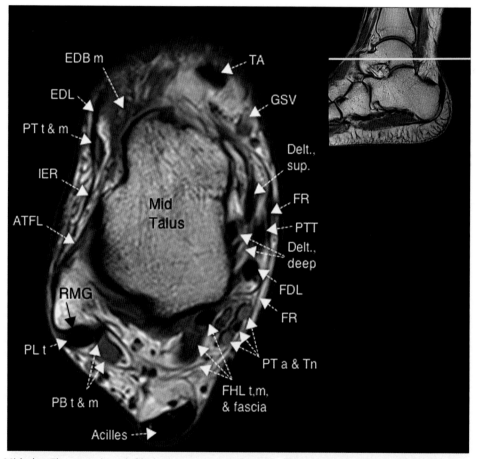

Fig. 4. Midtalus. The posterior talofibular ligament is not clearly visualized. The anterior talofibular ligament can be seen. The flexor hallucis longus muscle tapers into its fascia, seen as a fine curvilinear band through the posterior subcutaneous tissue. The deltoid ligament fans inferiorly from the medial malleolus. The deep deltoid ligament (anterior tibiotalar portion) attachment is visible along the medial tubercle of the talus. More superficially, the superficial deltoid fibers (tibionavicular, tibiocalcaneal, and posterior tibiotalar bands) are seen. The PTT courses over the superficial surface of the deltoid ligament. The peroneal tendons are situated within the retromalleolar groove (RMG). On axial view, the Achilles tendon is normally flat to concave along its anterior surface, and loss of this concavity suggests thickening and tendinitis. However, a portion of the anterior surface is convex, with this convexity shifting from lateral to medial near the insertion, representing the course of the merging soles fibers. Merging of fibers may also explain linear T2 signal, which is normally present within the tendon.

edema or possibly a marrow replacing process. Abnormalities detected on the T1 NFS sequences can then be compared with the T2 FS sequence to assess for fat-containing lesions such as an intraosseous lipoma, bone marrow edema, or replacement of normal fat signal within the sinus tarsi. T2 FS sequence in the axial plane also demonstrates excellent anatomic detail, while suppressing fat signal and accentuating fluid and bone marrow edema. Although time-consuming, STIR provides the most uniform fat suppression and is not subject to the heterogeneous effect observed on T2 FS sequences. In addition, the STIR sequence is useful in limiting susceptibility artifact related to adjacent metallic hardware.

Intravenous gadolinium contrast is typically used for cases involving mass or infection. Specific etiologies more commonly encountered in the foot and ankle requiring contrast-enhanced sequences include cellulitis, abscess, osteomyelitis, plantar fibroma, Morton neuroma, differentiating a solid from a cystic mass, or a synovial inflammatory processes (ie, rheumatoid or reactive arthritis). Gadolinium highlights the soft tissue changes seen in cellulitis as well as the bone marrow changes seen in osteomyelitis. However, contrast

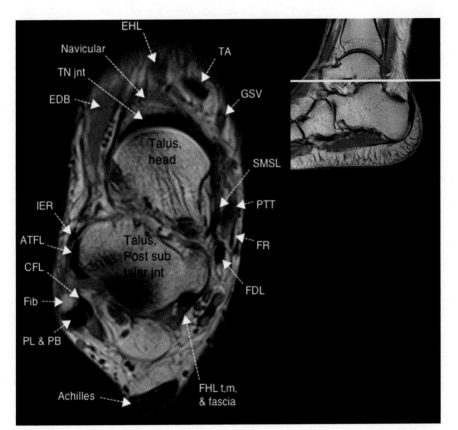

Fig. 5. Posterior subtalar joint. The extensor digitorum brevis muscle (EDB), arising from the inferior extensor retinaculum (IER) and proximal superior surface of the calcaneus, becomes prominent along the anterolateral ankle, deep to the extensor digitorum longus tendon (EDL). Immediately anterolateral to the posterior subtalar joint are the anterior talofibular ligament (ATFL) and the inferior extensor retinaculum (IER). The calcaneofibular ligament (CFL) becomes visible deep to the peroneal tendons (PL and PB) at its fibular attachment (fib). The flexor hallucis longus tendon (FHL) sits within the posterior talar sulcus, and the flexor retinaculum (FR) becomes visible overlying the tendons of the posterior compartment. The thick fan-shaped superomedial portion of the spring ligament (SMSL) or plantar calcaneonavicular ligament is reliably seen deep to the posterior tibialis tendon (PTT) from its attachment on the sustentaculum tali posteriorly to its attachment on the undersurface of the navicular anteriorly. Talonavicular (TN) joint is profiled.

is not essential for the diagnosis of either. Enhancement of a Morton neuroma may help to distinguish it from intermetatarsal bursitis or a ganglion cyst; however, anatomic location is a more reliable characteristic. Contrast enhancement patterns help to differentiate a solid from a cystic mass. Lastly, gadolinium will accentuate thickened and inflamed synovial tissue. If contrast is indicated, T1 FS

short-axis precontrast and 3 planes of T1 FS postcontrast imaging are added to the routine sequences.

Direct (intra-articular) MRI arthrogram studies are infrequently ordered by referring clinicians, but may be considered in specific clinical settings. Typical indications include assessment of intra-articular bodies, articular cartilage

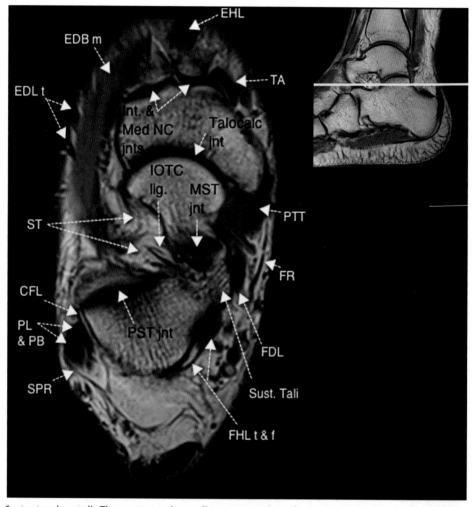

Fig. 6. Sustentaculum tali. The sustentaculum tali represents the calcaneal contribution to the middle subtalar joint. The flexor digitorum longus tendon (FDL) courses lateral to it and the flexor hallucis longus tendon (FHL) posterior to it. In addition to the spring ligament, the medial talocalcaneal ligament and the tibiocalcaneal fibers of the superficial deltoid ligament also attach to the sustentaculum tali. The posterior tibialis tendon (PTT) inserts onto the navicular tuberosity or the os naviculare. The extensor digitorum brevis (EDB m) muscle remains prominent anterolaterally. The calcaneofibular ligament (CFL) courses toward its attachment on the calcaneal tubercle. Fibers of the interosseous talocalcaneal (IOTC) ligament are visible coursing through the sinus tarsi (ST), which is profiled.

injuries, osteochondral defects, and postoperative cases in the setting of microfracture surgery or osteochondral implantation. Evaluation of the foot and ankle with direct MR arthrography primarily uses T1 FS imaging sequences secondary to the T1 shortening characteristics of gadolinium.

Sample protocols are presented (**Tables 1** and **2**) from the authors' institution using a 3 Tesla Siemens MRI machine (Erlangen, Germany). The parameters shown are used as a basic guideline, but are routinely optimized for patient specific factors such as area of interest, patient size, and time restrictions. These parameters will also vary widely with magnetic field strength (ie, 3T vs 1.5 T), as well as the specific make of the MRI machine.

PERFORMING THE EXAMINATION

At the authors' institution, MRI arthrograms and the majority of the conventional MRI examinations are performed on a 3 Tesla MRI magnet. MRI of the foot and ankle is performed with the

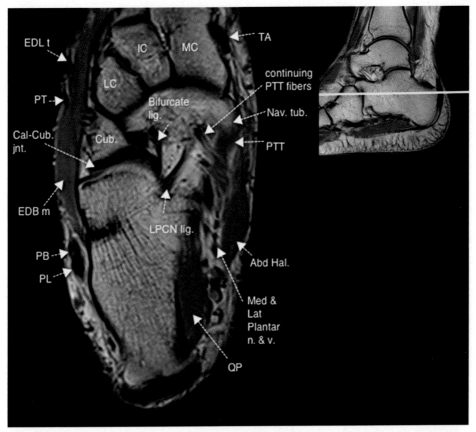

Fig. 7. Navicular tuberosity. The bifurcate ligament (calcaneocuboid and calcaneonavicular portions) and lateral plantar calcaneonavicular ligament (LPCN) are partially visualized. Majority of the PTT has been inserted onto the navicular tuberosity. Some continuing fibers of the PTT are seen extending to the cuneiforms or base of the second, third, or fourth metatarsls. The TA approaches its insertion on the medial plantar aspect of the medial cuneiform. Posteromedially, 2 additional intrinsic muscles are visible: the quadratus plantae (QP) along the medial surface of the calcaneous and the abductor hallucis muscle (Abd Hal.) more superficially. Between these 2 muscles, the medial and lateral plantar nerves and vessels become visible as low signal striated structures. Laterally, the flexor digitorum longus tendons (EDL), peroneus tertius tendon (PT), and extensor digitorum brevis muscle EDB remain along the lateral midfoot.

patient in a supine position, feet first, with the foot 90° to the lower leg. A standard smokestack foot and ankle coil (**Fig. 1**) is used, and the foot and ankle of interest are centered within the bore. Additional support is placed around the toes for immobilization purposes if necessary. Vitamin E markers may be placed outlining the region of interest as directed by the referring physician or patient. An initial localizer sequence is performed. MRI planes are then selected from the localizer images to identify 3 conventional anatomic planes including short axis, long axis, and sagittal (see **Fig. 1**), allowing the anatomy to be most easily be understood and consistently reproduced.

ANATOMY

Anatomy of the foot and ankle is detailed and complex. This discussion will be limited to a brief description of the anatomy that can be routinely and confidently visualized by conventional MRI.

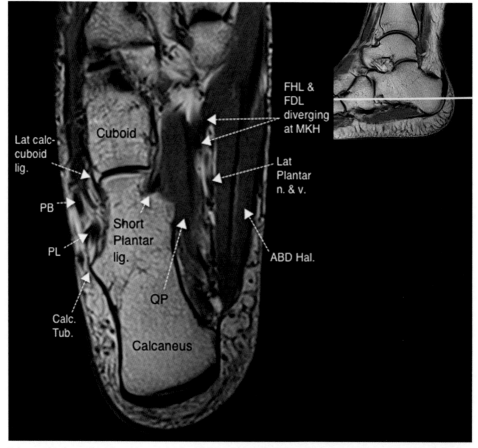

Fig. 8. Calcaneal tuberosity. The calcaneal cuboid joint is profiled and the lateral calcaneocuboid ligament can be seen along the joint space laterally. The plantar calcaneocuboid (short plantar) ligament is a striated structure along the inferomedial calcaneocuboid joint space. A prominent calcaneal tubercle is visualized, which separates the grooves for the peroneal tendons. The peroneal tendons begin to diverge, with the peroneus brevis tendon (PB) coursing anteriorly toward the fifth metatarsal base and the peroneus longus tendon (PL) coursing toward the cuboid tunnel along the undersurface of the cuboid. The flexor hallucis longus tendon (FHL) and flexor digitorum longus (FDL) tendons begin to diverge from the master knot of Henry (MKH), with the FHL coursing medially and the FDL continuing laterally.

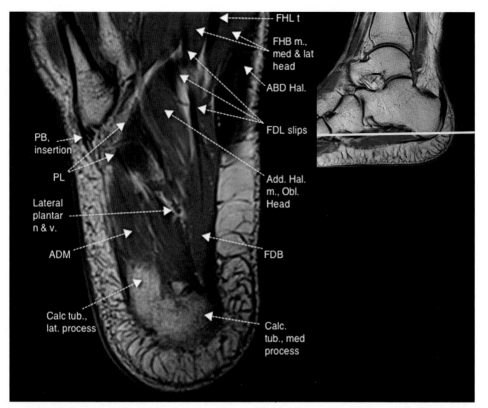

Fig. 9. Undersurface of cuboid. Peroneus brevis tendon (PB) inserts onto the fifth metatarsal base laterally. Peroneus longus tendon (PL) courses obliquely medially through the peroneal groove of the cuboid. The abductor digiti minimi muscle (ADM) arises from the lateral process of the calcaneal tuberosity and the flexor digitorum brevis muscle (FDB) from the medial process of the calcaneal tuberosity. The lateral plantar neurovascular bundle fibers can be seen between the ADM and the FDB.

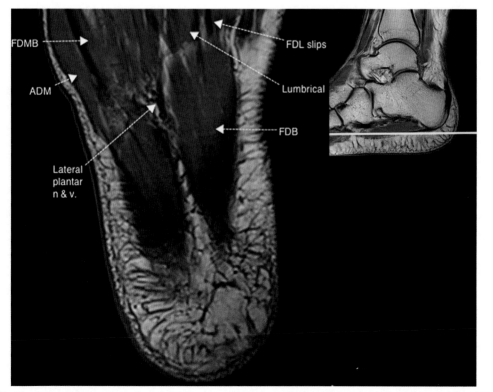

Fig. 10. Plantar soft tissue. More superficially, lateral plantar vessels and nerve course between the abductor digiti minimi muscle (ADM) and the flexor digitorum brevis muscle (FDB). Flexor digiti minimi brevis (FDMB).

Additional smaller structures of the foot and ankle are inconsistently visible and identifiable. Several of these smaller structures are labeled on **Figs. 2–26.** Routinely reported structures should be identifiable in multiple imaging planes and with multiple imaging sequences. The authors will illustrate the foot and ankle anatomy in the short axis for this article, and will use select sagittal and long-axis images to demonstrate specific structures optimally evaluated in those planes (**Figs. 27–29**).

Anterior/Dorsal Structures

The structures routinely assessed and reported along the anterior ankle and dorsum of the foot include the extensor tendons (tibialis anterior, extensor hallucis longus, and extensor digitorum longus), as well as the extensor digitorum brevis muscle and tendons.

Medial Structures

The structures routinely assessed and reported along the medial aspect of the ankle and foot include the medial flexor tendons (tibialis posterior, flexor digitorum longus, and flexor hallucis longus), the neurovascular bundle (posterior tibial artery, posterior tibial vein, and tibial nerve), the tarsal tunnel, the medial collateral (deltoid) ligament complex, and the spring ligament complex.

Lateral Structures

The structures routinely assessed and reported along the lateral ankle include the peroneus longus and brevis tendons, the anterior and posterior talofibular and tibiofibular ligaments, calcaneofibular ligament, the superior and inferior extensor retinacula, and the sinus tarsi.

Posterior Structures

The structures routinely assessed and reported along the posterior ankle include the Achilles tendon and adjacent bursae. The Achilles tendon, formed by a confluence of the gastrocnemius and soleus tendons, is located along the midline of the posterior ankle and inserts onto the posterior calcaneus. The Achilles tendon is not contained within a true tendon sheath; rather it is partially vested along its posterior medial and lateral margins by a paratenon. The retrocalcaneal bursa is present between the tendon and the posterior margin of the calcaneus, and the retro-Achilles bursa lies along the posterior margin of the Achilles at its insertion. These bursae are not typically visualized unless distended with fluid.

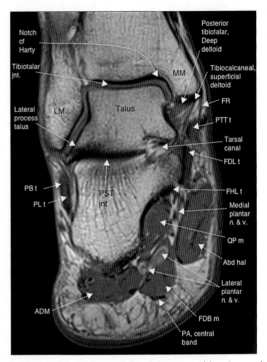

Fig. 11. Coronal T1 weighted image ankle. Coronal projection is particularly used to evaluate the osseous structure of the ankle including the talar dome and tibiotalar joint, deltoid ligament, calcaneofibular ligament, plantar aponeurosis (PA), tarsal canal, and sinus tarsi.

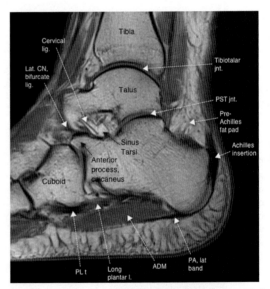

Fig. 12. Sagittal T1 weighted image ankle. Sagittal projection is particularly used to evaluate the osseous structure of the ankle including the talar dome, the tibiotalar joint, subtalar joints (posterior subtalar joint, PST shown), sinus tarsi, plantar aponeurosis (PA), and Achilles tendon.

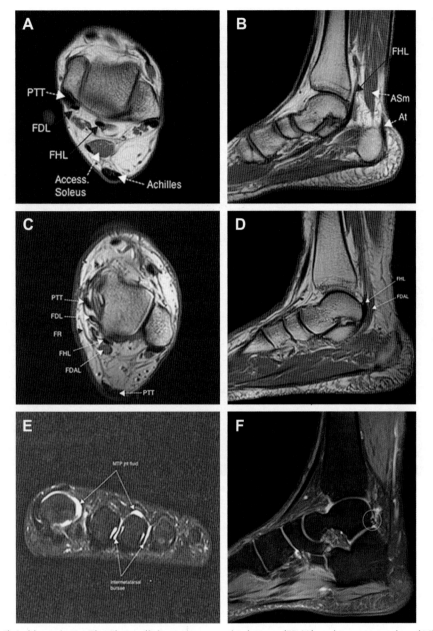

Fig. 13. (*A–F*) Ankle variants. The Flexor digitorum accessorius longus (FDAL) and accessory soleus (AS) are 2 of 5 anomalous muscles reported about the ankle, which are the first and second most common anomalous muscles along the medial ankle respectively.[9] (*A, B*) An accessory soleus muscle courses through the pre-Achilles fat and is distinguished by its course superficial to the flexor retinaculum (FR). (*C, D*) In contrast, the flexor digitorum accessorius longus (FDAL) courses deep to the flexor retinaculum. (*E*) Short axis T2 FS. Physiologic amount of fluid within the second and third intermetatarsal bursa. (*F*) Sagittal STIR. Pseudodefect of the talus, which represents a normal groove containing the posterior talofibular ligament.

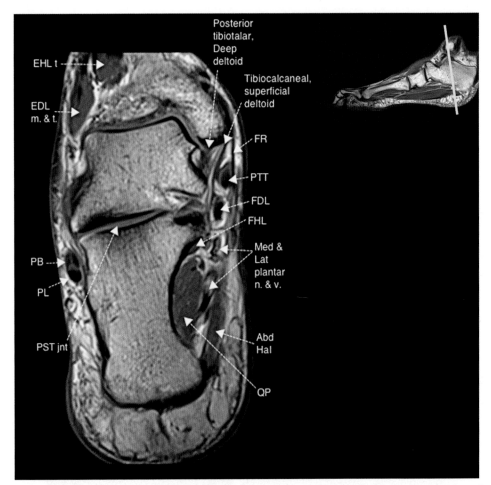

Fig. 14. Posterior talocalcaneal joint. Short axis (coronal) projection of the hindfoot with the posterior talocalcaneal/posterior subtalar (PST) joint profiled. Anatomy similar to coronal view of the ankle. Deltoid ligament is well-profiled. Note an apparent split tear of the peroneus brevis (PB) in this asymptomatic subject.

Plantar Structures

The structures routinely assessed and reported along the plantar surface of the foot include the plantar fascia as well as several flexor muscles (flexor digitorum brevis, quadratus plantae, abductor hallucis, and abductor digiti minimi).

Anatomic Variants

Accessory muscles of the foot and ankle are important to recognize, as they can be associated with compression neuropathies or may present as a palpable mass. Likewise, awareness and recognition of these structures may help the interpreting radiologist avoid misdiagnoses and possibly preclude further unnecessary tests. Along the posterolateral aspect of the ankle, a peroneus quartus may be present. The term peroneus quartus may be used to refer to a number of accessory peroneal muscles, the majority of which arise from the peroneus brevis (PB), and can be mistaken for split tear of the peroneus brevis. Along the medial

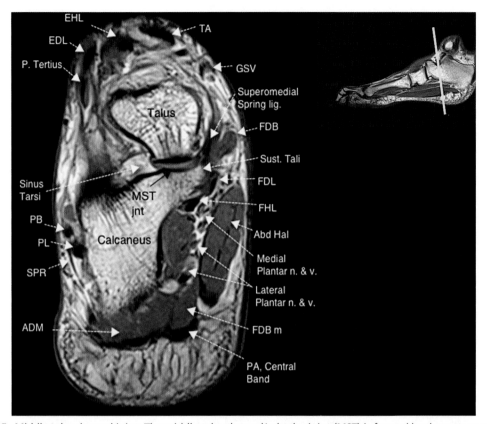

Fig. 15. Middle talocalcaneal joint. The middle talocalcaneal/subtalar joint (MST) is formed by the sustentaculum tali and the plantar surface of the talus. The cone-shaped sinus tarsi lies lateral to the anterior middle talocalcaneal joint. Dorsally, from medial to lateral, the greater saphenous vein (GSV), tibialis anterior tendon (TA), extensor hallucis longus tendon (EHL), extensor digitorum longus (EDL), and peroneus tertius (PT) are prominent structures. Laterally, the peroneus brevis tendon (PB) and peroneus longus tendon (PL) are deep to the superior peroneal retinaculum (SPR), and the lesser saphenous vein and sural nerve are superficial to the retinaculum. A subtle ridge, the peroneal trochlea can often be seen separating the grooves through which the peroneal tendons course. Four major intrinsic muscles course along the plantar and plantar–medial aspect of the foot. The abductor digiti minimi muscle (ADM) is the only muscle to arise from the lateral process of the calcaneal tuberosity. It courses along the plantar aspect of the foot laterally, ultimately inserting onto the lateral aspect of the base of the proximal phalanx of the didth digit. The flexor digitorum brevis muscle (FDB) arises from the medial process of the calcaneal tuberosity, courses along the central plantar aspect of the foot, and inserts distally onto both sides of the middle phalanx of the second through fifth digits. The quadratus plantae muscle (QP) predominantly arises just anterior to the medial calcaneal tuberosity, courses along the medial wall of the calcaneus, and inserts onto the lateral border of the flexor digitorum longus tendon (FDL), flexing the distal phalanges of the lateral 4 toes. Finally, the abductor hallucis muscle (Abd Hal) originates from the medial process of the calcaneal tuberosity and plantar aponeurosis and extends along the medial foot, inserting distally at the medial aspect of the base of the proximal phalanx of the great toe. The plantar aponeurosis (PA) forms the plantar margin of the FDB. Medial and lateral plantar vessels and nerves course between the abductor hallucis, flexor digitorum brevis, and quadratus plantae muscles. The inframalleolar portions of the medial flexor "Tom," "Dick" and "Harry" tendons: the PTTt, FDLt, and FHLt respectively, are seen medially.

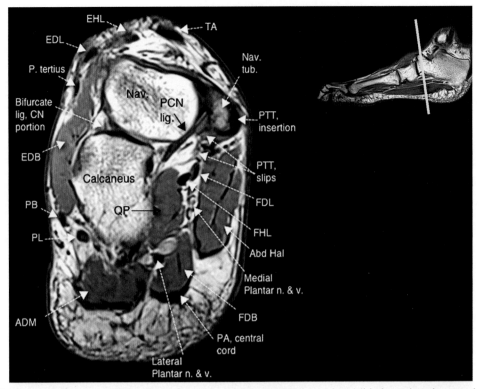

Fig. 16. Anterior talocalcaneal joint. A small portion of the sinus tarsi remains visible lateral to the anterior subtalar joint. The calcaneonavicular portion of the bifurcate ligament is visualized centrally at this level. Anterolaterally, the extensor digitorum brevis (EDB), which arises from the dorsum of the calcaneus, lies lateral to the sinus tarsi. The PTT begins its insertion onto the navicular tuberosity (or os naviculare). The plantar calcaneonavicular (spring, PCN) ligament is consistently seen deep to the flexor tendons, coursing from the navicular tuberosity to the calcaneus, forming a sling beneath the head of the talus. The lateral plantar nerves and vessels now course deep to the flexor digitorum brevis (FDB) muscle, while the medial plantar artery and nerve course between the quadratus plantae (QP) and the abductor hallucis muscle (Abd Hal).

aspect, a flexor digitorum accessorius longus (FDAL) muscle (see **Fig. 13**B) can be present in approximately 12% of individuals with tarsal tunnel syndrome[10] and is often associated with flexor hallucis longus tenosynovitis.[11] It descends immediately posterior and superficial to the tibial nerve and flexor hallucis longus, courses beneath the flexor retinaculum and through the tarsal tunnel, most commonly inserting onto the quadratus plantae or the flexor digitorum longus.

Additional accessory muscles include the peroneocalcaneus internus (PCI) as well as the tibiocalcaneus internus (TCI), which can be differentiated by their insertion onto the calcaneus. An accessory soleus muscle is distinguished by its course superficial to the flexor retinaculum (FR) (see **Fig. 13**A). Accessory ossicles and secondary ossification centers about the foot rarely pose a diagnostic dilemma due to their smooth corticated margins and typical locations. A small amount of

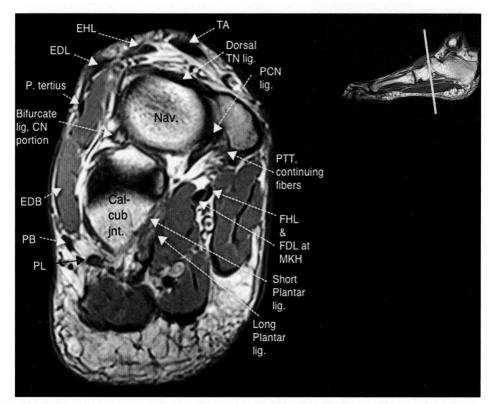

Fig. 17. Calcaneocuboid joint. The dorsal talonavicular ligament is seen along dorsum of talonavicular joint, closely applied to the joint capsule. A portion of the bifurcate ligament is seen. The flexor digitorum brevis (FDB) tendon closely approximates the QP muscle. The long plantar ligament (LPL), which attaches at the anterior plantar surface of the calcaneus, can be seen at this level coursing between the abductor digiti minimi muscle (ADM) and the flexor digitorum brevis muscle (FDB). It also attaches distally onto the plantar surface of the cuboid, converting the groove on the plantar surface of the cuboid (peroneal sulcus) into a canal for the peroneus longus tendon as it courses medially on its way to its insertion on the first metatarsal base.

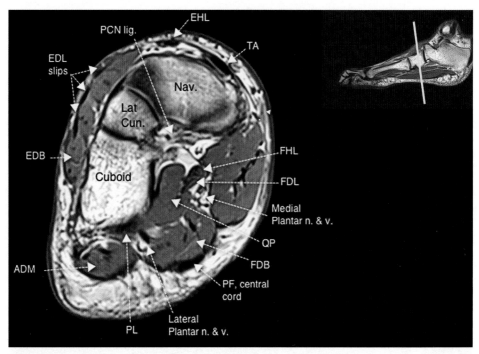

Fig. 18. Navicular–cuneiform joints. At this level, the cuboid, lateral cuneiform, and navicular are seen. The tibialis anterior tendon (TA) becomes progressively more flat and closely apposed to the navicular as it approaches its insertion onto the dorsomedial medial cuneiform and base of first metatarsal. Peroneus longus continues its medial oblique course through the calcaneal trochlea and peroneal sulcus of the cuboid. The plantar calcaneal-cuboid (short plantar) ligament and long plantar ligament are seen near their attachment. Flexor hallucis longus (FHL) is now dorsal to the flexor digitorum longus (FDL).

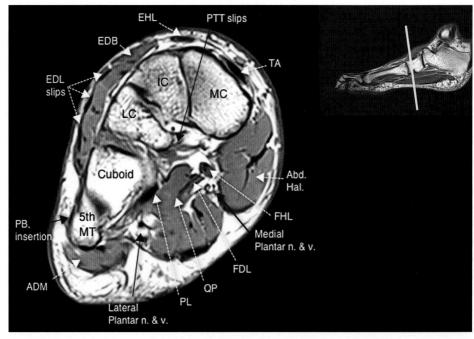

Fig. 19. Cuneiforms. The fifth metatarsal base, cuboid, and all 3 cuneiforms are demonstrated at this level. This is the level of the proximal transverse arch of the midfoot. The peroneus brevis tendon (PB) inserts onto the dorsolateral aspect of the fifth metatarsal base. The peroneus longus (PL) tendon exits the cuboid tunnel. Flexor digitorum longus tendon (FDL) is closely applied to the quadratus plantae muscle (QP) muscle and tendon. Slips of the posterior tibialis tendon (PTT) insert onto the lateral cuneiform (LC).

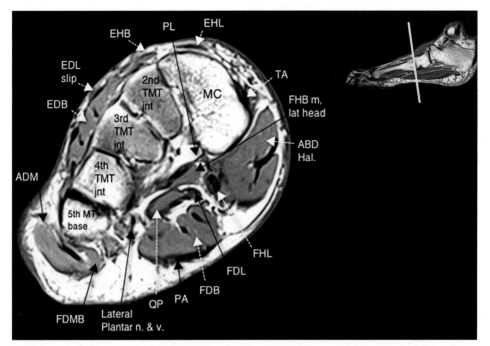

Fig. 20. Second through fourth tarsal–metatarsal joints. The tibialis anterior (TA) partially inserts onto the medial cuneiform (MC). Extensor hallucis brevis (EHB) becomes visible along the dorsum of the foot. Second through fifth extensor tendons fan over the dorsolateral aspect of the foot. Flexor digiti minimi brevis (FDMB) can be seen arising from the fifth metatarsal base. Later plantar nerve and vessels (n & v) are prominent structures between the abductor digiti minimi (ADM) muscle laterally and the flexor digitorum brevis muscle (FDB) and quadratus plantae (QP) medially. The QP tendon remains closely applied to the flexor digitorum longus tendon (FDL), which begins to branch into its digital tendons at this level. Flexor hallucis brevis (FHB) muscle and tendons arise from the distal slips of posterior tibialis tendon (PTT). The adductor hallucis muscle (AH) oblique head is seen centrally arising from its sheath, as well as the base of the second through fourth metatarsals.

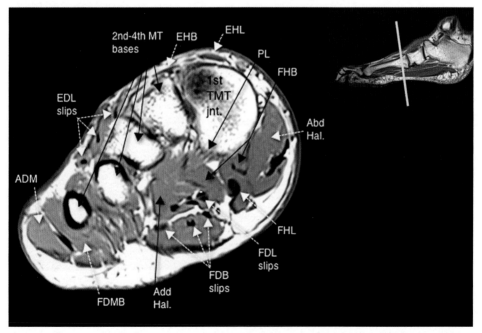

Fig. 21. Base of metatarsals/first tarsal-metatarsal joint. Tibialis anterior (TA) has completed its insertion onto the plantarmedial aspect of the base of the first metatarsal. The long and short extensor tendons of the great toe as well as the long and short second through fifth extensor tendons begin coursing together. Adductor hallucis (Add Hal) becomes prominent deep to the flexor digitorum longus (FDL) tendon slips within the plantar concavity of the forefoot. Flexor hallucis brevis (FHB) remains muscular at this level. The peroneus longus tendon (PL) inserts onto the lateral aspect of the first metatarsal base and plantar second metatarsal base.

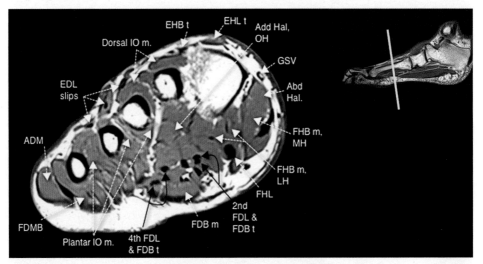

Fig. 22. Proximal metatarsal diaphysis. Dorsal and plantar interosseous (IO) muscles become visible. There are 4 dorsal interossei, which are bipennate, arising from the base of 2 consecutive metatarsals. The first inserts onto the medial aspect second proximal phalanx, and the remaining 3 insert at the lateral aspects of the corresponding phalanges. There are 3 plantar interossei, which arise from the medial aspect of the third, fourth, and fifth metatarsals and insert along the corresponding medial aspect of the proximal phalanges. Along the plantar lateral aspect of the foot, the abductor digiti minimi (ADM) and flexor digiti minimi brevis (FDMB) muscle are seen from lateral to medial. The adductor hallucis oblique head (Add Hal, OH) occupies the majority of the concavity of the forefoot. Lateral and medial heads of the flexor hallucis brevis (FHB) become prominent along the plantar aspect of the great toe.

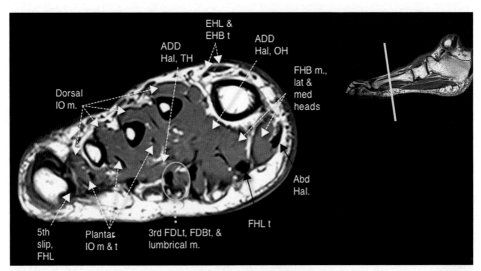

Fig. 23. Midmetatarsal shaft. The abductor digiti minimi (ADM) and flexor digiti minimi brevis (FDMB) muscle and tendon approach their insertion onto the base of the fifth proximal phalanx. The flexor digitorum longus tendons (FDL) and the lumbrical muscles course just deep to the flexor digitorum brevis tendons (FDB) along the plantar aspect of the foot. The adductor hallucis muscle (Add Hal), transverse head (TH) lies deep to the flexor tendons, supporting the metatarsals. Adductor hallucis muscle transverse and oblique heads join with the FHBt lateral head, which are shown coursing toward their attachment on the base of the first proximal phalanx. This common tendon will contain the lateral sesamoid of the great toe. The abductor hallucis tendon (Abd hal) and the medial head flexor hallucis brevis tendon (FHBt) converge toward their attachment on the base of the first proximal phalanx. Their common tendon will contain the medial sesamoid of the great toe.

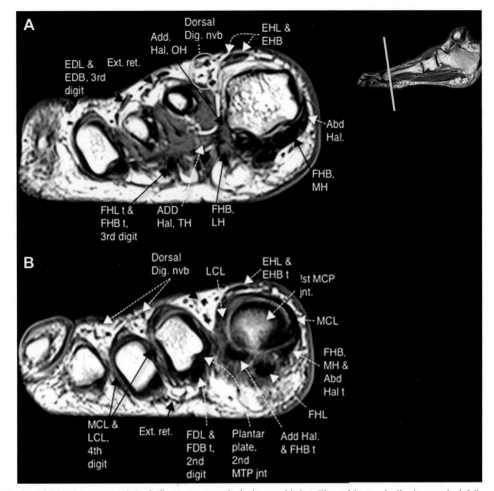

Fig. 24. (*A, B*) Distal metatarsal shaft/first metatarsal phalangeal joint. The adductor hallucis muscle (oblique and lateral head), along with the flexor hallucis brevis muscle lateral head (FHB, LH), are seen converging near the base of the first proximal phalanx. This common tendon contains the lateral sesmoid bone of the great toe. The flexor hallucis brevis muscle medial head (FHB, MH) and the abductor hallucis muscle (Abd Hal) converge onto the lateral aspect of the base of the first proximal phalanx and contain the lateral sesmoid. Dorsally, the extensor digitorum longus (EDL) tendons course medial to and in parallel with the EDB tendons over the metatarsal heads. The extensor retinaculum (Ext ret) of the second toe is seen. Dorsal digital neurovascular bundles are visible coursing through the interosseous fat. Along the plantar aspect, the flexor hallucis longus (FHL) and brevis (FHB) tendons are aligned over the metatarsal heads. The plantar plate, immediately deep to the flexor tendons, is formed by the plantar aponeurosis and plantar capsule, arising from the distal plantar aspect of the metatarsal neck and inserting onto the plantar aspect of the base of each proximal phalanx. Lumbricals may be seen coursing along the medial aspect of the distal metatarsals, before inserting onto the medial margins of the proximal phalanges. Note the plantar fascia (PF) and its fibrous septae.

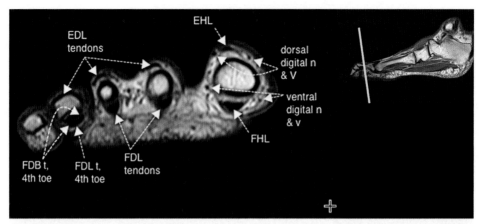

Fig 25. Proximal phalanges:. xtensor digitorum longus tendon (EDLt), extensor hallucis longus (EHL), flexor hallucis longus (FHL), flexor digitorum longus (FDL), flexor digitorum brevis tendon (FDBt).

fluid may be present within the first to third intermetatarsal joints within the intermetatarsal bursae in up to 49% of asymptomatic individuals (see **Fig. 13E**).[12] A groove along the posterior aspect of the talar dome, which contains the posterior talofibular ligament, is commonly refered to as a pseudodefect of the talar dome, and should not be mistaken for an osteochondral defect or erosion (see **Fig. 13F**).[9,13]

Although the majority of structures of the foot and ankle can be identified and evaluated in all 3 standard planes, certain imaging planes allow for optimal evaluation of certain anatomic structures. A checklist is included in **Boxes 1** and **2**.

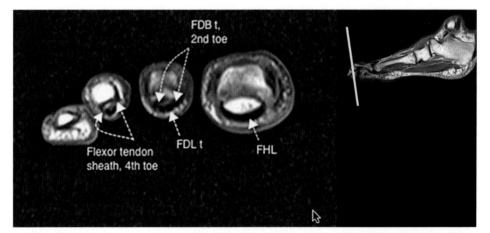

Fig 26. Middle phalanges. Flexor hallucis longus (FHL), flexor digitorum longus tendon (FDLt), flexor digitorum brevis tendon (FDBt).

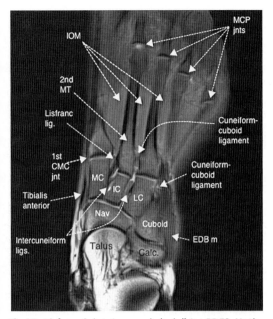

Fig 27. Lisfranc joint. Long axis (axial) Int PDFS. Notice the Lisfranc ligament attaching primarily to the lateral aspect of the medial cuneiform (MC) and the second metatarsal (MT) base. Metacarpal phalangeal (MCP) joints, interosseous muscles (IOM), carpalmetacarpal (CMC) joint, intermediate cuneiform (IC), lateral cuneiform (LC), navicular (Nav), calcaneus (Calc). Extensor digitorum brevis muscle (EDB m).

SUMMARY

MRI allows for optimal radiologic evaluation of the foot and ankle with its superior soft tissue contrast resolution, multiplanar capability, lack of ionizing radiation, and ability to do postcontrast imaging. The anatomy and mechanics of the foot and ankle are highly inter-related, and therefore can often be assessed and addressed as a single unit.

Selecting the appropriate imaging planes and sequences, based on the clinical indication and a variety of other factors, is crucial for obtaining optimal images. Understanding the anatomic relationships of structures of the foot and ankle is imperative for the accurate assessment of pathology. After reviewing this article, the interpreting radiologist should have a thorough understanding of the role of MRI, utility of imaging protocols, as well as the location and relationships of anatomic structures with regards to the foot and ankle.

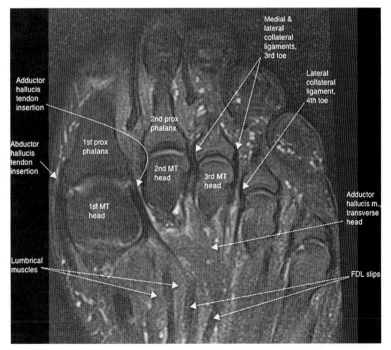

Fig. 28. Metatarsal phalangeal joints. Long axis (axial) Int PDFS. Metatarsal (MT), flexor digitorum longus (FDL), interosseous (IO).

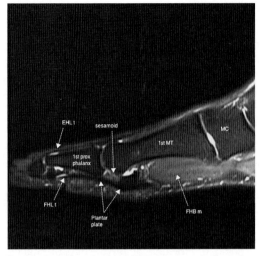

Fig. 29. Forefoot. Sagittal STIR. Extensor hallucis longus tendon (EHL t), flexor hallucis longus tendon (FHL t), flexor hallucis brevis (FHB m), metatarsal (MT), medial cuneiform (MC).

Box 2
Checklist for routinely evaluated structures of the foot in the most commonly utilized planes

1. Sagittal

   a. Osseous structures (phalanges, length of metatarsals, sesamoids)
   b. Plantar plates
   c. Plantar fascia
   d. Chopart and Lis Franc joints including osseous structures
   e. Flexor and extensor tendons

2. Short axis (coronal)

   a. Osseous structures (cross section metatarsals, sesmoids)
   b. Plantar plates
   c. Plantar fascia
   d. Intermetatarsal structures (interosseous muscles, bursae)
   e. Flexor and extensor tendons

3. Long axis (axial)

   a. Osseous structures (length of metatarsals)
   b. Chopart, Lis Franc, metatarsophalangeal, and interphalangeal joints, including osseous structures
   c. Intermetatarsal structures (interosseous muscles, bursae)

Box 1
Checklist for routinely evaluated structures of the ankle in the most commonly utilized planes

- Sagittal

  ○ Achilles tendon
  ○ Tibiotalar and subtalar joints including osseous structures (ie, talar dome and calcaneus)
  ○ Plantar fascia
  ○ Sinus tarsi

- Axial

  ○ Tendons

    ■ Medial flexor
    ■ Peroneal
    ■ Extensor
    ■ Achilles

  ○ Lateral ankle ligaments

    ■ Talofibular
    ■ Tibiofibular
    ■ Calcaneofibular

  ○ Spring ligament (superomedial)

- Coronal

  ○ Tibiotalar and subtalar joints with their respective osseous structures (including talar dome and tibial plafond)
  ○ Deltoid ligaments (superficial and deep)
  ○ Calcaneofibular ligament
  ○ Plantar fasci

ACKNOWLEDGMENTS

Special acknowledgment: Michael Tenzer, MD.

REFERENCES

1. Kaplan PA, Helms CA, Dussault R, et al. Basic principles of musculoskeletal MRI. In: Musculoskeletal MRI. 1st edition. Philadelphia: WB Saunders; 1995.
2. The ankle & foot. Stoller DW, editor. Stoller's atlas of orthopaedic and sports medicine. Baltimore (MD); Philadelphia (PA): Lippincott Williams & Wilkins; 2008. p. 425–90.
3. Foot, ankle, calf. Berquist TH, editor. MRI of the musculoskeletal system. 5th edition. Philadelphia (PA): Lipincott Williams & Wilkins; 2005. p. 430–6.
4. Farber JM, Buckwalter KA. MR imaging in nonneoplastic muscle disorders of the lower extremity. Radiol Clin North Am 2002;40:1013–31.
5. Sookur PA, Naraghi AM, Bleakney RR, et al. Accessory muscles: anatomy, symptoms, and radiologic evaluation. Radiographics 2008;28:481–99.
6. El-Khoury GY, Bergman RA, Montgomery WJ. In: Whitten CG, Walker CW, Montgomery WJ, editors.

Sectional anatomy by MRI. 2nd edition. Philadelphia: Churchill Livingstone Incorporated; 1995. p. 725–817.

7. Pfirrmann C, Zanetti M, Hodler J. Joint magnetic resonance imaging. Normal variants and pitfalls related to sports injury. Radiol Clin North Am 2002;40:177.

8. Manaster BJ, Andrews CL, Petersilge CA, et al, editors. Diagnostic and surgical imaging anatomy: musculoskeletal; managing. 1st edition. Salt Lake City: Amirsys; 2006. Section VII Ankle, p. 2–131; Section VIII Foot, p. 2–95.

9. Cheung YY, Rosenberg ZS, Colon E, et al. MR imaging of flexor digitorum accessorius longus. Skeletal Radiol 1999;28:130–7.

10. Kinoshita M, Okuda R, Morikawa J, et al. Tarsal tunnel syndrome associated with an accessory muscle. Foot Ankle Int 2003;24:132–6.

11. Eberle CF, Moran B, Gleason T. The accessory flexor digitorum longus as a cause of flexor hallucis syndrome. Foot Ankle Int 2002;23:51–5.

12. Zanetti M, Strehle JK, Zollinger H, et al. Morton neuroma and fluid in the intermetatarsal bursae on MR images of 70 asymptomatic volunteers. Radiology 1997;203:516–20.

13. Miller TT, Bucchieri JS, Joshi A, et al. Pseudodefect of the talar dome: an anatomic pitfall of ankle MR imaging. Radiology 1997;3:857–8.

Index

Note: Page numbers of article titles are in **boldface** type.

A

Abdominal anatomy, nonvisceral, 542–543
  normal and variant, on magnetic resonance imaging, **521–545**
Abdominal vasculature, anatomic considerations in, and MR imaging features of, 539–542
  MR imaging of, technical considerations in, 539, 540
Accessory abductor digiti minimi, 605
Acromial pseudospur, 589
Adrenal glands, anatomic considerations in, and MR imaging features of, 536–537
  MR imaging of, technical considerations in, 536
Anconeus epitrochlearis, 617
Ankle, and foot, anatomy of, 664–676
    coil, 657
    MR imaging of, protocol for, 655–663
    normal anatomy of, magnetic resonance imaging of, **655–679**
    performance of examination of, 663–664
    supramalleolar area of, 658
  coronal T1-weighted image of, 666
  sagittal T1-weighted image of, 666
  variants of, 667
Aorta, normal, MR imaging of, 492–494
Arm, muscle anatomy of, 570–573
  neurovascular anatomy of, 577–579
Arteries, coronary, MR imaging of, 502, 503–504
Atrium, left, MR imaging of, 501
  right, and superior and inferior vena cava, MR imaging of, 498–499, 500
  MR imaging of, 499–500

B

Biceps, tendon/pulley system, 585
Biceps tendon, accesssory head of, 591–592
Bile ducts, gallbladder and, anatomic considerations and MR imaging features of, 530–533
    MR cholangiopancreatography of, 528–530, 531
Bones, long, of upper extremity, anatomy of, 568–570
    magnetic resonance imaging of, **567–579**
      normal signal for, 568
      sequences in, advantages of, 568
Bowel, anatomic considerations and MR imaging features of, 538–539
  MR imaging of, technical considerations in, 537–538

Brachial plexus, imaging of, 470, 471–472
Brachialis, 571
Brachioradialis, 576
Brain, axial T2 images of, 436
  deep structures of, 433
  DW images of, 436
  lobes of, identifying of, 429–435
  midline structures of, 432–433
  nooks and crannies of, imaging of, 435–436
  normal anatomy of, on magnetic resonance imaging, **429–437**
    protocol for, 429
  sagittal T1 images of, 435–436
  superficial surface anatomy of, 430–432
Brainstem, anatomy of, 434–435
Breast, normal anatomy of, enhancement kinetics and, 516–518
    functional, MR imaging of, 514–516, 517
    MR imaging of, **507–519**
      protocol for, 507–512, 513, 514
    structural, MR imaging of, 511, 512, 513–514
Bronchi, MR imaging of, 491
Buccal space, 461
Buford complex, 591
Bursae, in shoulder, 587–589

C

Calcaneal tuberosity, 664
Calcaneocuboid joint, 671
Capitellum, pseudodefect of, 569, 570, 615
Carotid space, 467
Carpal boss, 604
Cerebellum, anatomy of, 434
Cervical space, posterior, 467–468
Cervix, anatomy of, 549–550
Chest wall, MR imaging of, 490, 491
Cholangiopancreatography, MR, of gallbladder and bile ducts, 528–530, 531
Clavicle, anatomy of, 583–584
Coracobrachialis, 571
Coracohumeral ligament, 587
Cranial fossae, anatomy of, 442–443
Cranial nerve(s), anatomy of, 447, 449–455
  I, anatomy of, 450
  II, anatomy of, 450
  III, anatomy of, 450–451
  IV, anatomy of, 451
  IX, anatomy of, 454

Magn Reson Imaging Clin N Am 19 (2011) 681–684
doi:10.1016/S1064-9689(11)00065-1

mri.theclinics.com